MW00574095

Emergency Care of the Elder Person

 Geriatric Emergency Medicine Task Force

Arthur B. Sanders, MD, Editor

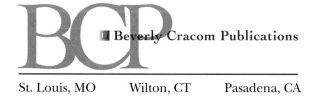

St. Louis, MO   Wilton, CT   Pasadena, CA

A joint venture between Beverly Foundation and Cracom Publishing, Inc.

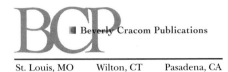
■ Beverly Cracom Publications

St. Louis, MO   Wilton, CT   Pasadena, CA

Publisher & Editorial Director: Barbara Ellen Norwitz
Developmental Editor: Marny Johnson
Design: Bill Drone
Production: Bill Drone, Bette Russ

Notice: The authors and the publisher of this volume have taken care to make certain that the doses of drugs and schedules of treatment are correct and compatible with the standards generally accepted at the time of publication. Nevertheless, as new information becomes available, changes in treatment and in the use of drugs become necessary. The reader is advised to carefully consult the instruction and information material included in the package insert of each drug or therapeutic agent before administration. This advice is especially important when using new or infrequently used drugs. The publisher and authors disclaim any liability, loss, injury, or damage incurred as a consequence, directly or indirectly, of the use and application of any of the contents of this volume.

Library of Congress Cataloging-in-Publication Data
Emergency Care of the Elder Person / Geriatric Emergency Medicine Task Force: Arthur B. Sanders, MD, Editor
        p.   cm.
   Includes bibliographical references and index.
   ISBN 1-886657-00-9
   1. Geriatrics. 2. Emergency medicine. I. Sanders, Arthur B. (Arthur Barry), 1947-
   II. Society for Academic Emergency Medicine (U.S.). Geriatric Emergency Medicine Task Force.
        [DNLM: 1. Geriatrics. 2. Emergency Medicine. 3. Emergencies—in old age.
        WT 100 E53 1996]
     RC952.5.E54 1996
618.97'025—dc20
DNLM/DLC
for Library of Congress   95-23015
                                                                                              CIP

Printed in the United States of America

10   9   8   7   6   5   4   3   2   1

GERIATRIC EMERGENCY MEDICINE TASK FORCE

Edward Bernstein, MD, FACEP

Rawden Evans, PhD, MD

David M. Habben, A.S., Paramedic

Gordon A. Ireland, PharmD

Jeffrey S. Jones, MD

Norm Kalbfleisch, MD, FACEP

Pamela Kidd, RN, PhD, CEN

Mark Lachs, MD, MPH

Joseph LaMantia, MD, FACEP

Robert M. McNamara, MD

John E. Morley, MB, BCh

David B. Reuben, MD

Kathleen M. Richmond, RN, BS

Arthur B. Sanders, MD, FACEP, FACP

Donald B. Witzke, PhD

Robert H. Woolard, MD

Contributors

Edward Bernstein, MD, FACEP
Associate Professor, Department of Sociomedical and Community Medicine, (Emergency Medicine), Boston University School of Medicine and
Associate Professor, Department of Social and Behavioral Sciences, Boston University School of Public Health, Boston, Massachusetts

Rawden Evans, PhD, MD
Lecturer, Section of Emergency Medicine, University of Michigan Medical Center, Ann Arbor, Michigan

Glenn Freas, MD, JD, FACEP
Director of Emergency Medicine Education, Temple University School of Medicine and
Assistant Director of Emergency Services, Temple University Hospital, Philadelphia, Pennsylvania

Darrin Fryer, MD
Kern Medical Center, Bakersfield, California

David M. Habben, A.S., Paramedic
EMS Instructor/Consultant, Boise, Idaho

Richard S. Hartoch, MD
Assistant Professor of Emergency Medicine, Portland Veterans Affairs Medical Center and Oregon Health Sciences University, Portland, Oregon

Gordon A. Ireland, PharmD
Associate Professor, St. Louis College of Pharmacy
and
Adjunct Associate Professor, Division of Geriatric Medicine, St. Louis University School of Medicine, St. Louis, Missouri

Jeffrey S. Jones, MD
Research Director, Department of Emergency Medicine and Associate Professor of Medicine, Butterworth Hospital, MSU College of Human Medicine, Grand Rapids, Michigan

Norm Kalbfleisch, MD, FACEP
Assistant Professor, Emergency Medicine and Assistant Chief, Emergency Medical Services, Portland Veterans Administration Medical Center and
Assistant Residing Director, Oregon Health Sciences University, Portland, Oregon

Pamela Kidd, RN, PhD, CEN
Associate Professor, College of Nursing, University of Kentucky, Lexington, Kentucky

Mark Lachs, MD, MPH
Assistant Professor of Medicine and Chief, Geriatrics Unit, Division of General Internal Medicine, Department of Medicine, Cornell University Medical College
and
Attending Physician, The New York Hospital, Amsterdam Nursing Home Corporation, New York, New York

Robert M. McNamara, MD
Associate Professor and Program Director, Emergency Medicine Residency, The Medical College of Pennsylvania and Hahnemann University, Philadelphia, Pennsylvania

John E. Morley, MB, BCh
Dammert Professor of Gerontology and Director, Division of Geriatric Medicine, St. Louis University Health Sciences Center
and
Director, Geriatric Research, Education and Clinical Center, St. Louis VA Medical Center, St. Louis, Missouri

Lidia Pousada, MD, FACP
Chief, Division of Geriatrics and Gerontology,
New Rochelle Hospital Medical Center, New
Rochelle, New York

David B. Reuben, MD
Chief, Division of Geriatrics, Director,
Multicampus Program in Geriatric Medicine
and Gerontology, and Associate Professor of
Medicine, UCLA School of Medicine, Los
Angeles, California

Kathleen M. Richmond, RN, BS
Clinical Supervisor, Sisters of St. Casimir
Infirmary, Chicago Illinois
and
Emergency Department Staff Nurse, Olympia
Fields Osteopathic Medical Center, Olympia
Fields, Illinois

Arthur B. Sanders, MD, FACEP, FACP
Professor, Section of Emergency Medicine,
Department of Surgery, University of Arizona
College of Medicine, Tucson, Arizona

Sharon Sheahan, PhD, CFNP
Associate Professor, University of Kentucky,
College of Nursing, Lexington, Kentucky

Donald B. Witzke, PhD
Associate Professor, Department of Pathology
and Laboratory Medicine and Director,
Student Testing and Evaluation, Office of
Education, College of Medicine, University of
Kentucky, Lexington, Kentucky

Preface

Emergency Care of the Elder Person is the culmination of a 5-year effort by the Geriatric Emergency Medicine Task Force of the Society for Academic Emergency Medicine (SAEM) to fill a gap in the knowledge base and practice of emergency medicine with regard to the care of elder persons. Gaps like this often go unrecognized for years until someone illuminates them by asking the right question.

In this case, the right question was asked in 1990 when Donna Regenstreif, PhD, Senior Program Officer of the John A. Hartford Foundation of New York, made inquiries of SAEM regarding the emergency care of older persons. Suddenly, it became apparent that there was a dearth of education, training, and research on care of the elderly in emergency departments. Some efforts had been made by a few visionary academicians, particularly Michael Eliastam, MD and Jeffrey Jones, MD. Overall, however, there was an obvious lack of in-depth information on the special emergency care needs of older persons. This area had largely been ignored in textbooks, journals, and educational programs. There was a similar dearth of education, training, and research on the emergency care of older patients in the geriatric subspecialty.

As we began to explore these issues and talk with our colleagues in geriatrics, it became clear that the two specialties — emergency medicine and geriatrics — were both rapidly developing with little communication about common problems. Geriatricians performed comprehensive assessments of their patients but gave little attention to emergency care needs. Most of their educational efforts focused on traditional primary care disciplines in family practice and internal medicine. Some geriatricians were unaware of the remarkable growth and sophisticated academic development of emergency medicine as a specialty. Likewise, although emergency medicine had achieved remarkable growth over the past 15 years, little attention had been paid to the discipline of geriatrics. The language and basic tools of each specialty were not even generally understood by practitioners of the other specialty.

Geriatricians often used standardized tools that assess a patient's functional status over a period of time. Abbreviations and terms such as ADL (Activities of Daily Living), IADL (Instrumental Activities of Daily Living), Mini-Mental State Score, and CAM (Confusion Assessment Method) Score are commonplace in the geriatric community but are unknown to emergency physicians. Similarly, many geriatricians were unfamiliar with the EMS system or with the mindset of emergency health care professionals in their focus on emergent and urgent conditions. This book attempts to optimize the emergency care of older patients by merging parts of both disciplines — geriatrics and emergency medicine.

With the generous support of the John A. Hartford Foundation of New York, SAEM formed the Geriatric Emergency Medicine Task Force, an interdisciplinary task force composed of emergency physicians, geriatricians, emergency nurses and paramedics. A series of studies were undertaken to define the status of geriatric emergency medicine, and recommendations were made to solve the identified problems. This report was published in a series of articles in the *Annals of Emergency Medicine* (July 1992: 792-841). The investigations included a survey of practicing emergency physicians, a multicenter study comparing the treatment of older and younger adult patients in six representative emergency departments, a multicenter survey of patients regarding their perception of emergency department care, interviews with older patients regarding emergency medical care, a multicenter database encompassing 70 hospitals regarding the emergency care of older patients, and a survey of residency programs regarding the extent of geriatric training for emergency medicine residents.

After analyzing the data from all of these studies, the Task Force concluded that older patients were a unique population with special needs that were not being met in the emergency care system.

Older persons have special concerns such as atypical disease presentations, polypharmacy, altered physiology, and altered diagnostic test standards, among others. Furthermore, the demographics of the aging population will make care of the elderly a major concern of emergency medicine for at least the next 50 years, with the number of elderly needing emergency care continuing to increase rapidly.

The Task Force further concluded that the care of elder persons can best be addressed by changing the traditional model of emergency care for this population. This precedent has been set for a number of other special populations such as children and trauma patients.
Similar principles for geriatric emergency medicine had to be developed that would take into account the unique physiology, atypical disease presentations, and psychosocial needs of older persons. These principles needed to be incorporated into the traditional emergency care model. *Emergency Care of the Elder Person* defines these principles in the context of emergency medicine, providing practical information for emergency health care and geriatric professionals.

Section I of the text establishes the special needs of the older population with discussions of demographics, physiology, pharmacology, diagnostic tests, ethical issues, and attitudes. Section II introduces the principles and implementation guidelines for a geriatric emergency care model. Section III gives the reader standardized instruments for assessing the elderly and explains the importance of using these instruments to improve the care older persons receive in the emergency health care environment. Section IV gives the reader practical information on how to approach specific clinical issues in older patients, including: trauma, infections, myocardial infarction, altered mental status, elder abuse and neglect, functional decline, abdominal pain, dizziness, and cerebrovascular accidents.

The content of each chapter was reviewed and revised by several contributors, then reviewed by the entire Task Force and presented as the focus of group discussions. Three Task Force Meetings as well as many conference calls were held to reach a consensus on the recommendations presented in this book.

Emergency Care of the Elder Person is accompanied by an Instructor's Manual. The Instructor's Manual provides the tools needed to apply the model of care and the principles of geriatric emergency medicine. Case-based discussions are presented using interactive, problem-oriented learning methodologies. The Instructor's Manual also contains transparencies, a video on Elder Persons in the Emergency Medical Care System, and a video on *Recognizing Delirium in the Elder Person, Perspectives for the Emergency Care Professional.*

The Instructor's Manual, transparencies, and the Elder Persons in the Emergency Medical Care System video are available through the Society for Academic Emergency Medicine, 901 N. Washington Avenue, Lansing, Michigan 98906 (telephone number: 517-485-5484).

The textbook and delirium video are available through Beverly Cracom Publications, 12131 Dorsett Road, Suite 109, St. Louis, Missouri 63043 (telephone number: 314-291-0880).

Acknowledgments

The material in this book represents the efforts of many people in addition to the chapter authors and Geriatric Emergency Medicine Task Force members who worked so diligently to complete this project. The John A. Hartford Foundation of New York has generously supported the efforts of the Task Force for the past 3 years. We especially would like to recognize the vision and efforts of Donna Regenstreif, PhD, Senior Program Officer of the Hartford Foundation, and Laura Robbins, Program Officer, for their encouragement and guidance throughout this project.

This consensus effort by the interdisciplinary Geriatric Emergency Medicine Task Force could not have taken place without the efforts of the Society for Academic Emergency Medicine. We would like to thank Mary Ann Schropp, Executive Director of SAEM, and Patty Miller, Administrative Assistant, for their tireless efforts on behalf of this project. Their organizational skills brought everything together and kept us on schedule. The officers and Board of Directors of SAEM from 1990-95 have been extremely supportive of this effort. We especially would like to thank Jerris Hedges, MD, who initiated the Geriatric Emergency Task Force as an SAEM project and actively participated in many of the studies. Steven Dronen, MD, was extremely helpful and influential in ensuring the relevance of the material to residents training in emergency medicine through the Council of Emergency Medicine Residency Directors. We also thank Drs. Bill Barsan, Louis Ling, Louis Binder, David Sklar, Lewis Goldfrank, and Marcus Martin for their leadership and support of this project.

Finally, we thank Barbara Norwitz and Craig Cuddeback, Publisher and Co-Director of Beverly Cracom Publications. Their vision, dedication, and commitment to this project were essential to its success. Marny Johnson, Developmental Editor at Beverly Cracom Publications, was the heart and spirit of both the textbook and instructor's manual. Ms. Johnson did a remarkable job of coordinating the efforts of the authors and Task Force and editing the manuscripts to ensure successful completion of the project.

Arthur B. Sanders, MD
Chair, SAEM Geriatric Emergency Medicine Task Force

Contents

A Special Population

1 Demographics, Aging, and Emergency Medical Care

LEARNING OBJECTIVES

1. Anticipate changes in emergency department (ED) utilization, including the frequency of visits and time requirements.
2. Correlate demographic changes to demands on ED and hospital resources, including bed space and ancillary services, health professional time and efforts, prehospital system utilization, and trauma systems.

CURRENT POPULATION TRENDS

Medical professionals are aware that the population is aging, but it is important to realize the exact scope of this trend to place the future of emergency medical care in a clear perspective. In the United States, persons aged 65 years and older represented 11.3% of the population, or 25.5 million persons, in 1980. By the year 2000 this figure will rise to 13.1% of the population, or 35 million elderly persons. In the year 2030 the predicted number is 20% of the population equaling over 55 million persons aged 65 years or older.[1,2] Thus the elderly population in raw numbers will have doubled in size from 1980 to 2030, a mere 50 years (Figure 1–1).

A further point of interest is the fact that the oldest persons of the elderly population represent the fastest growing segment of the population. The number of persons over the age of 85 years will increase at three to four times the rate of the general population between the years 1990 and 2010. In the 10 years from 1990 to 2000, it is predicted that the number of persons aged 75 years and over will increase 26%.

The number of persons over the age of 85 will increase at three to four times the rate of the general population between the years 1990 and 2010.

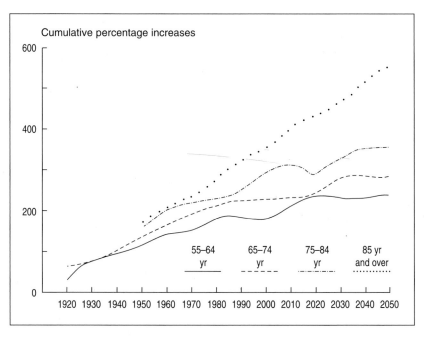

Figure 1–1 Percentage (%) increase of elderly population from 1920 to 2050. (From Eliastam M. Elderly patients in the emergency department. *Ann Emerg Med.* 1989;18:1222–1229.)

These trends can be attributed to the steadily increasing life expectancy for the population. Approximately 5 years have been added to the life expectancy for both sexes in the 25-year period ending in 1986.[1,2]

EMERGENCY DEPARTMENT UTILIZATION

Providers of emergency medical care can expect an increasing volume of geriatric patients. The aging of the population will be the major underlying cause for this, but other factors may further increase the flow of elderly patients into emergency care systems. Several studies indicate that the elderly utilize emergency services at a rate higher than expected for their numbers in the population. In a multicenter study of ED utilization, the elderly accounted for 15% of the visits, yet they only comprised 12% of the population[3] (Table 1–1 and Figure 1–2). Similar results have been obtained in two separate studies at single institutions.[4,5] A further factor that may directly influence the number of elderly patients encountered in the ED is the steadily increasing number of visits to these facilities by the population as a whole.[6]

The increasing number of elder patients will disproportionately tax the ED as they require more time and consume more resources. Their length of stay in the ED is nearly 20% longer than younger patients (Figure 1–3). Their visits are rated as high or intermediate urgency.[7] The rate of admission to the hospital is several fold higher for both general and intensive care unit beds[3,7] (Figure 1–4). Although account-

While accounting for only 15% of the ED visits, those over the age of 65 comprised 43% of all hospital admissions and 48% of all intensive care admissions from the ED.

Table 1–1 **Patient Visits in 1990 for Multihospital Data Base**

	Elderly (% of Total Elderly Patients)	Nonelderly (% of Total Nonelderly Patients)	Total Patients	Elderly Patients as % of Total Patients
Total visits	177,700 (100)	1,016,043 (100)	1,193,743	14.9
Age				
65-74 yr	81,900 (46.1)	—	—	5.8
75-84 yr	65,400 (36.8)	—	—	5.9
85 yr or older	30,400 (17.1)	—	—	2.6
Admissions	56,900 (32.0)	76,400 (7.5)	133,300	42.7
Critical care unit (CCU) admissions	12,300 (6.9)	13,400 (1.3)	25,700	47.9
Ambulance transports	52,800 (29.7)	93,100 (9.2)	145,900	36.2
Level of service				
Brief	400 (0.2)	4,400 (0.4)	4,800	8.3
Limited	15,100 (8.5)	306,500 (30.2)	322,600	4.7
Intermediate	30,700 (17.3)	372,600 (31.8)	353,300	8.7
Extended	28,000 (15.8)	149,300 (14.7)	177,300	18.8
Comprehensive	82,500 (46.4)	127,300 (12.5)	209,800	39.3

From Strange GR, Chen EH, Sanders AB. Use of emergency departments by elderly patients: projections from a multi-center data base. *Ann Emerg Med.* 1992; 21: 819–824.

ing for only 15% of the ED visits, persons over 65 years comprised 43% of all hospital admissions and 48% of all intensive care admissions from the ED in a multicenter study.[3] Ancillary services will also be strained as elderly patients undergo radiography and laboratory testing at a rate roughly 50% higher than for younger patients.[7]

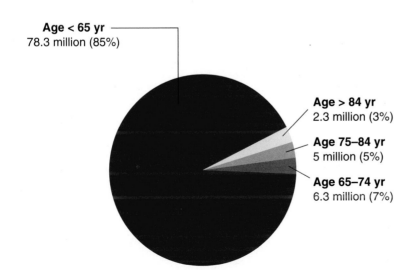

Age < 65 yr
78.3 million (85%)

Age > 84 yr
2.3 million (3%)

Age 75–84 yr
5 million (5%)

Age 65–74 yr
6.3 million (7%)

FIGURE 1–2   Age distribution for 1990 ED visits. (From Strange GR, Chen EH, Sanders AB. Use of emergency departments by elderly patients: projections from a multi-center data base. *Ann Emerg Med.* 1992;21:819–824.)

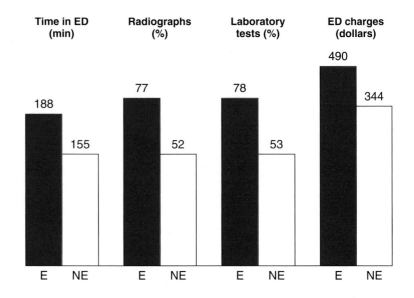

FIGURE 1–3 Patterns of ED resource use. *E,* Elderly; *NE,* nonelderly. (Data from Singal BM, Hedges JR, Rousseau EW, et al. Geriatric patient emergency visits, I: comparison of visits by geriatric and younger patients. *Ann Emerg Med.* 1992;21:802–807.)

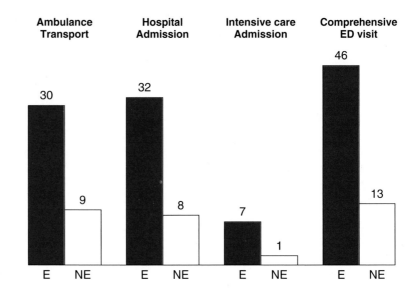

FIGURE 1–4 Acuity of illness. (Numbers represent percent [%] of patients.) *E,* Elderly; *NE,* nonelderly. (Data from Strange GR, Chen EH, Sanders AB. Use of emergency departments by elderly patients: Projections from a multi-center data base. *Ann Emerg Med.* 1992: 21:819–824.)

HEALTH PROFESSIONAL UTILIZATION

The increased length of stay and higher urgency level of visits already directly impact those caring for elderly persons in the ED. A large majority of emergency physicians indicate that caring for elderly patients is more time-consuming for the following major clinical presentations to the ED (Figure 1–5)[8]:

1. Abdominal pain
2. Altered mental status
3. Chest pain
4. Dizziness/vertigo
5. Fever without a source
6. Headache
7. Multi system trauma

In addition to time factors another significant issue is the mental energy required to handle older patients in the ED. Nearly half or more

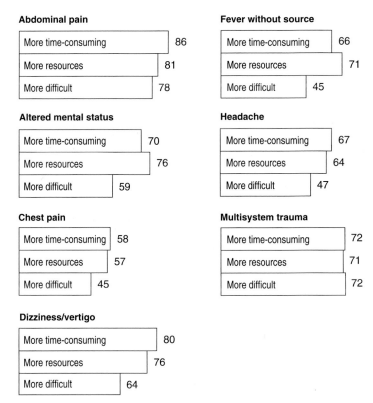

FIGURE 1–5   Evaluation of clinical symptoms in older compared to younger adult patients. (Numbers represent percent [%] of affirmative responses.) (Adapted from McNamara RM, Rousseau E, Sanders AB: Geriatric emergency medicine: a survey of practicing emergency physicians. *Ann Emerg Med*. July 1992;21:796–801.)

of emergency physicians report a higher level of difficulty in managing each of the clinical presentations mentioned above[8] (Tables 1–2 and 1–3). Further stressing emergency health care providers are frequent difficulties in communication with the older patient and the referring physician or nursing home.[8]

Table 1–2 **Reported Level of Difficulty Managing Older Compared with Younger Adult Patients**

Clinical Issue	Responses (%)		
	Less Difficult	Equal	More Difficult
Abdominal pain	1	21	78
Altered mental status	10	31	59
Chest pain	12	43	45
Dizziness and vertigo	4	32	64
Fever without a source	14	41	45
Headache	7	46	47
Multisystem trauma	3	25	72

From McNamara RM, Rousseau E, Sanders AB: Geriatric emergency medicine: a survey of practicing emergency physicians. *Ann Emerg Med*. July 1992; 21: 796–801.

PREHOSPITAL ISSUES

Prehospital resources currently are disproportionately used by older patients. This was recognized as early as 1982 in Akron, Ohio, where elderly people accounted for 22% of all emergency medical service (EMS) runs.[9] More recent data indicates that elderly persons use emergency ambulance services at rates three to four times higher than younger patients.[3,7] The rate of ambulance use increases steadily within the elderly subset of patients to the point where 55% of ED arrivals by those over the age of 85 years involve ambulance transport as compared to 32% of those aged 65 to 74 years.[7] Those responsible for planning and financing EMS systems will need to anticipate this future strain on resources.

TRAUMA SYSTEM IMPACT

Currently the 14- to 34-year-old age group is the most frequently injured, but their numbers are declining while those of the elderly age group are

Table 1–3 **Responses to Questions Comparing Evaluation and Management of Older vs. Younger Adult Patients**

	Affirmative Responses (%)		
Clinical Issue	**Elderly More Time-Consuming**	**Elderly Require More Resources**	**Better Standards of Care for Younger**
Abdominal pain	86	81	43
Altered mental status	70	76	44
Chest pain	58	57	31
Dizziness and vertigo	80	76	40
Fever without a source	65	71	29
Headache	67	64	37
Multisystem trauma	72	71	40

From McNamara RM, Rousseau E, Sanders AB: Geriatric emergency medicine: a survey of practicing emergency physicians. *Ann Emerg Med.* July 1992;21:796–801.

increasing. This change in demographics will alter the pattern of trauma presentations with a decline in penetrating injury and a rise in those injured by a blunt mechanism.[10] The majority of injuries in elder persons are related to falls, with assaults and work-related mishaps being very uncommon.[7,11] Older victims of trauma are more likely to have the following:

Of ED arrivals by those over the age of 85, 55% involve ambulance transport, compared to 32% among those aged 65 to 74.

1. Higher injury severity scores
2. Higher hospital charges
3. Longer lengths of stay
4. Longer ICU stays[11]

Further, when compared to younger patients with comparable severity of illness or injury, the elderly have a higher case fatality rate and are more likely to require placement in an intermediate or long-term care facility at the time of hospital discharge.[11] This change in the demographics of trauma may have a significant negative financial impact on the already-stressed trauma systems, because reimbursement for trauma in older persons is considered inadequate.[10]

SUMMARY POINTS

- The population is rapidly aging. By the year 2030 persons aged 65 years or older will comprise 20% of the population.
- Older adults utilize the ED at a higher rate than younger patients.
- Older patients in the ED require more time, resources, and mental energy than younger patients. They are more frequently admitted to both the general hospital and intensive care units.
- All systems of traditional care delivery will be challenged by the increasing number of elderly persons in our society.

CHAPTER AUTHOR

Robert M. McNamara, MD

REFERENCES

1. Sanders AB. Care of the elderly in the emergency department: where do we stand? *Ann Emerg Med.* 1992;21:792–795.
2. US Bureau of the Census. *Statistical Abstract of the United States: 1990.* 110th ed. Washington, DC: US Government Printing Office, 1990.
3. Strange GR, Chen EH, Sanders AB. Use of emergency departments by elderly patients: projections from a multi-center data base. *Ann Emerg Med.* 1992;21:819–824.
4. Lowenstein SR, Crescenzi CA, Kern DC, et al. Care of the elderly in the emergency department. *Ann Emerg Med.* 1986;15:528–535.
5. Baum SA, Rubinstein LZ. Old people in the emergency room: age related differences in emergency department use and care. *J Am Geriatr Soc.* 1987;35:398–404.
6. *AHA Hospital Statistics.* Chicago: American Hospital Association; 1990.
7. Singal BM, Hedges JR, Rousseau EW, et al. Geriatric patient emergency visits, I: comparison of visits by geriatric and younger patients. *Ann Emerg Med.* 1992;21:802–807.
8. McNamara RM. Geriatric emergency medicine: a survey of practicing emergency physicians. *Ann Emerg Med.* 1992;21:796–801.
9. Gerson LW, Skvarch L. Emergency service utilization by the elderly. *Ann Emerg Med.* 1982;11:610–612.
10. Fischer RP, Miles DL. The demographics of trauma in 1995. *J Trauma.* 1987;27:1233–1235.
11. Covington DL, Maxwell JG, Clancy TV. Hospital resources used to treat the injured elderly at North Carolina trauma centers. *J Am Geriatr Soc.* 1993;41:847–852.

2 *Physiology of Aging*

LEARNING OBJECTIVES

1. Apply an understanding of variability in functional longevity to perceptions and ED care of the elderly.
2. Define physiologic aging.
3. Explain the concepts of functional reserve capacity and critical threshold for development of clinical symptoms.
4. Identify physiologic changes occurring with age in regard to the following:
   a. Homeostasis
   b. Body composition
   c. Oxygen conductance
   d. Cardiovascular function
   e. Central nervous system (CNS) function
   f. Immune system function
5. Identify diagnostic tests that may be altered by the aging process and those that are not affected.

In the most simple and unbiased terms, aging can be defined as any process that involves change over time. Americans tend to view aging negatively and associate the process with decline in function, vitality, and worth. Other societies have a more balanced attitude toward aging and emphasize more desirable qualities of maturity such as wisdom accrued by experience and the attainment of equanimity. This chapter will delineate the physiology of aging as an objective physiologic process, with specific changes in physiology related to the clinical presentation and management of the older patient in the ED.

It is important to distinguish between chronologic and biologic age when considering physiologic aging. Everyone has encountered vital octogenarians who appear decades younger than their birth dates imply, as well as morbidly senescent persons younger than 60 years with a depressing array of infirmities. As a species, humans display a surprising variability in functional longevity. This is due largely to a diversity of genetic determinants influenced to varying degrees by environment, occupation, lifelong disease experience, and cultural and socioeconomic background. Health behaviors also have a material influence on the aging process. Diet, tobacco, alcohol, drug use, exercise and conditioning, rest, stress, outlook, and attitude all impact the well-being of the individual and contribute to longevity. The following discussion will by necessity deal in generalities regarding aging and focus on aging as a normal phenomenon independent of coexisting disease.

ALTERED FUNCTIONAL CAPACITIES

CRITICAL THRESHOLDS

From a strictly physiologic standpoint it is evident that few things improve with age (Figure 2–1). After the fourth decade there is an inexorable decline in most parameters of function, although we remain by and large healthy and robust for decades to come. Built into most major organ systems is a *functional reserve capacity* that allows the individual to adapt to and survive a variety of challenges encountered through-

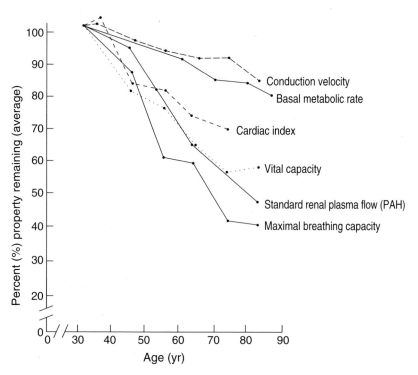

FIGURE 2–1 Changes in physiologic function that accompany normal aging. (Reprinted with permission of Simon & Schuster, Inc. from *Developmental Physiology and Aging* by Paola S. Timiras. Copyright © 1972 P.S. Timiras.)

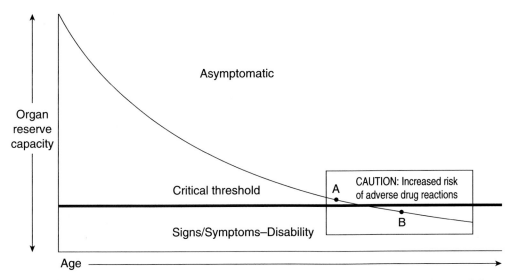

FIGURE 2–2   Decline of organ reserve with age. Incidence of adverse drug reactions and drug-disease interactions increases as the largest organ system approaches the critical threshold. A drug may act as a provocative stressor, in some cases moving impaired organ system below the critical threshold (Point *A* to Point *B*). (From Sloan RW. Principles of drug therapy in geriatric patients. *Am Fam Physician.* 1992;45: 2709–2718.)

out life. Physiologic aging can thus be characterized as a predictable decline in the functional reserve capacity of major organ systems and a resultant limit in the ability to adapt. The decline in reserve function of organs such as the heart, lungs, and kidneys may be clinically inapparent in an otherwise healthy person. This decline becomes evident only when the individual is faced with a major physiologic challenge such as an acute change in environment, an injury, an infection, or exposure to potentially toxic materials or medications. A *critical threshold* of organ function exists above which the individual functions normally and below which signs and symptoms of organ failure become manifest (Figure 2–2). For example, congestive heart failure may develop in the patient with marginal but compensated cardiac function who is prescribed a beta-adrenergic antagonist (i.e., propranolol, metoprolol, atenolol) for angina. Similarly, acute renal failure can be precipitated by the angiotensin converting enzyme (ACE) inhibitors (i.e., enalapril, captopril, lisinopril) prescribed to an elderly hypertensive person with clinically silent renal insufficiency. The importance of diminishing functional reserve and critical thresholds will be evident in the following discussions of organ system aging.

A critical threshold of organ function exists above which the individual functions normally and below which signs and symptoms of organ failure become manifest.

HOMEOSTASIS

Homeostasis is a term originally coined to describe the remarkable ability of an organism to maintain the constancy of its internal environment in the face of a changing external environment. In general, homeostasis is achieved by a system of feedback loops made up of receptors located in the internal and external environments that constantly provide input to a central regulatory system dedicated to the protection of a physiologic set point. Output from this central regula-

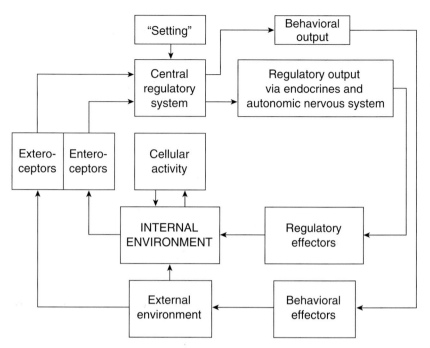

FIGURE 2–3   Homeostasis is achieved by a series of feedback loops that regulate the internal environment. (From Kenney RA. Physiology of aging. *Clin Geriatr Med.* 1985;1:37–59.)

Aging is characterized by a narrowing of the environmental limits within which an individual is able to maintain homeostasis.

tory system alters voluntary and involuntary output to effector organs whose activity reestablishes the physiologic equilibrium (Figure 2–3).

Thermoregulation is perhaps one of the best studied and understood homeostatic mechanisms. Control of body temperature depends on the operation of a complex series of feedback loops. To illustrate, a decrease in cellular metabolic activity or external temperature causes a drop in the temperature of the internal environment that is then detected by internal and external thermoreceptors. These receptors provide input to thalamic centers that maintain a temperature set point. Output from these centers influences behavioral output from cortical areas governing behavior and output from the autonomic nervous system and endocrine glands. Behavioral output could consist of the individual turning up a thermostat, putting on a sweater, or leaving a cold environment. Output from the autonomic nervous system results in shunting of cutaneous blood flow to preserve heat and shivering to generate more heat. Endocrine output influences basal metabolic activity through changes in pituitary, thyroid, and adrenal hormone secretion. Speed and accuracy characterize these feedback systems to such an extent that even minute alterations within the internal environment normally produce instantaneous compensation and prevent wide excursions about the set point.

Defective thermoregulation manifested by a predisposition to hypothermia and hyperthermia is a special problem. While the basic components of homeostasis are intact, the ability to detect changes in external and internal environments and the rapidity and adequacy of response to these changes are often diminished. Thermal, chemical, and mechanical receptor density and sensitivity tend to decline with aging. The older individual has a decreased appreciation of temperature changes in the external environment. Degenerative changes in the skin lead to loss of cutaneous thermal receptors and diminished sensitivity of those remaining receptors. Control centers in the hypothalamus and brain stem become less precise in integrative function. Although set points such as basal body temperature are not significantly altered by aging, larger deviations from those set points are often required to activate a homeostatic adjustment. Effector systems are affected by aging as well. Basal metabolic heat production may be compromised by decreased muscle mass, voluntary activity, peripheral insulation, and cardiac output. Aging skin has a lower density of sweat glands, which may compromise heat dissipation. Undershoot, overshoot, and response delay are typical changes in homeostatic mechanisms seen with aging. Involuntary responses become attenuated, and voluntary responses are often influenced by dementia, deconditioning, and immobility.

BODY COMPOSITION

Body weight is not greatly affected by aging; however, important changes occur in body composition. With the unfortunate exception of the prostate, most organs decrease in size or in the content of functional tissue or in both parameters with age. Lean body mass and bone mass tend to decrease in proportion to an increase in adipose tissue. Adipose tissue redistributes from the extremities to more central sites such as the omentum and perinephric area, contributing to somatic changes that characterize the aging body. Solid organs tend to accumulate adipose tissue, which replaces functional parenchyma. Adipose tissue is anhydrous and accounts for an age-related decrease in total body water as a percent of total body weight. Water is lost to a greater extent from the intracellular than from the extracellular fluid space. These changes in body composition significantly affect the volume of distribution of many commonly prescribed drugs and intoxicants such as alcohol. Drugs such as digoxin, theophylline, and aminoglycoside antibiotics distribute in lean tissue and must have their dosages adjusted downward to avoid potential toxicity. Conversely, drugs that distribute in adipose tissue such as benzodiazepines, barbiturates, phenothiazines, and phenytoin may have a prolonged duration of action in elderly persons and have a greater potential for toxicity as a result of accumulation.[1]

> *Digoxin, theophylline, and aminoglycoside antibiotics distribute in lean tissue. Adjust dosages downward to avoid potential toxicity.*

OXYGEN CONDUCTANCE

Changes in body composition result in a net decrease in oxygen-consuming lean tissue mass. However, oxygen uptake and delivery are affected by aging as well. Oxygen conductance is influenced by age-related changes in respiratory, cardiac, and red blood cell (RBC) function as outlined here.

Maximum breathing capacity declines, along with the loss of thoracic muscle mass, diminished airway and lung compliance, and increased airway resistance. Ventilatory drive decreases, reflecting a loss of chemoreceptor sensitivity to hypercapnia and hypoxemia. Changes in the shape of the thorax because of skeletal aging and de-

> *Benzoidiazepines, barbiturates, phenothiazines, and phenytoin distribute in adipose tissue. Watch for toxicity resulting from accumulation.*

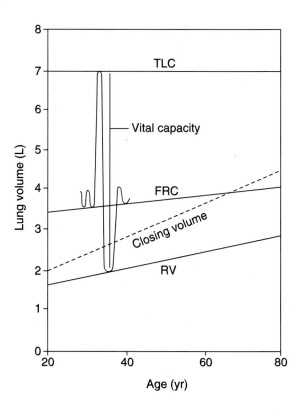

FIGURE 2–4 Effect of age on the subdivisions of lung volume. *TLC,* Total lung capacity; *FRC,* functional residual capacity; *RV,* residual volume. As closing volume approaches FRC, resulting ventilation-perfusion mismatch causes a predictable decline in arterial Po₂. (From Tackman MS. Aging of the respiratory system. In: Hazzard WR, Bierman EL, Blass JP, Ettinger Jr WH, Halter JB, eds. *Principles of geriatric medicine and gerontology.* 3rd ed. New York, NY: McGraw-Hill; 1994:555–564. Copyright 1994. Reproduced with permission from McGraw-Hill, Inc.)

creased lung elasticity contribute to a decline in respiratory functional reserves. Although total lung capacity is relatively constant, vital capacity declines as the residual volume increases. Changes in elastic recoil of the lungs cause the airway closing volume to increase and gradually approach the functional reserve capacity (Figure 2–4). In well-perfused areas of the lungs, airway closure then creates ventilation-perfusion mismatch, resulting in a predictable decline in arterial Po_2. These changes all combine to increase the metabolic cost of breathing and contribute to respiratory insufficiency and failure when the person is challenged by disease.[2,3]

Resting cardiac output decreases at a rate of approximately 1% per year after 30 years of age.

The heart undergoes gradual histologic and biochemical change with aging that influences function. Resting cardiac output decreases at a rate of approximately 1% per year after 30 years of age. Maximum output, or cardiac reserve, declines as well. These age-related changes ultimately result in decreased blood flow and oxygen delivery to all organ systems both at rest and especially with the stress of exercise, work, or serious illness (Figure 2–5).[4]

Anemia is not a natural consequence of aging.

Anemia is not a natural consequence of aging, and the oxygen-carrying capacity of the blood does not change appreciably. Although hemoglobin concentration is relatively constant, the RBC oxygen dissociation curve may be shifted leftward by an age-related depletion of 2-3 diphosphoglycerate (DPG). Decreased oxygen dissociation from RBCs may further compromise oxygen delivery to tissues. Any toxin or drug causing further depletion of DPG is likely to have an even greater effect.[5]

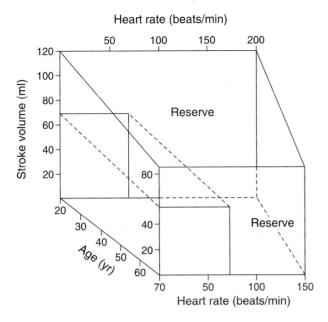

FIGURE 2–5   Changes in resting cardiac output and reserve that occur with aging. (From Kenney RA, Physiology of aging. *Clin Geriatr Med.* 1985; 1:37–59.)

FLUID VOLUME AND ELECTROLYTES

Total body water declines with aging as lean body mass is replaced by anhydrous adipose tissue. Although electrolytes and osmolarity are normal in otherwise healthy older adults, abnormalities in fluid and electrolyte balance commonly occur in the face of acute illness or physiologic stress (Table 2–1). Homeostatic regulation of extracellular fluid volume and composition depends on neuroendocrine communication between the CNS and the kidneys. The principal CNS controls of fluid balance operate through changes in thirst and vasopressin (antidiuretic hormone [ADH]) secretion. Although the reason is unclear, it is well documented that older persons have a diminished thirst response to water deprivation, placing them at risk of dehydration under a variety of circumstances. Vasopressin secretion is stimulated by elevated plasma osmolarity and by hypovolemia. In the elderly, baseline vasopressin secretion is normal; however, the response of vasopressin secretion to an osmolar challenge or water deprivation is markedly increased. However, the enhanced secretion of vasopressin does not translate into greater water conservation, because the renal response to vasopressin is generally diminished with aging and results in the decreased ability to produce concentrated urine. The combination of blunted thirst, decreased access to water secondary to immobility or cognitive impairment, and diminished renal response to vasopressin can further predispose the elderly to dehydration (Table 2–2).

Total body water declines with aging as lean body mass is replaced by anhydrous adipose tissue.

Table 2–1 **Causes of Increased Fluid Loss in Elderly Patients**

Chronic or acute infections	Gastrointestinal losses
Excessive urinary losses	Upper gastrointestinal
Diuretic misuse	Vomiting
Glycosuria	Nasogastric drainage
Hypercalciuria	Lower gastrointestinal (diarrhea)
Mannitol	Laxative abuse or bowel
Radiographic contrast agents	preparations
Elevated blood urea nitrogen	Infectious or secretory
(BUN)	Surgical bypass or fistulas
Diabetes insipidus	Ischemic bowel
Central (pituitary)	Colectomy
Nephrogenic	Excessive blood loss
Hypoaldosteronism	Environment-related fluid loss
Addison's disease	Heat wave
Hyporeninemic	Hypothermia
hypoaldosteronism	Compartmental fluid shifts
Suppressed vasopressin	Hypoalbuminemia
Alzheimer's disease	Pancreatitis
Phenytoin	Ascites
Ethanol	Anaphylaxis
Postatrial tachyarrhythmia	Burns
Postobstructive diuresis	Hypertonic peritoneal dialysate

Davis KL, Minaker KL. Disorders of fluid balance. In: Hazzard WR, et al, ed. *Principles of Geriatric Medicine and Gerontology.* 3rd ed. New York, NY: McGraw-Hill, Inc; 1994: 1185. Copyright 1994. Reproduced with permission from McGraw-Hill, Inc.

Table 2–2 **Causes of Decreased Fluid Intake in Elderly Patients**

Limited access to fluids	Gastrointestinal disorders
Physical restraints	Swallowing disorders
Mobility restriction	Bowel obstruction
Poor visual acuity	Mechanical
Fluid restriction	Metabolic
Preprocedure	Ischemic
Prevention of incontinence or	Anticholinergic medication
nocturia or aspiration	Alteration in thirst mechanism
Therapy for edema or	Primary adipsia
hyponatremia	Medication-related
Altered sensorium	Cardiac glycosides
Decreased consciousness level	Amphetamines
Sedatives, neuroleptics,	Associated with focal CNS
narcotics	pathologic condition
Structural and metabolic CNS	
insults	
Febrile illness	
Decreased level of awareness	
Dementia, delirium	
Mania, psychosis, depression	

Davis KL, Minaker KL. Disorders of fluid balance. In: Hazzard WR, et al, ed. *Principles of Geriatric Medicine and Gerontology.* 3rd ed. New York, NY: McGraw-Hill, Inc; 1994: 1185. Copyright 1994. Reproduced with permission from McGraw-Hill, Inc.

Table 2–3 **Factors Associated with Hypernatremia**

Factor	Patients (%)
Febrile illness	70
Infirmity	40
Surgery	21
Nutritional supplementation	20
Intravenous solutes	18
Diabetes mellitus	15
Diarrhea	11
Gastrointestinal bleeding	9
Diuretics	9
Diabetes insipidus	7
Dialysis related	3

Davis KL, Minaker KL. Disorders of fluid balance. In: Hazzard WR, et al, ed. *Principles of Geriatric Medicine and Gerontology.* 3rd ed. New York, NY: McGraw-Hill, Inc; 1994:1184. Copyright 1994. Reproduced with permission from McGraw-Hill, Inc.

Hypernatremia often accompanies dehydration in the acutely ill elderly patient and indicates a poor prognosis in those hospitalized (Table 2–3). Hypernatremic dehydration is especially prevalent in older residents of extended care facilities and has been suggested as an indicator of neglect[6]. The prevalence of hyponatremia increases with age as well. Problems with sodium conservation are generally equated to defects in the renin-aldosterone system. Hypovolemic hyponatremia may result from chronic diarrhea or may complicate diuretic use. Hypervolemic hyponatremia often accompanies edematous conditions with excess total body sodium, such as nephrosis, cirrhosis, and congestive heart failure. Normovolemic hyponatremia is especially common because of the prevalence of diseases associated with the syndrome of inappropriate antidiuretic hormone secretion (SIADH). These include chronic lung disease, cancer, and CNS disease. A number of commonly prescribed drugs can produce SIADH. Indomethacin and chlorpropamide increase renal sensitivity to ADH, whereas opiate narcotics, carbamazepine, and tricyclic antidepressants increase central ADH release.

An age-related decline in glomerular filtration and responsiveness of the renin-aldosterone system make the elderly more prone to hyperkalemia. The aging kidney is often unable to cope with extra potassium derived from prescribed dietary supplements, sodium-restricted salt substitutes, gastrointestinal bleeding, or an accelerated catabolism that occurs in various disease states. Drugs that interfere with potassium excretion are the most common cause of hyperkalemia. These drugs include the ACE inhibitors prescribed for hypertension, nonsteroidal antiinflammatory drugs (NSAIDs), and the so-called potassium-sparing diuretics (triamterene, amiloride, and spironolactone). Hypokalemia is also prevalent. Diuretic-induced renal potassium wasting is likely the most common cause and is worsened by decreased dietary potassium intake. Recent studies suggest that the elderly are at a particularly higher risk of malignant cardiac dysrhythmias precipitated by drug-induced hypokalemia.

Table 2–4 **Factors That Affect Susceptibility to Postural Hypotension**

Predisposing Factors	Protective Factors
Decline in baroreflex sensitivity	Impaired beta-adrenergic–mediated vasodilation
Decreased arterial compliance	
Increased venous tortuosity	Normal alpha-adrenergic–mediated vasodilation
Decreased cardiac compliance	
Decreased renal sodium conservation	Elevated norepinephrine levels
Decreased plasma volume	
Blunted vasopressin release to standing	
Decreased renin, angiotensin, and aldosterone levels	

From Mader SL. Aging and postural hypotension. *J Am Geriatr Soc.* 1989;37(2):129–137. Reprinted with permission.

CARDIOVASCULAR STATUS

Cardiac output and reserve decline with age, reflecting a decline in ventricular contractility, compliance, and distensibility. There is a greater reliance on endogenous catecholamines for inotropic support in the aging heart. Sinus node dysfunction and conduction abnormalities are more common in aged persons. In this setting beta-adrenergic blocking agents and certain calcium channel blockers (such as verapamil), alone or in combination, may precipitate congestive heart failure or varying degrees of heart block. The incidence of occlusive coronary artery disease increases with age. The elderly have a higher mortality from acute myocardial infarct and are more prone to complications of infarct management (Chapter 12).[4]

Hypertension is common. Characteristically, systolic blood pressure rises to a higher extent than does diastolic. Age-related increases in blood pressure are thought to be a consequence of changes in arterial connective tissue structure resulting in generalized loss of elasticity. Atherosclerosis has a higher prevalence and also contributes to hypertension but should be considered as a specific disease entity rather than a natural consequence of aging.

Maintenance of blood pressure and cerebral perfusion during postural changes depends on the coordinated response of the autonomic nervous system through the baroreflex (Table 2–4). On assuming an upright position reflex sympathetic discharge and parasympathetic inhibition increase peripheral vascular tone, heart rate, and contractility to preserve orthostatic blood pressure. Diminished responsiveness of the autonomic nervous system is reflected by the increased frequency of orthostatic hypotension . Orthostasis can become particularly severe with the use of certain antihypertensives, tricyclic antidepressants, and phenothiazines.[1]

Diminished responsiveness of the autonomic nervous system is reflected by the increased frequency of orthostatic hypotension.

NEUROLOGIC INTEGRITY

The weight of the brain declines with age, reflecting characteristic regional loss of neurons from the cortex, cerebellum, and hippocampus. In certain areas the density of dendritic connections is reduced as well. In otherwise healthy individuals, however, brain function remains largely intact. Although somewhat variable, language skills, memory, attention, and general intelligence do not decline appreciably until quite late in life. Dementia should not be thought of as a natural consequence of aging, but rather as the result of a potentially alterable disease process. And while a cure remains elusive, considerable progress has been made in understanding the genetic and biochemical derangements of Alzheimer's disease.

Language skills, memory, attention and general intelligence do not decline appreciably until quite late in life. Dementia is not a natural consequence of aging.

The extrapyramidal system may be affected by aging, with decreased dopamine production by neurons in the substantia nigra. In the absence of overt Parkinson's disease extrapyramidal symptoms may be precipitated by drugs that affect dopamine action such as commonly prescribed psychotropics.

The special senses of touch, sight, hearing, taste, and smell are to varying degrees adversely affected by aging. These changes contribute to the isolation and immobility that often accompany aging. Emergency physicians should try to recognize potentially correctable defects in vision and hearing and make appropriate referrals.[7]

RESISTANCE TO INFECTION

In general, the immune system of the elderly is intact but sluggish in its response to infection. Cell-mediated immunity is influenced primarily by changes in T-cell function. T-cell number is not significantly reduced by aging; however, the response of various T-cell subsets to infection is materially altered. Interleukin II is a T-cell–derived lymphokine that stimulates the proliferation and differentiation of other T-cell lines (clones). T-cell production of interleukin II is diminished in aging, which accounts in part for the reduced response of cell-mediated immunity to infection. T cells dedicated to immune memory become depleted, reducing the immune systems' ability to respond to new antigens and keep other latent infections, such as tuberculosis and herpes zoster, in check.

Humoral immunity is relatively intact, and total immunoglobulin levels generally remain constant. However, the production of new immunoglobulin in response to new antigens is diminished by the decline in helper T-cell function. These changes tend to decrease the efficacy of vaccinations in older persons.

Phagocytosis and antigen processing functions of macrophages and monocytes are largely preserved. However, production by these cell types of the monokines interleukin I and tumor necrosis factor are diminished. These monokines mediate the nonspecific responses to serious infection and sepsis, including fever, various acute phase reactants, and depletion of the trace metals iron and zinc. Other nonspecific responses to infection remain essentially intact. Neutrophil number and function are unchanged by aging. Opsonization, complement levels, and activity also remain intact.

Physical barriers to infection are altered by aging. Atrophic skin is dry and less acidic secondary to decreased eccrine gland secretion, which also alters normal skin flora. The skin becomes thinner and more prone to injury by shearing forces. Loss of subcutaneous fat contributes to decubitus ulcer formation over bony prominences. A number of factors contribute to decreased saliva production, including autoimmune disease, endocrine disturbances, medications, and radiation exposure during cancer therapy. Xerostomia promotes dental caries and changes in normal oral flora. Colonization of the oropharynx with gram-negative enteric organisms is common. Aspiration pneumonia occurs frequently when decreased mucociliary clearance, inefficient cough, and swallowing disorders are combined. Atrophic changes in the gastric mucosa result in decreased acid production. Elevated gastric pH inhibits the clearance of various enteric pathogens such as *Salmonella* and *Listeria*. Cell surface changes in the genitourinary mucosa make colonization with pathogenic bacteria more likely, especially with *Escherichia coli*. Other factors that predispose the elderly to urinary tract infection include urinary tract obstruction, which increases the likelihood of instrumentation, nephrolithiasis, and dehydration.

Nutrition is important to the maintenance of immune competence, and protein malnutrition is common in elder persons. Malnutrition is accompanied by lymphoid tissue involution and secondary lymphopenia. Resultant defects in T-cell number and function contribute to anergy, and a higher incidence of intracellular infections by such organisms as *Mycobacterium tuberculosis*, *Listeria*, and *Salmonella*.[8,9]

DIAGNOSTIC TESTING

The effect of aging on routine laboratory test results and pitfalls in laboratory testing have been investigated and reported extensively (Table 2–5). As a rule, laboratory test results in a healthy elderly population do not fall outside of normal ranges. However, a number of routine tests can be influenced by aging.[10–12]

HEMATOLOGY

In the past a degree of anemia was accepted as a natural consequence of aging and grouped with the anemias of chronic disease. However, studies of normal elderly populations have found this generalization to be false (Table 2–6). Total mass of hematopoietic marrow tissue declines with age, which may affect blood cell proliferation in response to a significant challenge. The lowest acceptable normal hemoglobin values in the elderly are 11.0 g/dl in women and 11.5 g/dl in men. White blood cell (WBC) number and differential are not consistently influenced by aging; however, the proliferation of neutrophil cell lines in response to infection or sepsis is frequently attenuated. Platelet number and function remain intact.

Erythrocyte sedimentation rate (ESR) is a nonspecific test used most commonly to detect or monitor the progression of an inflammatory process, either infectious or rheumatologic. The ESR depends on RBC rouleaux formation. Rouleaux formation is influenced by a number of factors, including RBC number, shape, and electrical charge, and by

Table 2–5 **Laboratory Assessment of the Elderly**

Laboratory Parameters Unchanged*

Hemoglobin and hematocrit
White blood cell count
Platelet count
Electrolytes (sodium, potassium, chloride, bicarbonate)
Blood urea nitrogen
Liver function tests (transaminases, bilirubin, prothrombin time)
Free thyroxine index
Thyroid-stimulating hormone
Calcium
Phosphorus

Common Abnormal Laboratory Parameters†

Parameter	Clinical Significance
Sedimentation rate	Mild elevations (10–20 mm) may be an age-related change
Glucose	Glucose tolerance decreases
Creatinine	Because lean body mass and daily endogenous creatinine production decline, high-normal and minimally elevated values may indicate substantially reduced renal function
Albumin	Average values decline (< 0.5 g/ml) with age, especially in hospitalized elderly, but generally indicate undernutrition
Alkaline phosphatase	Mild elevations common in asymptomatic elderly; liver and Paget's disease should be considered if moderately elevated
Serum iron and iron-binding capacity	Decreased values are not an aging change and usually indicate undernutrition and/or gastrointestinal blood loss
Prostate specific antigen	May be elevated in patients with benign prostatic hyperplasia. Marked elevation or increasing values when followed over time should prompt consideration of further evaluation in patients for whom specific therapy for prostate cancer would be undertaken if cancer were diagnosed.
Urinalysis	Asymptomatic pyuria and bacteriuria are common and rarely warrant treatment; hematuria is abnormal and needs further evaluation
Chest radiographs	Interstitial changes are a common age-related finding; diffusely diminished bone density should generally indicate advanced osteoporosis
Electrocardiogram	ST-segment and T-wave changes, atrial and ventricular arrhythmias, and various blocks are common in asymptomatic elderly and may not need specific evaluation or treatment

Kane RL, Ouslander JG, Abrass IB. *Essentials of Clinical Geriatrics.* 3rd ed. New York, NY: McGraw-Hill, Inc;1994:60–61. Copyright 1994. Reproduced with permission from McGraw-Hill, Inc.
*Aging changes do not occur in these parameters; abnormal values should prompt further evaluation.
†Includes normal aging and other age-related changes.

serum fibrinogen, immunoglobulin, and albumin levels. Numerous studies have demonstrated an age-related increase in ESR in otherwise healthy individuals. Isolated Westergren ESR values up to 40 mm/hr may be normal and not indicative of disease. As with any laboratory test, an elevated ESR must be interpreted in the light of other clinical signs and symptoms.[5,12]

Table 2–6 **Hematologic Values in Ambulatory Healthy Adults***

	MEN			WOMEN		
	Elderly (*n = 19*)	Young (*n = 25*)	*p*	Elderly (*n = 25*)	Young (*n = 25*)	*p*
Red blood cell count in $10^6/mm^3$	4.8 ± 0.4	5.1 ± 0.2	.009	4.5 ± 0.3	4.6 ± 0.3	.309
Hemoglobin in g/dl	14.8 ± 1.1	15.6 ± 0.7	.009	13.6 ± 1.0	14.0 ± 0.8	.155
Hematocrit %	43.8 ± 3.3	45.3 ± 2.2	.08	40.7 ± 2.9	41.6 ± 2.3	.266
Serum iron in µg/dl	74 ± 19	99 ± 23	.002	73 ± 18	90.5 ± 27	.016
Erythrocyte sedimentation rate in mm/hr	12 ± 9	4 ± 2	.007	20 ± 11	10 ± 6	.001
Mean corpuscular volume in µm³	91.3 ± 5.4	87.8 ± 2.8	.017	90.5 ± 4.1	90.5 ± 5.0	.951
Mean corpuscular hemoglobin in pg	31 ± 2	30.1 ± 1.6	.195	30.2 ± 1.2	30.3 ± 2.1	.854
Mean corpuscular hemoglobin concentration in g/dl	33.7 ± 1.5	34.2 ± 1.6	.301	33.4 ± 1.2	33.5 ± 1.5	.883
White blood cell count in mm³	7400 ± 1900	6600 ± 1700	.122	6900 ± 1000	7500 ± 1800	.116

From Zauber NP, Zauber AG. Hematologic data of healthy very old people. *JAMA.* 1987;257:2181–2184. Copyright 1987, American Medical Association. Reprinted with permission.
*Values expressed as mean ± SD.

SERUM GLUCOSE

Carbohydrate metabolism is altered by aging, especially when accompanied by obesity, inactivity, acute and chronic disease, or familial predisposition to diabetes. Fasting blood glucose tends to increase at a rate of 2 mg/dl per decade of life. Thus a fasting blood glucose range of 135 to 150 mg/dl may be normal in an older person. Relative glucose intolerance is common, and 1-hour postprandial blood glucose values increase approximately 10 mg/dl for each decade.

CREATININE AND BLOOD UREA NITROGEN

In healthy young adults a normal serum creatinine is a relatively sensitive indicator of normal renal function because creatinine clearance is roughly equal to glomerular filtration rate. With aging, glomerular filtration rate declines, reflecting a gradual loss of functioning renal parenchyma. However, there often are parallel declines in the rate of creatinine production with aging as lean body mass contracts. Thus a normal serum creatinine may be seen in an older individual in the face of a significant reduction in renal function. To arrive at a more accurate estimate of renal function in elderly persons it is useful to estimate the creatinine clearance by the following equation.

$$\text{Creatinine clearance} = \frac{(140 - \text{age in yr}) \times \text{body weight in kg}}{72 \times \text{Serum creatinine (mg/dl)}}$$

(Multiply by 0.85 to correct this value for women.)

This calculated creatinine clearance value can be used to adjust the dosing of potentially toxic drugs such as aminoglycoside antibiotics and digoxin.[1]

There is no consensus on the effect of aging on blood urea nitrogen (BUN) values; however, there appears to be an upward trend. BUN values are influenced by renal function, dietary protein content, liver function, and the presence of gastrointestinal bleeding. A normal upper limit of 28-35 mg/dl is probably useful.[3,5,13]

SERUM ALKALINE PHOSPHATASE

Alkaline phosphatase is commonly elevated in elder persons, especially in older women. The range of normal may be expanded 2.5 times in an otherwise healthy older adult. Alkaline phosphatase is derived from both liver and bone. In the absence of other abnormal liver function tests, an elevated serum alkaline phosphatase most likely originates from bone and may be related to subclinical Paget's disease, bone fracture, or minor trauma in an osteoporotic individual. Less frequent causes of an elevated alkaline phosphatase include conditions of malabsorption and renal insufficiency.[5]

ARTERIAL OXYGEN CONTENT

Arterial blood oxygen tension (P_aO_2) declines in a predictable fashion with aging. This decline reflects an increase in the alveolar-arterial oxygen gradient ($P_{A-a}O_2$) resulting from physiologic changes in ventilation-perfusion relationships in the aging lung. This decline can be roughly estimated as follows: $P_aO_2 = 109 - 0.43 \times \text{Age (yr)}$.[3]

Arterial blood oxygen tension (P_aO_2) declines in a predictable fashion with aging.

ELECTROCARDIOGRAM

Age-related changes in the conduction system of the heart are often manifested as non-specific ST-segment and T-wave changes and by fascicular blocks on electrocardiogram (ECG) tracings. The prevalence of sinus node arrhythmias, atrial and ventricular premature systoles, axis deviations, and first-degree AV node block increase with age as well (Table 2–7). In non-selected individuals 65 years and older ECGs were abnormal in more than 50%. However, subtle indicators of ischemia and infarction can be difficult to distinguish from normal variations that occur with aging, and a diagnosis based soley on ECG interpretation is not recommended (Table 2–8). A previous ECG tracing may be invaluable in an emergency setting but is commonly lacking. The emergency physician must be aware of atypical clinical presentations of ischemia and infarction and be prepared to make a diagnosis without the benefit of a definitively diagnostic ECG.[4,14]

Table 2–7 **Prevalence of ECG Abnormalities in Subjects 65 Years or Older**

Entity	Percent (%)
Abnormal ECG	54
First-degree AV block	9
Left axis deviation (> −30 degrees)	36
Right axis deviation (≥ +120 degrees)	2
ST–T wave changes	17
Left bundle branch block	3
Right bundle branch block	6
Intraventricular conduction delay	2
Premature atrial systole	10
Premature ventricular systole	9
Atrial fibrillation	7

From Jones J, Strodulski ZM, Romisher S. The aging electrocardiogram. *Am J Emerg Med.* 1990;8:240.

Table 2–8 **Characteristic ECG Changes with Aging**

1. The incidence of abnormal ECG increases with age and heart disease.
2. Probable insignificant ECG findings in the elderly include left axis deviation without evidence of left anterior hemiblock, lower wave amplitudes, longer intervals, and isolated premature contractions.
3. T-wave inversions and ST-segment depression have too many noncardiac causes to be specific.
4. Bradycardias (sinus bradycardia, sinus arrest, exit block, and second- or third-degree AV block) are rare in normal subjects.
5. The specific ECG abnormalities that correlate strongly with heart disease are atrial fibrillation, left bundle branch block, and nonspecific intraventricular conduction delay.
6. Myocardial infarction patterns, left anterior hemiblock, and right bundle branch block do not correlate with presence of clinical disease but may reflect anatomic disease.
7. With the exception of left ventricular hypertrophy, prognosis of a specific ECG abnormality remains that of the underlying disease.

From Jones J, Strodulski ZM, Romisher S. The aging electrocardiogram. *Am J Emerg Med.* 1990;8:240.

RADIOLOGY

Routine x-ray studies pose few problems. Occasionally, however, decreased bone density may make a non-displaced fracture difficult to appreciate on a radiograph. Multiple views and careful attention to cortex outlines will demonstrate fractures most of the time. However, if the examiner is in doubt, immobilization of a suspect extremity may be indicated with arrangements for follow-up x-ray studies or nuclear bone scan. Age-related histologic changes in the parenchyma of the lung result in enhanced interstitial markings on routine chest radiographs, which may be misinterpreted as pulmonary edema or, when asymmetric, pathologic infiltrates. Generally, clinical correlation is sufficient to interpret such findings.[15]

SUMMARY POINTS

- Aging in an otherwise healthy individual is a subtle process and often does not become clinically apparent until there is a significant physiologic challenge such as acute illness or injury. It is then that the silent decline in major organ reserve function and homeostatic responsiveness may become evident and place the elderly at increased risk of excess morbidity and mortality.
- Care should be taken to recognize important differences in chronologic and physiologic age and the impact of an individual's environment, health behaviors, lifelong disease experience, and heredity on the aging process.
- The emergency health care provider should appreciate the physiologic changes and limitations that accompany aging to optimize the care of this rapidly growing segment of our population.

CHAPTER AUTHOR

Rawden Evans, PhD, MD

REFERENCES

1. Sloan RW. Principles of drug therapy in geriatric patients. *Am Fam Physician.* 1992;45:2709–2718.
2. Comfort A. Physiology, homeostasis and aging. *Gerontologia.* 1968;14:224–234.
3. Sparrow D, Weiss ST. Respiratory physiology. *Annu Rev Gerontol Geriatr.* 1986;6:197–214.
4. Kennedy RD, Caird FI. Physiology of the aging heart. *Cardiovasc Clin.* 1981;12:1–8.
5. Kelso T. Laboratory values in the elderly (are they different?). *Emerg Med Clin North Am.* 1990;8:241–254.
6. Himmelstein DU, et al. Hypernatremic dehydration in nursing home patients: an indicator of neglect. *J Am Geriatr Soc.* 31:466;1983.
7. Kenney RA. Physiology of aging. *Clin Geriatr Med.* 1985;1:37–59.
8. Haddy RI. Aging, infections and the immune system. *J Fam Pract.* 1988;27:409–413.
9. Terpenning MS, Bradley SF. Why aging leads to increased susceptibility to infection. *Geriatrics.* 1991;46:77–80.
10. Coodley EL. Laboratory tests in the elderly: what is abnormal? *Postgrad Med.* 1989;85:333–338.
11. Corman LC. The interpretation of laboratory tests. *Emerg Med Clin North Am.* 1980;7:691–702.
12. McCabe JB. Decision making in laboratory test studies. *Emerg Med Clin North Am.* 1986;4:1–13.
13. Lindeman RD. Overview: renal physiology and pathophysiology of aging. *Am J Kidney Dis.* 1990;16:275–282.
14. Jones J, Srodulski ZM, Romisher S. The aging electrocardiogram. *Am Emerg Med.* 1990;8:240–245.
15. Loberant N, Rose C. Imaging considerations in the geriatric emergency department patient. *Emerg Med Clin North Am.* 1990;8:361–397.

SELECTED READINGS

Abrass IB. The biology and physiology of aging. *West J Med.* 1990;153:641–645.

Baum N, Dichoso CC, Carlton CE. Blood urea nitrogen and serum creatinine: physiology and interpretations. *Urology.* 1975;5:583–588.

Lowentahl DT, Kim KE, Affrime MB, Faulkner B. Overview of physiology in senescence. *Chest.* 1983;83:408–409.

Weg RB. Biology and physiology of development and aging. *Gerontol Geriatr Educ.* 1989;9:9–16.

Williams ME. Clinical implications of aging physiology. *Am J Med.* 1984;76:1049–1054.

Zoller DP. The physiology of aging. *Am Fam Physician.* 1987;36:112.

3 *Pharmacology and Aging*

LEARNING OBJECTIVES

1. Define the term *polypharmacy,* and identify factors contributing to the problem among the elderly.
2. Identify changes in pharmacokinetics and pharmacodynamics that may affect responses to medication.
3. Identify factors affecting compliance among the elderly.
4. Identify types of medications that carry the greatest risk of undesirable side effects.
5. Explain criteria for appropriate medication-prescribing strategies.

The elderly consume approximately 33% of all medications prescribed in the United States, with a projected increase to 50% by the year 2020. The average older American takes 4.5 prescription drugs and 2.1 over-the-counter drugs. It is not surprising that they suffer a disproportionately high incidence of adverse drug reactions. Up to one third of older persons develop undesirable side effects to medications, and they are at least twice as likely to have adverse outcomes related to medication as are their younger counterparts. Recent studies have pointedly suggested that physicians' prescribing practices contribute significantly. One large study of community-dwelling persons aged 65 years or older found that almost one fourth were taking 1 of 20 drugs considered by an expert panel to be inappropriate for use in this patient population. It is estimated that adverse outcomes to drug therapy result in 1 in 20 hospital admissions. Thus, with demographic trends

The average elderly American takes 4.5 perscription drugs and 2.1 over-the-counter drugs.

toward an aging society, emergency health professionals will likely see an increased incidence of medication-related problems among this population and must be prepared to respond appropriately.

Although it is clear that everyone benefits from modern advances in applied pharmacology, there is growing concern that polypharmacy with attendant adverse drug reactions and interactions has become a significant threat to the health and well-being of the elderly population. A number of factors place the elderly at increased risk of adverse drug reactions. Multiple medical problems may result in care from a number of different physicians with different specialties and differing prescribing practices. This predisposes to the prescription of multiple medications. Subsequent medication side effects may be interpreted as manifestations of new or worsening disease and prompt the addition of yet more medications. Without question, aging results in changes in pharmacokinetics and pharmacodynamics that affect potential drug toxicities. However, a growing body of evidence suggests that the number of drugs administered to an individual is a more important determinant of adverse drug reactions than is the age of the individual alone.

The emergency health care provider does not assume the role of extended primary care provider for any patient, but rather becomes a short-term medical advocate in times of need. This is particularly true when dealing with the frail elderly who suffer multiple medical problems. It is more important that the emergency physician be familiar with the special features of geriatric therapeutics that affect management of acute medical crises. Sorting through the medication histories of some older patients is time consuming and complex, but doing so provides an opportunity to identify reversible conditions and avoid iatrogenic complications; *primum non nocere*. This chapter highlights the pharmacology of aging, with an emphasis on the medication pitfalls in the emergency setting and practical suggestions to optimize drug-prescribing practices.

AGING AND ORGAN SYSTEM FUNCTIONAL RESERVE

Major organ systems have significant functional reserves that provide individuals with the capacity to adapt and survive a variety of physiologic challenges. In otherwise healthy, young adults, cardiac, pulmonary, hepatic, and renal functional reserve exceeds that required to maintain resting homeostasis by 4- to 10-fold. Normal aging is characterized by the progressive loss of organ system functional reserve at a rate of just less than one percent per year after 30 years of age. This decline is silent until an organ system is challenged and pushed beyond a critical threshold at which signs and symptoms of organ dysfunction become evident. Acute illness or injury may result in organ system decompensation, but so can certain therapeutic interventions. Several important examples illustrate this concept. The ability of the cardiovascular system to augment cardiac output diminishes with aging, and the heart increasingly depends on the inotropic support of endogenous catecholamines. In this setting the administration of beta-adrenergic blocking agents to an elderly hypertensive patient can precipitate symptoms of congestive heart failure. The dopamine-synthesizing capacity of neurons within the substantia nigra declines with age, predisposing the elderly to symptoms of parkinsonism when treated with phenothiazine psychotropics. Acute renal failure can occur with the prescription of nonsteroidal antiinflammatory drugs (NSAIDs) for pain in patients with marginal renal function and dependence on prostacyclin-mediated renal afferent arteriolar vasodilatation to maintain glomerular blood flow. Similarly, angiotensin converting enzyme (ACE) inhibitors can cause renal insufficiency in individuals with hypertensive renovascular disease in which renal perfusion becomes dependent on elevated renin-angiotensin level.

Aging is also accompanied by a decline in mucosal function that protects the stomach from drugs commonly associated with ulcer formation. There is a general reduction in gastric mucous and bicarbonate secretion, blood flow, and epithelial cell regeneration. These factors together with decreased gastric emptying time combine to increase the probability of significant gastrointestinal bleeding from an overuse of aspirin and NSAIDs.

PHARMACOKINETICS AND PHARMACODYNAMICS

An individual's clinical response to a medication depends on a number of factors that affect the tissue concentration of the active drug as well as the responsiveness of target cells to the drug (Figure 3–1). Tissue concentrations of a drug are influenced by the pharmacokinetic para-

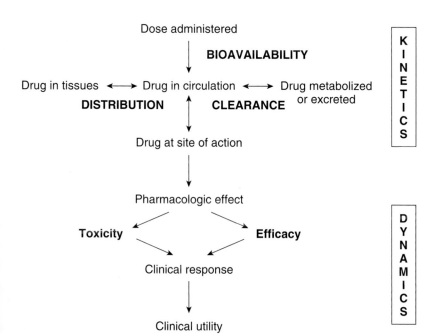

FIGURE 3–1

Pharmacokinetic and pharmacodynamic processes that relate a drug to the effects produced. (Schwartz JB. Clinical pharmacology. In: Hazzard WR, et al. eds. Principles of geriatric medicine and gerontology. 3rd ed. New York, NY: McGraw-Hill, Inc; 1994:266–267. Copyright 1994. Reproduced with permission from McGraw-Hill, Inc.)

meters of bioavailability, distribution, and clearance. Target cell response to a drug depends on the pharmacodynamics of drug-receptor interactions. All of these processes are altered to varying degrees by aging, as outlined below.

BIOAVAILABILITY

The overall bio-availability of most drugs is not significantly reduced.

Aging of the gastrointestinal system is characterized by decreases in gastric acid production and intestinal perfusion, motility, and active membrane transport. Despite these changes, the overall bioavailability of most drugs is not significantly reduced. The antifungal agent keto-conazole (Nizoral) is an exception, because its dissolution and absorption depend on an acid environment, which may be affected by an age-related increase in gastric pH. Drug bioavailability is more likely to be influenced by drug-drug interactions. Absorption of the fluoro-quinolone antibiotics, such as ciprofloxacin (Cipro) and ofloxacin (Floxin), is reduced by coadministration of the antiulcer medication sucralfate (Carafate) and the antacid-containing salts of aluminum and magnesium (Maalox and Mylanta). The antihypertensive ACE inhibitor quinapril (Accupril) contains a high concentration of magnesium, which may decrease the absorption of fluoroquinolone antibiotics and tetracycline. Drugs with anticholinergic effects delay gastric emptying and can decrease the absorption of other medications. Such drug-drug interactions can generally be circumvented by prescribing a dose-spacing interval of several hours.

DISTRIBUTION

While the extent of absorption does not change for most drugs, the rate of absorption for most medications decreases with aging.

Once absorbed or infused, drugs become distributed among the various extracellular and intracellular fluid compartments. Peak concentration of a drug after its administration, which often influences side effects and toxicity, is determined by the volume and rate of distribution of the drug. Major determinants of the volume of distribution of a drug include the degree of plasma protein binding, solubility characteristics in water and lipid, and the extent of tissue uptake and binding. Highly protein-bound drugs such as warfarin and phenytoin have volumes of distribution that approximate the intravascular space. Drugs such as digoxin (Lanoxin) that are extensively bound to tissue proteins have correspondingly large volumes of distribution. Drug distribution rates largely depend on differences in blood flow through various organs and tissues. Thus, in adipose tissue, drug distribution tends to occur slowly because fat is not as well perfused as lean tissues and organs such as the kidney and the heart.

Distribution of drugs is affected by age-related changes in body composition. Lean body mass declines with age. In young adults lean body mass may comprise 82% of ideal body weight but then slowly declines to approximately 64% in the average geriatric patient. Drugs distributed primarily in lean tissues such as aminoglycoside antibiotics, digoxin, and theophylline have reduced volumes of distribution, and dosages must be adjusted downward to avoid potential toxicity. In contrast to lean tissue, aging results in a proportionate increase in adipose tissue. The higher proportion of adipose tissue increases the volume of distribution of drugs such as phenytoin, benzodiazepines, barbiturates, and phenothiazines and prolongs their duration of action. Adipose tissue, being relatively anhydrous, contributes to a net decrease in total body water. Extracellular fluid volume may be contracted as a result of diuretic therapy. These factors contribute to higher blood levels of alcohol per drink consumed and an enhanced potential for intoxication.

CLEARANCE

Drug clearance depends primarily on hepatic metabolism and renal elimination. The efficiency of hepatic drug metabolism is influenced by hepatic blood flow, functional hepatocyte number, and the activity of the cytochrome P_{450} mixed-function oxidase system. Certain drugs are so rapidly and efficiently metabolized by the liver that hepatic blood flow is the main variable affecting their clearance. Examples of drugs that undergo rapid first-pass hepatic metabolism include lidocaine, calcium channel antagonists, beta-adrenergic receptor blockers, narcotics, nitrates, tricyclic antidepressants, hydralazine, and labetalol. The combination of diminished hepatic blood flow and portal-systemic shunting which is more common in older adults increases the potential toxicity of the aforementioned drugs. The metabolism of other drugs depends more on hepatic enzyme activity than on blood flow. Liver size decreases with aging, reflecting a decline in functional hepatocyte number and enzyme content. Chronic hepatocellular and fibrotic (cirrhotic) liver disease can significantly affect the clearance of drugs such as phenytoin.

Diazepam and alprazolam may cause excess sedation in the elderly.

Hepatic biotransformation of drugs involves synthetic (conjugation) and non-synthetic (oxidation-reduction and hydrolytic) reactions. Non-synthetic enzymatic processes are affected to a greater extent by aging than the synthetic reactions, which explains the differing side-effect profiles of benzodiazepines in the elderly. Thus diazepam (Valium) and alprazolam (Xanax), which undergo oxidative metabolism, are more likely to cause excess sedation than lorazepam (Ativan) and oxazepam (Ativan), which are metabolized by conjugation reactions.

Consider the impact of diminished renal function when administering digoxin and aminoglycoside antibiotics.

Drug elimination by the kidney depends on rates of glomerular filtration, tubular secretion, and tubular reabsorption. Aging is accompanied by a decline in renal blood flow and functional renal mass. Creatinine clearance and hence glomerular filtration rate decrease by approximately 10% per decade after 20 years of age. However, serum creatinine ceases to be a reliable indicator of renal function, because creatinine production by a diminishing lean body mass declines in parallel with creatinine clearance. It is important to consider the impact of diminished renal function when administering drugs such as digoxin and the aminoglycoside antibiotics, which have narrow therapeutic ranges and considerable toxic potential.

DRUG-RECEPTOR INTERACTIONS

Changes in dynamic responses to certain drugs suggest that the drug-receptor number or the coupling of drug-receptor systems with cellular effector systems is altered by aging. Dynamic responses are studied by considering drug concentrations at their sites of action rather than simple dose-response curves to circumvent variations in pharmacokinetics. A given concentration of the beta$_1$-adrenergic drug isoproterenol causes a decreased response in heart rate, contractility, and vasodilation in older subjects, suggesting an age-related decrease in receptor number. Such a decline in receptor number has been suggested as the basis for defective baroreflex response to hypotension. Serum concentrations of the calcium channel antagonists verapamil and diltiazem required to produce PR interval prolongation are increased, suggesting decreased sensitivity of the cardiac conduction system to these agents. Cardiovascular sensitivity and responses to parasympathetic agonists and antagonists tend to be blunted in aging; however, the frequency and severity of central nervous system (CNS) side effects suggest an underlying alteration in receptor-effector systems. In contrast to declines in drug responsiveness, the elderly have an increased sensitivity to warfarin and benzodiazepines.

The elderly have an increased sensitivity to warfarin and benzodiazepines.

Pharmacodynamics and aging currently constitute an area of considerable research interest.

Table 3–1 summarizes the physiologic changes in aging that can alter drug action. Table 3–2 lists commonly prescribed drugs in elderly patients with reported age-related alterations in pharmacokinetics.

PRACTICAL CONSIDERATIONS

Adverse outcomes to medications are common, occurring twice as frequently as in younger persons. Medication side effects are similar to those experienced by younger patients but are more likely to in-

Table 3–1 **Physiologic Changes That Can Alter Drug Action**

Drug Action	Physiologic Change
Bioavailability	Achlorhydria
	Delayed gastric emptying time
	Decreased gastrointestinal blood flow
	Alterations in gastric mucosa
Distribution	Decreased lean mass
	Increased (young old) and decreased (old old) adiposity
	Decreased body water
	Decreased cardiac output
Metabolism	Decreased liver size
	Decreased liver blood flow
	Decreased phase I enzyme function (oxidation, reduction, hydrolysis)
Clearance	Decreased cardiac output
	Decreased renal blood flow
	Decreased glomerular filtration rate
	Decreased tubular secretion
Altered receptor/ postreceptor function	Decreased beta-adrenergic function
Altered neurologic function	Decreased cognition

Table 3–2　**Commonly Prescribed Drugs in Elderly Patients and Reported Age-Related Alterations in Pharmacokinetics**

	Route of Elimination	Age Effects*			
		Clearance	Volume	$t_{1/2}$	Dose Adjustment
Cardiovascular					
Furosemide	Hepatic, renal	↓	↓	↑	↓§
Hydrochlorothiazide	Renal	NA	NA	NA	↓§
Chlorthalidone	Renal	NA	NA	NA	↓§
Digoxin	Renal	↓	↓, ↔	↑	↓
Quinidine	Hepatic	↓		↑	↓
Lidocaine	Hepatic	↓, ↔	↔, ↑	↑	↓
Procainamide + NAPA	Renal	↓	NA	↑	↓
Beta-blockers					
Propranolol	Hepatic	↓ (males)	↔	↑	↓
Metoprolol	Hepatic	↑, ↔	NA	↑, ↔	↓, ↔
Atenolol	Renal	Slight ↓	NA	↔	↔
Calcium antagonists					
Verapamil	Hepatic	↓, ↔	↔	↑, ↔	↓
Diltiazem	Hepatic	↓, ↔	↔	↑, ↔	↓
Nifedipine†	Hepatic	↓	↔	↑	↓
Nisoldipine	Hepatic	↓, ↔	NA	↑, ↔	↓, ↔
Amlodipine	Hepatic	↓	↔	↑	↓
Nicardipine	Hepatic	↔, ↑	↔	↔	↔, ↓
Alpha-adrenergic blockers					
Clonidine	Renal, hepatic	↓	NA	NA	↓§
Prazosin	Hepatic	↓, ↔	↔	↑	↓, ↔§
Terazosin	Hepatic, renal	↓, ↔	NA	↔, ↓	↔, ↓§
Alpha-methyldopa	Hepatic, renal	↓	NA	↑	↓
Labetalol	Hepatic	↓, ↔	NA	↑, ↔	?↓
ACE inhibitors					
Captopril	Renal	↓	NA	↑	↓
Enalapril†	Hepatic	↓	NA	↑	↓
Lisinopril	Renal	↓	NA	↑	↓
Hypoglycemic Agents					
Glipizide	Hepatic	↔	NA	↔	↔
Chlorpropamide	Renal	↓	↑	↑	↓
Glyburide	Hepatic, renal	↔	↑	↑	↔
Sedative/Hypnotics					
Lorazepam	Hepatic	↔	NA	↔	↓§
Diazepam	Hepatic	↓		↑	↓
Triazolam	Hepatic	↓	NA	↔	↓
Antituberculous					
Isoniazid (INH)					
Slow acetylators	Hepatic	↔	↔	↔	↔
Rapid acetylators	Hepatic	↓, ↔	↔	↑	↓
Rifampin	Hepatic	NA	NA	NA	

Schwartz JB. Clinical pharmacology. In: Hazzard WR, et al., eds. *Principles of Geriatric Medicine and Gerontology.* 3rd ed. New York, NY: McGraw-Hill, Inc; 1994:266–267. Copyright 1994. Reproduced with permission from McGraw-Hill, Inc.

Continued on following page.

Table 3–2 **Commonly Prescribed Drugs in Elderly Patients and Reported Age-Related Alterations in Pharmacokinetics—*Continued***

	Route of Elimination	Age Effects*			
		Clearance	Volume	$t_{1/2}$	Dose Adjustment
Antibiotics					
Erythromycin	Hepatic	↓	↔	↑	↓
Gentamycin	Renal	↓, ↔	↑, ↔	↑, ↔	↓
Ampicillin	Renal	↓	↔	↑	↓
Amoxicillin	Renal	NA	NA	NA	↓
Ciprofloxacin	Renal	↓		↑	↓
Antiarthritics					
Acetaminophen	Hepatic	↔, ↓	↓, ↔	↔	↔
Aspirin	Hepatic	↑, ↔	↑	↑	↓, ↔
Naproxen	Renal	↓	NA	↑	
Ibuprofen	Renal	↔, or ↓ in males	NA	↔ in males	↔ or ↓ in males
Salicylic acid	Hepatic	↔	NA	↔ or ↑	↔
Histaminergic Blockers					
Cimetidine	Hepatic, renal	↓	NA	↑	↓
Ranitidine	Hepatic, renal	↓	NA	↑	↓
Terfenadine	Hepatic	↑	NA	↑	↓
Antiulcer					
Misoprostol	Renal	↔	NA	Slight ↑	↔
Miscellaneous					
Levothyroxine	Hepatic	NA	NA	NA	§
Conjugated estrogen	Hepatic	NA	NA	NA	NA
L-dopa	Hepatic + other	↓	↓	↔	↓
Lithium	Renal	↓		↑	↓
Warfarin	Hepatic	↔	↔	↔	↓‡,§

*NA, Not available.
†Active drug is metabolite enalaprilat, which is renally excreted.
‡Decreased plasma binding → ↑ effect.
§Aging effects on specific pharmacokinetic parameters have not been well studied, but clinical efficacy has been observed with reduced doses in elderly persons.

One in 20 hospital admissions among the elderly are for adverse reactions to medications.

clude delirium, depression, worsening dementia, orthostatic hypotension, falls, and incontinence. These symptoms, although not always subtle, tend not to be recognized as medication side effects by physicians and caregivers, which is unfortunate because they are readily reversible. The following section discusses factors placing the elderly at increased risk for medication-related illness and complications.

RISK FACTORS

Polypharmacy and drug interactions probably represent more significant threats to the health and well-being of the elderly than do age-related changes in pharmacokinetics and dynamics. Sadly, aging is frequently accompanied by an increase in the number and severity of many disease processes. Aging begets illness, illness begets physicians, physicians beget medications, and medications beget cures *and* side effects. Some elderly patients are promiscuous in their pursuit of medical care and shop around. The patient with multiple medical problems may seek care from multiple physicians whose prescribing practices differ and who may remain unknown to the other care providers. The presenting complaint to physician C may be a side effect to drugs prescribed by physicians A and B, unknown to one another. Physician C, with good intention, prescribes yet another medication. Physician D is often an emergency practitioner who now faces a case of *iatrogenesis fulminans.*

The patient may also contribute to the problem of polypharmacy. It is not uncommon for elderly persons to share medications . . . "Your ankles are swollen just like mine! Why don't you try a few of my Lanoxin and Lasix?" A variety of over-the-counter medications interact with prescription medications and can cause significant side effects. Cold medications can produce postural hypotension and cognitive disorders. The NSAIDs can worsen renal insufficiency and promote gastrointestinal bleeding. Herbal medicines and excessive vitamin supplementation carry risks as well. Popular ginseng root preparations can produce or aggravate hypertension, and other herbs may cause diarrheal disturbances. Megadoses of vitamins A and D can produce hypercalcemia. Vitamin C interferes with stool guaiac detection of occult blood and with rapid serum and urine glucose determinations. The elderly patient may be less than forthright in revealing experimentation with nonconventional medicines and over-the-counter drugs. Herbals and vitamins are often not considered medications, and use of these substances must be assessed by direct questioning.

The conventional model for medical care calls for prescription of medications for each disease symptom suffered. The geriatric model takes a more pragmatic approach by first considering the functional status of the patient and then a risk-benefit analysis to balance therapeutic interventions with realistic expectations of outcome. For example, coronary artery disease risk factor modification in an 80-year-old person would probably not stress long-term management of hypercholesterolemia. Fine tuning of blood glucose in the elderly diabetic patient may result in dangerous bouts of hypoglycemia. Similarly, the treatment of chronic lower extremity stasis edema with a diuretic may place a patient at greater risk of adverse drug effects (i.e., volume depletion, orthostatic hypotension, hypokalemia) than is warranted by the minimal inconvenience of moderately swollen ankles. Diseases change over time as well and require a reassessment of therapeutics. For example, digoxin may improve cardiac function in one stage of congestive heart failure but become ineffective at a later stage and place the patient at increased risk of malignant arrhythmias. At times, one medication may be effective in the treatment of two or more conditions. A patient with hypertension experiencing urge incontinence might be treated effectively by a calcium channel antagonist alone instead of a variety of medications aimed at each condition.

In many cases, appropriate dosing can be determined only by checking drug steady-state levels.

Paradoxical drug combinations are yet another therapeutic problem (Table 3–3). In this situation one drug is either employed to treat symptoms caused by a primary drug or inadvertently antagonizes the beneficial effects of that drug.

COMPLIANCE ISSUES

Patient noncompliance is a chancre that plagues all areas of medicine and is especially problematic in elderly patients. It is a complicated issue that is affected by demographic, social, and economic factors over which physicians have very little control. However physicians do have control over two very important aspects of compliance: *communication* and *education.* The reality of modern emergency medicine does not always provide the emergency physician with the time needed for effective patient communication and education. This being the case, responsibility should be delegated to discharge personnel specifically trained to educate patients and field their medication questions. Basic information to provide includes drug dosages, dosing intervals, and duration of therapy. Whether to take medications with meals or between, and potential drug-drug interactions, side effects, and how and when to report these should also be included. Instructions must be legible and not abbreviated or in medical jargon. If the patient has significant visual, auditory, or cognitive impairment, medication instructions must be provided to a competent care provider. Preprinted instructions for medications commonly prescribed can be especially beneficial as well as time saving. Table 3–4 reviews factors affecting compliance, all of which depend on the effectiveness of communication and patient education.

It is worth mentioning the potential confusion that is created by generic medications and generic and trade drug names. Generic medication can be a two-edged sword. Generics are usually less expensive, which is an important consideration affecting compliance of older persons on fixed incomes and without insurance to defray medication costs. On the other hand, the cheaper generic drug may have clinically significant differences in bioavailability. Generic thyroid hormone preparations are illustrative of this variance and should be avoided. If a

Patient Teaching
- *Dosage*
- *Schedule*
- *Length of therapy*
- *Potential food or drug interactions*
- *Potential side effects*
- *How to report problems*

Table 3–3 **Paradoxical Drug Combinations**

Physiologic States or Actions	Drug That Increases State or Action	Drug That Decreases State or Action
Central dopamine	Levodopa-carbidopa (Sinemet)	Haloperidol (Haldol)
Myocardial contractility	Digoxin (Lanoxin)	Atenolol (Tenormin)
Airway resistance	Propranolol (Inderal)	Albuterol (Proventil, Ventolin)
Serum triglycerides	Nadolol (Corgard)	Gemfibrozil (Lopid)
Peripheral circulation	Pentoxifylline (Trental)	Propranolol
Blood sugar	Phenylpropanolamine	Glyburide (DiaBeta, Micronase)
Colonic motility	Bisacodyl (Dulcagen, Dulcolax, Fleet)	Verapamil (Calan, Isoptin)

From Sloan RW. Principles of drug therapy in geriatric patients. *Am Fam Physician* 1992;45:2709–2718.

Table 3–4 **Factors Affecting Compliance**

Improved Compliance	Decreased Compliance
Careful explanation by physician of medication purpose	Number of drugs
Belief by patient that disease is serious	Prolonged length of therapy
Belief by patient in effectiveness of medication	Fear of medication toxicity
Belief by patient that disease will develop if not prevented, e.g., hypertension treatment	Complex scheduling
	Difficulty opening medication bottles

generic brand is chosen, it should be used for the long term to avoid variation in potency and toxicity. Generic and trade names are confusing to physicians as well as to patients, especially as more prescription drugs become available over-the-counter. It is entirely possible to discover that an elderly arthritic patient is taking aspirin and several preparations of ibuprofen (Motrin, Advil, and generic) for joint pain. The potential for toxicity is staggering.

DRUGS TO AVOID

Some experts in geriatric medicine have established lists of drugs they believe should be entirely avoided in elderly patients. Other more moderate authorities acknowledge the heterogeneity of human aging and emphasize the importance of distinguishing between chronologic and physiologic age when prescribing medication. In general, drugs with anticholinergic and sedative properties, along with commonly prescribed diuretic agents, carry the greatest risk of undesirable side effects for the greatest number of older persons. Drugs with appreciable anticholinergic side effects not commonly recognized include amitryptyline, disopyramide, digoxin, theophylline and cimetidine. Paradoxical drug reactions occur in geriatrics as well as in pediatrics. For example, diphenhydramine prescribed as a sedative may surprisingly produce excitation. The antipsychotic/tranquilizer haloperidol may paradoxically increase agitation. Although controversial, a list of medications considered inappropriate for use in older persons is compiled in Table 3–5.

Drugs with anticholinergic and sedative properties, as well as diuretics, have the greatest potential for undesirable side effects.

MEDICATION-PRESCRIBING STRATEGIES

The goal of medication prescribing must be to achieve maximal therapeutic benefit, least possible adverse effects, good compliance, and minimal economic hardship. The value of a drug with the theoretic potential of increasing longevity must be balanced against its harmful effects on the quality of life. A clear therapeutic endpoint must be established at the outset. If the drug fails its therapeutic assignment it should be discontinued before the introduction of an alternative medication. Polypharmacy can be prevented by eliminating

Table 3–5 **Drugs Considered Inappropriate for use in Older Persons**

Sedative/Hypnotics	Platelet Inhibitor	Analgesics
Diazepam	Dipyridamole	Propoxyphene
Chlordiazepoxide		(Darvon,
Flurazepam	**Antiemetic Agent**	Darvocet-N)
Meprobamate	Trimethobenzamide	Pentazocine
Pentobarbital		
Secobarbital	**Antidepressant**	**Muscle Relaxants**
	Amitryptyline	Cyclobenzapine
Oral Hypoglycemic		Methocarbamol
Chlorpropamide	**NSAIDs**	Carisoprodol
	Indomethacin	Orphenadrine
Dementia Treatments	Phenylbutazone	
Isosuxprine		
Cyclandelate		

From Willcox et al. Inappropriate drug prescribing for the community dwelling elderly. *JAMA*. 1994;272:292–296. Copyright © 1994, American Medical Association.

A useful axiom to remember when prescribing to elderly patients is "Start low, and go slow!"

drug redundancy and antagonism, as in paradoxical drug combinations. Drug side effects should be monitored closely and every effort made to avoid treating side effects with further medication. One should be mindful of age-related changes in drug pharmacokinetics and responsiveness. A useful axiom to remember when prescribing to elderly patients is "Start low and go slow!"

SUMMARY POINTS

- Whenever an elderly patient presents with an acute illness or worsening chronic condition, a complete drug list should be carefully obtained and reviewed to exclude drug toxicity as a cause of the presenting complaint.
- Aging decreases the functional reserve capacity of major organ systems, placing the elderly patient at increased risk of physiologic decompensation in response to certain medications, particularly those potentially affecting cardiac and renal function.
- Drugs with narrow therapeutic ranges should be monitored closely. These include digoxin, theophylline, warfarin, lithium, lidocaine, quinidine, and aminoglycoside antibiotics.
- Drugs with CNS effects may significantly affect the quality of life, mentation, and functional status. These include long-acting hypnotics, histaminergic- and alpha-blocking agents, and drugs with anticholinergic effects such as disopyramide and antihistamines.
- Drug-related adverse effects may present atypically as a subtle change in mental status or an acute functional decline. A high index of suspicion must be present at all times.
- Drugs should only be prescribed with therapeutic endpoints clearly defined and with care to avoid drug-drug interactions. When possible, medications should be started at low doses and increased slowly and in small increments while signs and symptoms of toxicity are carefully monitored.

• Effective prescribing practices must encourage patient compliance by careful attention to communication, patient education, and timely follow-up.

CHAPTER AUTHORS

Rawden Evans, PhD, MD
Gordon Ireland, PharmD
John E. Morley, MB, BCh
Sharon Sheahan, PhD, CFNP

SELECTED READINGS

Beers MH. Medication use in the elderly. In: Callans E, Ford AB, Katz PR, eds. *Practice of geriatrics*. 2nd ed. Philadelphia, PA: WB Saunders; 1992:33–49.

Feely J, Coakely D. Altered pharmacodynamics in the elderly. *Clin Geriatr Med.* 1990;6:269.

Ireland GA. Principles of prescribing medications. In: Yoshikawa TTR, Cobbs EL, Brummer-Smith K, eds. *Ambulatory geriatric care*. St. Louis, MO: Mosby–Year Book; 1993:18–25.

Schwartz JB. Clinical pharmacology. In: Hazzard WR, Bierman EL, Blass JP, Ettinger Jr WH, Halter JB, eds. *Principles of geriatric medicine and gerontology*. 3rd ed. New York, NY: McGraw-Hill; 1994:259–275.

Sloan RW. Principles of drug therapy in geriatric patients. *Am Fam Physician.* 1992;45:2709–2718.

Yuen GJ. Altered pharmacokinetics in the elderly. *Clin Geriatr Med.* 1990;6:257.

4 *Ethical Issues in Geriatric Emergency Medicine*

LEARNING OBJECTIVES

1. Define advance directives; list types of advance directives; and explain their use in the emergency care of elderly patients.
2. Define the principles and proper exercise of durable power of attorney for health care.
3. Explain ethical concerns when applying the concept of medical futility in the emergency care setting.
4. Identify factors in medical decision making in the care of elderly patients and the role of the family in this process.
5. Explain ethical issues associated with the concepts and practice of rationing and resource allocation in the emergency care of elderly persons.

ADVANCE DIRECTIVES

An advance directive is an instrument that allows an individual to express autonomous decisions at some point in the future when the individual is no longer competent to do so.[1] The US Supreme Court landmark decision in the 1990 case of Nancy Beth Cruzan reaffirmed the right of competent patients to refuse life-sustaining treatment and also recognized that this right survives the loss of decision-making capacity.[2] Also known as "living wills," advance directives have been endorsed by the courts, state legislatures, physicians, and the President's Commission for the Study of Ethical Problems in Biomedical and Behavioral Research.[3] The Patient Self-Determination Act of 1990 is federal legislation that requires any health care facility that receives federal funding to inform patients of their right to limit medical care under state

In the hierarchy of medical decision-making in care of the incompetent patient, a properly executed advance directive is to be considered first.

law and to record their wishes regarding an advance directive at the time of their admission.[3,4] It is hoped that this legislation will increase the use of these currently underutilized documents.

Ideally, state legislation will allow prehospital care providers to honor these documents, but this is not clear in many jurisdictions.[1] The ideal advance directive clearly expresses the patient's wishes, delineates the goals of treatment, clarifies the "do not resuscitate" status, and designates a single proxy for decisions in circumstances where the patient's preferences are not clear.[3,5] In the hierarchy of medical decision making in care of the incompetent patient, a properly executed advance directive is to be considered first.[6] It should be noted that the patient can change his or her mind and overrule any advance directive regarding health care. Thus, even in the presence of an advance directive, the patient, whenever possible, should be questioned regarding treatment preferences.

Emergency health care providers can expect to encounter these documents with increasing frequency and must be aware of the issues surrounding their use. The right to self-determination exercised by the competent patient in the execution of an advance directive is a basic principle of American law and medical ethics.[3] Autonomy holds a preeminent position in health care decisions. Advance directives are an accepted and reliable expression of autonomy.

DURABLE POWER OF ATTORNEY FOR HEALTH CARE

In many states a competent person may appoint a surrogate decision maker for health care–related issues in the event of future incapacity by the person as a patient. The durable power of attorney for health care is an instrument to allow patients more flexibility by expressing their wishes to the designated proxy, who is usually a relative or close

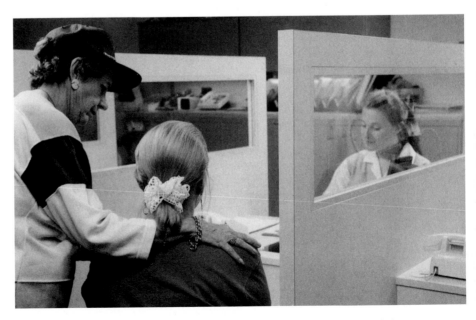

The proxy's decision should be consistent with the patient's wishes, and the proxy must decide in the patient's best interest.

friend. Decisions can then be made by the proxy based on the values and preferences of the patient. Emergency care providers may therefore encounter situations in which a previously designated proxy becomes involved in care decisions regarding an older patient. Points of importance include the following:

1. Patients' preferences are foremost as expressed by the patients themselves either through their retention of decision-making capacity or in a previously executed advance directive.[3,5]
2. The proxy's decision should be consistent with the patient's wishes, and the proxy must decide in the patient's best interest. If the physician feels that the proxy's decisions are not in keeping with the above then this conflict must be addressed. For example, the proxy does not have the right to insist on treatment that is apparently futile, particularly if there is no clear evidence that the patient, if competent, would request the treatment. The first step is to discuss the issue with the proxy, and, if this does not produce resolution, other professionals, an ethics committee, and, as a last resort, legal counsel may be called.[7]

MEDICAL FUTILITY IN EMERGENCY CARE

Emergency care providers frequently deal with critically ill older patients and are confronted with the dilemma of just how much care to provide and how aggressive this care should be. The patient is frequently unable to guide treatment decisions, and currently advance directives are only occasionally available. Most of the time, emergency physicians must strike the proper balance among patient/family autonomy, beneficence, and non-maleficence (do no harm).

Resuscitation decisions are a prime example of this dilemma. In the emergency setting the health care provider is hampered by the lack of a prior relationship with the patient and resulting unfamiliarity with the patient's values, beliefs, and wishes. This is further complicated by the need for quick action in situations where clinical information regarding prognosis is often unclear or unavailable.[1] There is also little ethical difference between withdrawing or withholding care. Therefore the recommendation is to offer full medical treatment to all patients who do not have specific documentation of wishes to the contrary.[8]

In recent years the concept of withholding treatments that are futile has gained increased attention.[8-10] The concept of medical futility may directly clash with patient autonomy when the patient or the surrogate requests care that is considered worthless by the treating physician. The physician is not obligated to provide treatments that obviously offer no benefit such as antibiotics for a cold, but many of the more difficult decisions have no absolutes. The probability that a treatment will help is rarely zero, and therefore certain value judgments come into play.

Many ethicists distinguish between quantitative and qualitative futility standards. A quantitative futility standard (also known as a strict or physiologic futility standard) is one that articulates a statistical probability of survival that is so low as to be incalculable or below an ac-

The probability that a treatment will help is rarely 0%, and therefore certain value judgments come into play.

cepted threshold of likelihood of restoration of physiologic parameters even with the proper treatment.[11] Qualitative futility standards (or disproportionate burden analysis) say that treatment is futile if it will not serve any useful purpose for the patient, may cause the patient needless pain or suffering, and does not achieve the goal of restoring the patient to an acceptable quality of life.[12]

Those who support the increased application of the principle of withholding futile treatment make the following points:

1. Physicians are not morally or legally obligated to offer treatment that is physiologically futile.
2. Physicians should not be required to obtain consent for "do not resuscitate" orders in every case.
3. It is best to inform the family of these decisions and the reasoning behind them.[8-10]

The environment of emergency care makes application of the concept of medical futility quite difficult.

The emergency care environment makes application of the concept of medical futility quite difficult.[1] In situations where resuscitation has already been initiated it is usually possible for the care provider to realize when there is no hope for a reasonable outcome and to cease the efforts. Decisions regarding the initiation or withholding of resuscitation are much more difficult. In the prehospital setting and in the ED the development of protocols to guide the provider in foregoing resuscitation can alleviate some of this burden.[13] Until reliable guidelines are developed to aid in some cases, emergency care providers will continue to face these difficult ethical problems and must strive to balance autonomy, beneficence, and non-maleficence.

Despite the appropriate emphasis on autonomy, patients and families still expect physicians to clarify the burdens and benefits of certain interventions and to help determine the proper goals of medical care. Decisions regarding medical futility will often be quite difficult for those involved in emergency care, and they should seek early assistance from the patient's personal physician when feasible.

DECISION-MAKING CAPACITY AND EMERGENCY CARE

The major issue confronting the emergency care provider regarding medical decision making is to determine the extent of the patient's abilities to make medical decisions, at what point to turn to others for assistance, and who exactly to turn to for this aid.

Treatment decisions are best made on an individual rather than a "population" basis.

The patient who retains decision-making capacity and the ability to communicate preferences regarding treatment should always be turned to first. Likewise, a properly executed advance directive should be honored if either of the above two criteria is not met.[3,5] To seek guidance from the family when the patient's wishes can be known is a major violation of the patient's right to self-determination.

In determining the patient's capacity to make decisions four basic standards are commonly used:

1. The ability to communicate a choice
2. The ability to understand fundamental information about a treatment decision

3. The ability to understand the current situation and the consequences of any decisions regarding treatment
4. The ability to process information rationally so as to weigh the benefits and risks of various treatment options[14]

A major point is that the fulfillment of all four of these criteria is not necessary for every treatment decision. In general, the more significant the decision the more important it is for the physician to have all four criteria fulfilled.[14]

When the patient's wishes cannot be determined the proper line of authority for medical decision making would be a legally appointed surrogate or guardian, followed by the spouse, the adult children, siblings, and then other family members.[14]

> *It cannot be assumed that because a patient is elderly the outcome or quality of life will be poor for any given treatment.*

RESOURCE ALLOCATION AND RATIONING

Decisions regarding the provision of care cannot be based on broad generalizations about the aged population.[15] It cannot be assumed that because a patient is elderly the outcome or quality of life will be poor for any given treatment.[15-17] The elderly have been shown to be quite responsive to intensive care and aggressive trauma care with substantial benefit.[16,17] Treatment decisions are therefore best made on an individual rather than a "population" basis.[15]

In emergency care the denial of care to an individual patient on the basis of better resource utilization or for cost reasons is currently ethically unacceptable.[18] Distributive justice is a societal principle that cannot be applied to individual bedside decisions. Distributive justice says that comparable individuals and groups in society should share comparably in the benefits and burdens of society. Resources, especially scarce resources, ought to be allocated fairly.[19] In the future, political decisions may affect the extent of care we are able to provide for patients but at this point the physician should choose what is in the patient's best interest. Such decisions are best guided by the patients wishes and the efficacy of the medical care.[20]

> *In emergency care the denial of care to an individual patient on the basis of better resource utilization or for cost reasons is currently ethically unacceptable.*

SUMMARY POINTS

- In the incompetent patient a properly executed advance directive should be honored.
- Proxy decisions should be in the best interest of the patient, and the proxy cannot insist on futile treatment.
- Physicians are not obligated to provide treatment that is physiologically futile.
- The competent patient should always be turned to first regarding treatment decisions regardless of the presence of advance directives.
- Standards exist for determining the patient's decision-making capacity.

CHAPTER AUTHORS

Robert M. McNamara, MD
Glen Freas, MD, JD, FACEP

REFERENCES

1. Adams J, Wolfson AB. Ethical issues in geriatric emergency medicine. *Emerg Med Clin North Am.* 1990;8:183–192.
2. Arras JD. Beyond Cruzan: individual rights, family autonomy and the persistent vegetative state. *J Am Geriatr Soc.* 1991;39:1018–1024.
3. Emanuel LL, Emanuel EJ. The medical directive: a new comprehensive advance care document. *JAMA.* 1989;261:3288–3293.
4. Goldstein MK, Shadlen M. Misuse of durable power of attorney for health care. *J Am Geriatr Soc.* 1991;39:730–733. Letter.
5. Emanuel L. The health care directive: learning how to draft advance care documents. *J Am Geriatr Soc.* 1991;39:1221–1228.
6. Molloy DW, Clarnette RM, Baum EA, et al. Decision making in the incompetent elderly: the daughter from California syndrome. *J Am Geriatr Soc.* 1991;39:396–399.
7. Abuse of durable power of attorney for health care: case report. *J Am Geriatr Soc.* 1991;39:806–809.
8. Hackler JC, Hiller FC. Family consent to orders not to resuscitate. *JAMA.* 1990;264:1281–1283.
9. Youngner SJ. Who defines futility? *JAMA.* 1988;260:2094–2095.
10. Tomlinson T, Brody H. Futility and the ethics of resuscitation. *JAMA.* 1990;264:1276–1280.
11. Schneiderman LJ, Jecker NS, Jonsen AR. Medical futility: its meaning and ethical implications. *Ann Intern Med.* 1990;112:949–950.
12. Nelson LJ, Nelson RM. Ethics and the provision of futile, harmful, or burdensome treatment to children. *Crit Care Med.* 1992;20:427–433.
13. Bonnin MJ, Pepe PE, Kimball KT, Clark PS. Distinct criteria for termination of resuscitation in the out-of-hospital setting. *JAMA.* 1993;270:1457–1462.
14. Applebaum PS, Grisso T. Assessing patients' capacities to consent to treatment. *N Engl J Med.* 1988;319:1635–1638.
15. Wetle T. Age as a risk factor for inadequate treatment. *JAMA.* 1987;258:516.
16. DeMaria EJ, Kenney PR, Merriam MA, et al. Agressive trauma care benefits the elderly. *J Trauma.* 1987;27:1200–1205.
17. Wu AW, Rubin HR, Rosen MJ. Are elderly people less responsive to intensive care? *J Am Geriatr Soc.* 1990;38:621–627.
18. Lo B, Jonsen AR. Clinical decisions to limit treatment. *Ann Intern Med.* 1980;93:764–768.
19. Kapp MB. Futile medical treatment: a review of the ethical arguments and legal holdings. *J Gen Intern Med.* 1994;9:170–177.
20. Pawlson LG, Glover JJ, Murphy DJ. An overview of allocation and rationing: implications for geriatrics. *J Am Geriatr Soc.* 1992;40:628–634.

5 *Attitudes and Ageism*

LEARNING OBJECTIVES

1. Define the term *ageism,* and describe examples of potential bias in the clinical management of elderly patients.
2. Explain the significance of demographic trends to an appreciation of attitudes about aging.
3. Define the term *new ageism,* and explain potential clinical implications.

The term *ageism* was coined by the noted geriatrician and champion of older persons, Robert N. Butler, MD, to describe an insidious and largely unacknowledged form of bigotry.[1] Ageism is formally defined as "discrimination based on age; especially discrimination against middle-aged and elderly people." The term is relatively new, but the reality of ageism is far from a modern phenomenon. Attitudes held toward older members of any given society are variable. From an anthropologic perspective, the aged of nomadic peoples tend not to be highly revered and are more likely to be viewed as burdens. In these societies mobility may be the key factor to survival, and any member less than robust could be a detriment to the whole. The older members of more geographically fixed societies are more likely to occupy positions of influence and respect. The wealth of knowledge and experience that accompanies aging becomes of greater value in such societies.

In the last half century US society has undergone rather dramatic change. Although not nomadic in the anthropologic sense, we are anything but geographically fixed. Economic and lifestyle imperatives have placed great value on mobility. Children grow up and move elsewhere

The elderly are constant reminders of our own mortality.

to seek education and employment and to establish families of their own. Older members of families become long-distance abstractions who come to mind at birthdays and holidays. If children do remain proximate as adults, their parents may pack up at retirement and migrate to a more favorable climate. Older family members often become members in absentia.

In more recent years social and economic changes have reversed some of these trends. Maintaining certain standards of living, established in what we perceive to have been simpler times, has become increasingly challenging. Dual-income families are more the rule than the exception to meet modern lifestyle expectations. The number of single-parent families has increased dramatically as well. Child care needs have in many circumstances brought older family members back into the picture. Grandparents have become more important as providers of low-cost child care and are now increasingly becoming the primary care providers of their grandchildren. Middle-aged persons facing the challenges of raising a family today may look at the eventual infirmity of their parents with dread.

AGEISM IN AMERICA

At the turn of the century Sir William Osler expressed his views on the "... comparative uselessness of men above 40 years of age ... the uselessness of men above 60 years of age, and the incalculable benefit it would be in commercial, political, and professional life if, as a matter of course, men stopped work at this age."[2] Although the mean life expectancy at the time was approximately 46 years, and Osler was well into his fifties, his comments brought considerable stir and general outrage. Osler later protested that his remarks were largely in jest, reminding his listeners that he had dedicated much of his professional life to the treatment of diseases that plague older adults. Nevertheless, this attitude regarding the older members of our society persisted well into this century. The U.S. attitude has been youthful, strong, and aggressive toward our country's development and expansion. Theodore Roosevelt, in purging the US Navy of its senior officers, said "Weaklings and those who feared hard work and war [should] vanish from the earth." It became common practice in industry to shut out workers over the age of 40 years. Quotas existed limiting the immigration of older individuals when industry was in need of foreign workers.[3]

The U.S. attitude has been youthful, strong, and aggressive toward our country's development and expansion.

Over the years a stereotype of elderly persons evolved that is almost entirely negative in connotation.

> An older person thinks and moves slowly. He does not think as he used to or as creatively. He is bound to himself and to his past and can no longer change or grow. He can learn neither well nor swiftly and, even if he could, he would not wish to. Tied to his personal traditions and growing conservatism, he dislikes innovations and is not disposed to new ideas. Not only can he not move forward, he often moves backward. He enters a second childhood, caught up in increasing egocentricity and demanding more from his environment than he is willing to give to it. Sometimes he becomes an intensification of himself, a caricature of a lifelong personality. He becomes irritable and cantankerous, yet shallow

and enfeebled. He lives in his past; he is behind the times. He is aimless and wandering of mind, reminiscing and garrulous. Indeed he is a study in decline, the picture of mental and physical failure. He has lost and cannot replace friends, spouse, job, status, power, influence, income. He is often stricken by diseases which, in turn, restrict his movement, his enjoyment of food, the pleasures of well-being. He has lost his desire and capacity for sex. His body shrinks, and so does the flow of blood to his brain. His mind does not utilize oxygen and sugar at the same rate as formerly. Feeble, uninteresting, he awaits his death, a burden to society, to his family and to himself.[4]

The above composite stereotype assembled by Robert Butler in 1975, like most stereotypes, contains just enough accurate generalizations to be taken as true in its entirety.

THE LANGUAGE OF AGEISM

A whole language of ageism exists with the number of disparagements, a partial list of which is given here, far exceeding that used in reference to any other group.[5]

Act one's age	Dotage	Lawrence Welk generation
Anecdotage	Dotard	Little old lady
Anile	Eccentric	Maid
Anility	Fart	Miser
Bag	Feebleminded	Obsolete
Bat	Fogy	Old
Battle ax	Fool	Old-fashioned
Beldam	Fossil	Outmoded
Biddy	Fuddy-duddy	Overage
Caducity	Gaffer	Over the hill
Cantankerous	Garrulous	Peevish
Codger	Geezer	Rambling
Constipated	Generation gap	Rickety
Convalescent center	Geriatric generation	Rambling
Coot	Geritol generation	Second childhood
Crank	Goat	Senile
Cranky	Golden age	Senility
Crone	Granny	Senior citizen
Crotchety	Graybeard	Spinster
Debility	Grimalkin	Superannuated
Declining years	Grump	Toothless
Decrepit	Grumpy	Twilight years
Decrepitude	Hag	Withered
Dirty old man	Infirm	Wisened
Doddering	Infirmity	Wrinkled

The medical profession has added its own descriptives, including gomer, gork, and crock, to name but a few. For some reason, political correctness has lagged far behind in the treatment of older persons. Go to any greeting card store and peruse the birthday selections to see how aging is portrayed. The fortieth year is a particularly woeful celebration with black balloons popular and such sayings as "It's better to be over the hill than under it!" printed on T-shirts and caps. Of course, this is all in good fun, but can one imagine a similar treatment of an ethnic or racial group? One can still generally get away with poking fun at the elderly, but that day may soon be gone.

DISMANTLING THE STEREOTYPE

On average the lot of the United States' older citizens has improved significantly in the last several decades. In large part these improvements are a result of the elderly population gaining a louder voice in the political mainstream. Major advances include the Age Discrimination and Employment Act championed by the late congressman Claude Pepper, a virtual end to mandatory retirement, improved health care, and a general elevation in social image. Trailblazing organizations such as the Gray Panthers and more recently the American Association of Retired Persons and the National Council on Senior Citizens have helped to create political solidarity among older citizens. Regardless of one's ideology, former president Ronald Reagan served as a potent symbol of the possibilities and opportunities that can accompany aging. The elevation of geriatric medicine to specialty status has certainly had an important impact on our awareness of issues important to the health and well-being of our older patients.[3]

The "peripheral" older character has given way to older characters who are central to the story.

One can never be sure whether the media of television and cinema merely reflect changing attitudes or actually create them. Regardless, it is clear that the characterization of older persons in film and television has radically changed. The old-fashioned, benign, charmingly senile, dottering, quaint, marginally competent, and usually peripheral elderly personification has given way to older characters who are central to the story, intelligent, powerful, influential, frequently affluent, healthy, and active both physically and socially.[6] Today older characters are more often portrayed in positive ways and actually admired and looked up to by the more youthful characters. Several examples of popular television shows include "Murder, She Wrote," "Matlock," "Golden Girls," "Jake and the Fatman," and "In the Heat of the Night." Movies carried by the strength of their older performers include *Harold and Maude, Atlantic City, On Golden Pond, Driving Miss Daisy, Fried Green Tomatoes,* and most recently *Grumpy Old Men* and *Nobody's Fool,* to name some personal favorites.

Changing demographics have undoubtedly contributed to the overall improvement in the status of the older person. Our nation is aging, and with aging comes the development of new emphases. Our older members of society have a greater sense of entitlement than ever before and are not shy about letting their needs be known. Both their numbers and their assertiveness can be expected to increase in the coming decades as the baby-boomers leave middle age behind. Tolerance is giving way to acceptance and the critical realization that the growing elderly population will be an increasingly important consumer market.

A dubious testament to the recent successes of our older population is the emergence of so-called *new* ageism. There are those who feel elderly persons have made too many advances and see a growing disparity between the "truly needy" and the "truly greedy." Although it is a fact that fewer older Americans are now living at or below the poverty level, only 6% of those over 65 years of age have incomes in excess of $50,000. Older people still remain the poorest of all adults, and those living alone have poverty rates of approximately 20%. Other age-related myths deserve closer scrutiny. The elderly are not bankrupting the Social Security system as many individuals fear. It is projected that Social Security trust funds will reach approximately 1 trillion dollars by the end of the century and 12 trillion dollars will have accumulated by the time the average baby-boomer reaches 65 years of age. The number of retired persons is increasing steadily; however, the so-called dependence ratio in our population, that is, the number of individuals under 18 years and over 65 years, continues to decline because of a low overall birthrate that approaches zero population growth. Some persons point out that the economic condition of our nation's children has deteriorated steadily as the elderly population has gained and suggest that resources are not being allocated fairly. In terms of federal expenditures, the elderly receive more than the young. However, at the local level costs of education, which are enormous, are borne in large part by community-based property taxes. Further, it is unjust to argue that older people should be faulted for their gains while failing to address the complex problems facing our young persons, which are clearly more than economic. Studies show that the aged do not contribute to rising health care costs as much as advances in certain technologies such as organ transplantation, of which the elderly are seldom recipients. Only 6% of Medicare beneficiaries use in excess of $15,000 in their last illness, equivalent to approximately 30 days of hospitalization.[7]

Older people still remain the poorest of all adults, and those living alone have poverty rates of approximately 20%.

TOWARD HEALTHIER ATTITUDES

Despite advances, certain attitudes toward the elderly seem to be firmly ingrained in our attitudes about life in general. Certainly, the realization that we all share death as a common fate is an issue, and uneasiness or fear of aging and death does not cultivate positive imagery. The very old are constant reminders of our own mortality. In some cases they may come to symbolize unmet obligations, regrets, and anxieties we feel toward older members of our own families. A phenomenon referred to in psychoanalytic terms as *unresolved countertransference issues* has been described in physicians who deal extensively with aged persons. Thus superimposition and confusion of parent and child roles may complicate physician-patient relationships in a negative way.

The elderly are constant reminders of our own mortality.

The attitude one develops toward any group of people over time reflects to some degree the cultural and socioeconomic background of that individual. However, knowledge and experience are probably even more important to the development of one's attitude. Generalization is an important part of learning, and a degree of stereotypical thinking can

The realization that we all share death as a common fate is an issue, and uneasiness or fear of aging and death does not cultivate positive imagery.

be useful. The individual who becomes sick after drinking outdated milk and generalizes to avoid all outdated food products has gained useful knowledge from the experience. The individual suffering a similar intoxication who then swears off all milk products forever has not profited similarly. This exemplifies a rational vs. an irrational response.

More often than not stereotypes are built on factually incorrect perceptions. Having incomplete or inaccurate information about aging and elderly persons correlates well with the formation of negative attitudes. The converse holds true as well. Medical students and residents with exposure to outpatient clinics serving the well elderly population are more likely to develop and keep positive attitudes toward the elderly.[8-10] The inference is that these physicians in training have the opportunity to learn more about normal aging rather than subsisting on a steady diet of the infirm. Tests have been constructed to assess the degree of knowledge about aging for both research and educational purposes. One such test, Palmore's Facts on Aging Quiz, is presented in Table 5-1.[11,12] This quiz is short and easily graded, because the even-numbered questions are true and the odd numbered questions are false. The facts supporting each answer can be found throughout this book, or the interested reader may refer to Palmore's original work referenced here.

Worth mentioning is an interesting relationship between the opinions and attitudes of younger individuals about aging and those of the aged about themselves and about their peers. In a 1974 Harris survey older persons tended to agree with their younger counterparts on the seriousness of a host of problems faced by the aged population, including finances, health, housing, crime, loneliness, and social isolation; but, when asked what impact these problems had on them personally, the majority stated that they were little affected. The inference was that the perceived impact of aging on well-being depends highly on one's frame of reference. It was further concluded that people contribute significantly to their own well-being by making adjustments in their expectations as they grow older. In other words, although the older person may experience a decline in financial and health status, the overall sense of well-being is not necessarily affected adversely, because there is often a parallel adjustment in expectations. Although the public may think that old people have rather unsatisfactory lives, and old people believe other old people have lives almost as unsatisfactory, the view that old people have of their own lives is very much more positive.[13]

The perceived impact of aging on well-being depends highly on one's frame of reference.

SUMMARY

It is hazardous to generalize and jump to conclusions in medical practice. Much of the health professionals' education is dedicated to looking beyond the obvious to generate as broad a differential diagnosis as possible when faced with a clinical diagnostic challenge. Stereotyping the elderly, or any group for that matter, stands in the way of health professionals being effective clinicians by not allowing them to see the elderly's diversity as unique individuals with unique problems.

Emergency medical providers have the opportunity to observe the human condition at its best and, all too frequently, its worst. They do not often have the pleasure of interacting with the healthy, independent, and

Table 5–1 **Palmore's Facts on Aging Quiz**

1. The majority of old people (age 65+) are senile (defective memory, are disoriented, demented).
2. The five senses (sight, hearing, taste, touch and smell) all tend to weaken in old age.
3. The majority of old people have no interest in, nor capacity for, sexual relations.
4. Lung vital capacity tends to decline in old age.
5. The majority of old people feel miserable most of the time.
6. Physical strength tends to decline in old age.
7. At least one tenth of the aged are living in long-stay institutions (such as nursing homes, mental hospitals, homes for the aged, etc.).
8. Aged drivers have fewer accidents per driver than those under 65.
9. Older workers usually cannot work as effectively as younger workers.
10. Over three-fourths of the aged are healthy enough to carry out their normal activities.
11. The majority of old people are unable to adapt to change.
12. Old people usually take longer to learn something new.
13. It is almost impossible for the average old person to learn something new.
14. Older people tend to react slower than younger people.
15. In general, old people tend to be pretty much alike.
16. The majority of old people say they are seldom bored.
17. The majority of old people are socially isolated.
18. Older workers have more accidents than younger workers.
19. Over 15% of the population are now age 65 or over.
20. The majority of medical practitioners tend to give low priority to the aged.
21. The majority of old people have incomes below the poverty line (as defined by the federal government).
22. The majority of old people are working or would like to have some kind of work to do (including housework and volunteer work).
23. Old people tend to become more religious as they age.
24. The majority of old people say they are seldom irritated or angry.
25. The health and economic status of old people will be about the same or worse in the year 2000 (compared to younger people).

Reprinted with permission. Palmore E. The facts on aging quiz: a handbook of uses and results. 1988. Copyright © The Gerontological Society of America.

robust members of the elderly population. EDs by definition attract acutely and chronically ill patients, who present with varying degrees of decompensation and functional decline. Emergency physicians' view of this population may be skewed toward a more negative stereotype: the elderly tend to present to the ED with greater urgency and a variety of co-morbid conditions; require more physician and nursing time; more laboratory, x-ray, and other diagnostic tests; they stay longer and consume more resources; and they require hospitalization more frequently than their younger counterparts. Further, interviews with emergency physicians have revealed a general discomfort in dealing with the various clinical problems and challenges presented by older patients.

Emergency physicians' views of the elderly may be skewed toward a negative stereotype.

Attitude stems from experiences and knowledge. If experience creates an attitude that is dysfunctional, it can in theory be balanced by education. Emergency health care providers must have a more accurate and balanced frame of reference to avoid the depersonalization that comes with negative stereotypes and ultimately hurts all members of society. It is incumbent that emergency medical personnel be educated about the reality of aging and the special needs of elderly patients. Armed with knowledge, they can form a more balanced attitude toward elderly persons and in so doing become more effective clinicians.

SUMMARY POINTS

- Ageism is formally defined as "discrimination based on age; especially discrimination against middle-aged and elderly people."
- The elevation of geriatric medicine to specialty status has had an important impact on our awareness of issues important to the health and well-being of our older patients.
- Medical students and residents with exposure to outpatient clinics serving the well older population are more likely to develop and keep positive attitudes toward elderly persons. The inference is that these physicians in training have the opportunity to learn about normal aging rather than subsisting on a steady diet of the infirm.
- Stereotyping the elderly, or any group, stands in the way of our being effective clinicians by not allowing us to see their diversity as unique individuals with unique problems.

CHAPTER AUTHOR

Rawden Evans, PhD, MD

REFERENCES

1. Butler RN. Age-ism: another form of bigotry. Gerontologist. 1969;9:243–246.
2. Berk SL. Sir William Osler, ageism, and "The fixed period." *J Am Geriatr Soc.* 1989;37:263–266.
3. Tibbitts C. Can we invalidate negative stereotypes of aging? *Gerontologist.* 1979;19:10–20.
4. Butler RN. Why survive? Being old in America. New York, NY: Harper & Row; 1975.
5. Nuessel FR Jr. The language of ageism. *Gerontologist.* 1982;22;273–276.
6. Bell J. In search of a discourse on aging: the elderly on television. *Gerontologist.* 1992;32:305–311.
7. Butler RN. A disease called ageism. *J Am Geriatr Soc.* 1990;38:178–180..
8. Spence DL, Feigenbaum EM, Fitzgerald F, Roth J. Medical student attitudes toward the geriatric patient. *J Am Geriatr Soc.* 1968;16:976–983.
9. Adelman RD, Fields SD, Jutagir R. Geriatric education, II: The effect of a well elderly program on medical student attitudes toward geriatric patients. *J Am Geriatr Soc.* 1992;40:970–973.
10. Intrieri RC, Kelly JA, Brown MM, Castilla C. Improving medical students' attitudes toward and skill with the elderly. *Gerontologist.* 1993;33:373–378.
11. Palmore E. *The facts on aging quiz: a handbook of uses and results.* Springer Publishing Co., Inc., New York, NY. 1988.
12. Thomas WC. The expectation gap and the stereotype of the stereotype: images of old people. *Gerontologist.* 1981;21:402–407.

Geriatric
Emergency
Care Model

Principles of Care and Application of The Geriatric Emergency Care Model

---

LEARNING OBJECTIVES

1. Demonstrate use of a geriatric model for emergency treatment of elderly patients.
2. Apply principles of geriatric emergency medicine to the clinical evaluation and management of elderly patients.
3. Describe the impact of attitudes and misperceptions about aging on health care decisions.
4. Identify methods for improving level of comfort for elderly patients in the ED environment.
5. Demonstrate how pre-hospital emergency care providers can facilitate assessment and treatment of elderly patients.
6. Demonstrate unique aspects of the history and physical examination for the elderly ED patient.
7. Explain the importance of cognitive and functional assessment of elderly patients.
8. Demonstrate appropriate discharge planning for elderly ED patients.

Optimal emergency care involves altering the traditional medical model with consideration of the special needs of elderly patients. The traditional emergency medicine approach to patients focuses on a single presenting complaint as described in Table 6–1. The process begins in the pre-hospital care environment with the emergency medical services (EMS) system and continues through triage, initial assessment, and stabilization. A focused history and physi-

Table 6–1 **Principles of Emergency Care**

- The emergency medical system (EMS) focuses on caring for acutely ill or injured patients.
- Emergency medicine focuses on the patient's chief complaint.
- Emergency health care providers try to anticipate and monitor patients for life or limb threatening illness or injury.
- Beyond life threatening processes, emergency health care professionals focus on acute disease processes which need prompt attention and common diseases.
- Making a diagnosis is not as important as ruling out life or limb threatening processes.
- The emergency department must always be ready to divert its staff and resources to new patients with acute injuries or illnesses.
- Emergency health care professionals are constantly making priority decisions regarding multiple patients and ED resource availability because of the constantly changing emergency department.
- Emergency health care professionals often must make immediate decisions based on limited data.
- Time pressures and limited resources are important elements in the care of emergency department patients.

Reprinted by permission of Blackwell Science, Inc. Sanders AB. Emergency care. In: Schrier RW, Jahnigan D. Eds. Geriatric Medicine. 3rd ed. Cambridge, MA: Blackwell Scientific; 1995.

cal examination are done and a differential diagnosis is developed based on the following questions:

1. Is a life- or limb-threatening process causing this patient's complaint?
2. Is there an urgent disease process or injury that needs prompt attention?
3. What common conditions can cause the patient's symptoms?

Vague complaints— for example, weakness or decreased functional ability— may indicate serious diseases such as myocardial infarction, congestive heart failure, or sepsis.

The ED assessment attempts to answer these questions with a reasonable degree of certainty. The subsequent diagnostic decisions, treatment, and management plans focus on ruling out serious diseases and treating common conditions.[1]

The emergency medicine model of care (Figure 6-1) differs from the traditional medical model used in a clinic or office setting. A patient with the same complaint will be treated differently based on the model of care used. Emergency health care providers tend to focus on a single complaint rather than on comprehensive assessments. The history and physical examination are limited and focused on the specific complaint. The important goal is to reasonably rule out life-threatening processes. The final diagnosis, however, is not always determined. Emergency health care providers are constantly prioritizing complaints of multiple patients and making quick decisions based on limited data. The emergency medicine environment is one of high pressure and limited resources.[1,2]

This traditional emergency medicine, biomedical model is efficient and works well for most ED patients. It does not work well, however, for special populations such as children or the elderly. The ED model used for children routinely evaluates their caretakers and social environ-

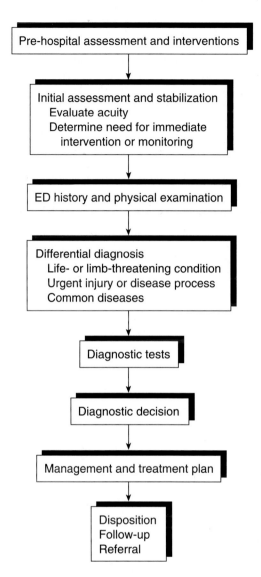

FIGURE 6-1 Emergency medicine model of care.

ment. Information about feeding and immunizations is frequently sought and evaluated. A 1-year-old infant who is seen in the ED with a fractured femur is assessed for child abuse as well as for the fracture.

Similarly, the approach to the patient who sustains major trauma in many communities uses an alternate model of emergency care. Trauma patients are approached with a team instituting a protocol of diagnostic procedures and monitoring. Evaluation is done using standardized tools such as the Glasgow Coma Scale or Injury Severity Score.

The elderly also represent a special population for emergency medicine. Key differences include the following principles (Table 6–2).

The patient's presentation is frequently complex.
There is often not one discrete presenting complaint. Older patients may give vague, imprecise, or ambiguous symptoms such as

Table 6–2 **Principles of Geriatric Emergency Medicine**

1. The patient's presentation is frequently complex
2. Common diseases present atypically in this age group
3. The confounding effects of co-morbid diseases must be considered
4. Polypharmacy is common and may be a factor in presentation, diagnosis, and management
5. Recognition of the possibility for cognitive impairment is important
6. Some diagnostic tests may have different normal values
7. The likelihood of decreased functional reserve must be anticipated
8. Social support systems may not be adequate, and patients may need to rely on caregivers
9. A knowledge of baseline functional status is essential for evaluating new complaints
10. Health problems must be evaluated for associated psychosocial adjustment
11. The emergency department encounter is an opportunity to assess important conditions in the patient's personal life

weakness or "not feeling right" or multiple complaints. This frustrates emergency health care professionals because it does not fit neatly into the ED model of care. Nevertheless, vague complaints such as weakness or decrease in functional ability may indicate serious diseases such as myocardial infarction, congestive heart failure, or sepsis.

Common diseases present atypically in this age group.

The traditional emergency medicine model focuses the history and physical examination on the chief complaint. Elderly patients, like children, often give atypical symptoms for common diseases. Acute appendicitis is often missed because medical professionals do not realize that the classic signs and symptoms such as localization of pain to the right lower quadrant may not occur in the elderly.[3,4] Similarly, only a minority of patients older than 85 years will have chest pain with an acute myocardial infarction.[5,6]

The confounding effects of co-morbid diseases must be considered.

The elderly frequently will have co-morbid diseases that may influence disease presentation, ED workup, and management strategy.[7-12]

Polypharmacy is common and may be a factor in presentation, diagnosis, and management.

Symptoms may reflect the effects of medications or medication interactions. There needs to be a heightened awareness of the effect of recently prescribed medications and their possible interactions.[7-12]

Recognition of the possibility for cognitive impairment is important.

It is important that emergency health care professionals be capable of systematically evaluating cognitive function in elderly patients. Impaired cognitive function can interfere with the evaluation of the patient as well as have important implications for patient workup and disposition.[12,14]

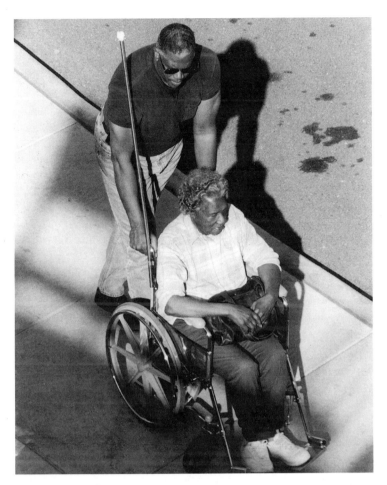

Care given by family and friends can be provided at several levels, from emotional support to actual physical care and ADLs.

Some diagnostic tests may have different normal values.

A knowledge of which values are altered is necessary to interpret test results accurately. For example, arterial blood oxygen tension declines in a predictable fashion with age; however, normal hemoglobin values do not change.[7,8]

The likelihood of decreased functional reserve must be anticipated.

Cardiac output, for example, declines with age. This physiologic change may not be important for persons performing their daily activities. However, when older persons are stressed by acute injury or illness, the lack of cardiac reserve can result in rapid deterioration as well as significant complications.[7-10]

Social support systems may not be adequate, and patients may need to rely on caregivers.

Apparently uncomplicated tasks such as making appointments and transportation to clinics may be major obstacles to obtaining adequate care. The elderly patient must be viewed in the context of the home environment and social support system. An assessment of the caretaker's ability to help the patient in light of acute illness or injury should be made.[7-12]

A knowledge of baseline functional status is essential for evaluating new complaints.

The elderly patient's complaints, ED workup, management, and disposition will depend on the ability to manage activities of daily living (ADLs), self-care, and meeting personal needs. Emergency health care professionals must assess the ability to function in light of the presenting problem and change in health.[11,12]

Health problems must be evaluated for associated psychosocial adjustment.

Elderly men have the highest rates of successful suicide attempts. The patient's presenting complaint and disease must be viewed in terms of the patient's emotional status and psychosocial functioning. Although depression is less common in older persons than in younger persons, it is often misdiagnosed; depression may present with atypical symptoms such as weight loss, jaw pain, or shoplifting.[7,10,15-17]

The emergency department encounter is an opportunity to assess important conditions in the patient's personal life.

A number of conditions may not be obvious if emergency health care professionals only focus on the chief complaint.[13-15] For example, the majority of elderly patients who are abused or mistreated by family caretakers or others are seen in EDs but do not complain of the abuse.[18,19] It is easy for emergency health care professionals to focus on the specific presenting condition such as a broken arm, contusions, or ankle sprain rather than on the circumstances surrounding the event. Screening for high-risk conditions such as elder abuse should be a general concern of emergency health care professionals.[15]

HEALTHY AGING

Falls, incontinence, and confusion are not normal deteriorations of the human body; treat aggressively.

It is unfortunate that some emergency health care professionals have a negative view of the elderly and the aging process. In the ED, older patients are frequently seen with severe illnesses and disabilities. Many emergency health care professionals see a large number of nursing home patients who are transferred for evaluation and treatment. Dealing with elderly patients who have multiple medical conditions as well as cognitive and functional disability can be very frustrating and produce a slanted view of the aging process.[20]

One can view aging as a process in which the body and organs gradually deteriorate. An alternative view is to see aging as another stage in life with its own joys, pains, and experiences. Healthy aging requires a positive attitude on the part of the patient as well as by health care providers. Many older people are productive, active, and able to enjoy the benefits of advanced age. They see it for the grace, respect and privileges that it can bring. The elderly are complex, diverse, and wise. They often can devote more time and energy than younger persons to important parts of their lives.[7,10,21]

It is most important that emergency health care professionals avoid stereotyping and acknowledge the heterogeneity and diversity of elderly patients as they would any other population. Underlying all emergency medical care must be a respect for an older person's belief systems, values, and personal preferences.

Society has promulgated many misperceptions about aging, which leads to stereotypes and colors attitudes toward the elderly. For example, illness and disability are not inevitable consequences of growing old. Only 5% of the elderly require nursing home placement.[7,10] Major stumbling blocks in providing health care for older persons are the attitudes and biases of health care professionals. Conditions such as falls, incontinence, and confusion are not normal deteriorations of the human body; they should be aggressively treated.[7,10] The elderly have been needlessly excluded from the initial trials of thrombolytic agents in the United States for patients with acute myocardial infarction despite having the highest mortality for this condition.[22] Data have clearly shown that the efficacy of thrombolytics for acute myocardial infarction is greater for older patients than for younger patients.[23,24] It is thus crucial that emergency health care professionals understand these issues as they treat elderly patients.

GERIATRIC EMERGENCY CARE MODEL

This model for the ED evaluation and treatment of the elderly patient places the presenting symptoms in the context of a more comprehensive evaluation. The ED presentation is viewed in the context of comorbid diseases, medications, the patient's cognitive function, functional status, emotional status, and social and bioethical considerations (Figure 6–2).

There is a great deal of heterogeneity among persons 65 years and older. Physiologic age for a variety of reasons may differ from biologic age. A 55-year-old patient may demonstrate a higher physiologic age than another patient who is 75 years of age. One must adopt a flexible attitude about characterizing all patients based on a numeric chronologic age. Some authorities divide the elderly into the younger elderly (65-74 years), middle-aged elderly (75-84 years), and the oldest elderly (85 years and older). Demographically the oldest elderly persons are the fastest growing segment of the population. Patients over 85 years also will present the most difficult challenges for emergency health care professionals.

EMERGENCY DEPARTMENT ENVIRONMENT

The ED environment does not lend itself easily to the care of elderly patients.[8] Most EDs see a high volume of patients with little time for lengthy individual encounters. There is a great deal of pressure to make quick decisions regarding patient assessment and disposition so that new patients can be seen. The ED is an uncomfortable, stressful environment for most persons. Patients present with a perceived acute change in their health status; they are often anxious and may be in

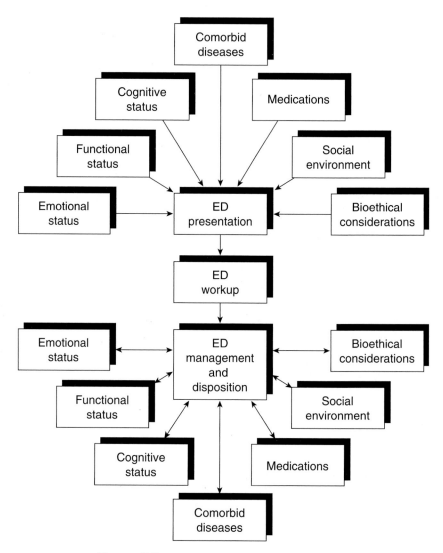

FIGURE 6-2 Geriatric emergency care model.

pain. Although elderly patients frequently have primary care physicians, in the ED setting they must interact with unfamiliar health care professionals with whom they have not built relationships of trust and confidence.[25]

The physical environment of many EDs can be unpleasant as well. Many EDs provide little privacy and thus little confidentiality. The beds are hard and uncomfortable. The lighting is poor, and ambient noise is high, making it especially difficult for older patients with vision or hearing disorders. Whereas children are often accommodated with special rooms to meet their needs, few EDs provide special environments for older patients.[25]

The ED environment can be made more comfortable for older patients.[26] A quiet, private room can enhance communication, decrease anxiety, and show respect for patient privacy. Hearing amplification devices can be a useful adjunct for communication with some patients. It is often difficult for elderly patients to step up to an examination bed; beds can be lower to the floor and wider for greater comfort. Simple amenities such as pillows and warm blankets can make a significant difference in providing comfort and respect. The room should be warm for comfort. Many elderly patients have cataracts and have difficulty seeing. Glare and shadows intensify the problem. Indirect lighting is optimal. Direct light, if used, should not be directed toward the patient's face.[7] The patient's family or caregiver can be welcomed into the patient's room as soon as feasible to provide comfort and support and decrease the sense of isolation. Finally, the emergency care team should try to provide the patient and family with information and updates regarding medical findings and course of management. The elderly may be anxious and unfamiliar with the emergency health care system. They need to know why tests are being done, what diseases are being considered, and what will happen. Reassuring dialogue with the emergency health care team can help address these anxieties.[25,26]

COMMUNICATIONS

Emergency health care professionals have noted that communication barriers are a significant problem in dealing with elderly patients.[27] Many of these issues can be addressed by making the ED environment user-friendly. Fundamentally, however, it is the professional interaction that will set the tone for the ED encounter. Sensitivity, empathy, and respect are conveyed in choice of words, tone of voice, and body language. It is essential to take the time and make the effort to convey respect and dignity in all communications. One should speak slowly, clearly, and in deep tones while facing the patient. It is best to interview the patient at eye level rather than speaking over the bed or from the foot of the bed. Noises, monitors, and other activity in the room can be distracting, increase anxiety, and decrease one's ability to obtain an accurate history. Respect is shown by addressing the patient by title (Mr., Ms., Dr.) and last name. Touch can be especially reassuring and can impart a sense of connection and confidence. If possible, contact can be made with the patient's primary care physician. This not only provides the emergency physician with valuable information about the patient, but also reassures the patient and family that the health care team is working together. All procedures, tests, and treatments should be carefully explained to the patient, accommodations made for the patient's privacy during the physical examination.

PRE-HOSPITAL CARE

The emergency evaluation of the elderly patient frequently begins in the pre-hospital environment. Approximately 30% of elderly patients seeking care in EDs use ambulance transport.[28] Pre-hospital care professionals must be familiar with the special needs of the elderly. Elderly patients are four times more likely to arrive in the ED by ambulance compared to non-elderly patients. Thirty-six percent of all ambulance transports to the ED are for patients 65 years or older.[28]

In one study, the detection of a social problem by paramedics had a 98% positive predictive value when compared to follow-up assessments.

Most elderly patients are transported to the ED from their home; this gives pre-hospital care professionals an important opportunity to assess the home environment. One study demonstrated that paramedic assessment of the home environment of elderly patients was extremely useful for detecting elderly persons at risk.[18] In 98% of cases, detection of a social problem by paramedics was confirmed by a professional assessment from a social service agency. Paramedics evaluated the patient's living conditions with regard to environmental conditions, social support systems, and medical and mental issues.[18] Figure 6-3 shows the report form used by Gerson et al. in Akron, Ohio. Reports that indicated a problem were referred to the area agency on aging, prompting a home visit assessment. Modifications of this form can be incorporated into local EMS protocols in conjunction with social service agencies.[18]

In addition to screening at-risk elderly in the home environment, pre-hospital care professionals must be aware that elderly individuals may present with atypical manifestations of serious diseases. Vague symptoms such as weakness or dyspnea may indicate an acute myocardial infarction.[5] Non-specific abdominal pain without rebound or guarding may indicate a bowel infarction or dissecting abdominal aneurysm.[29-31] The history is not always easy to obtain, especially in light of possible cognitive impairment, acute anxiety, and underlying disabilities.

It is important that pre-hospital care professionals realize that the elderly may have hearing losses and visual changes that impair the ability to communicate. Sensitivity to their needs by demonstrating a demeanor of respect is key to effective communication. Making sure the patient brings physical aids such as glasses or hearing aids can facilitate patient comfort and communication as well. The patient is given a sense of control during this stressful time. Pre-hospital care professionals should always identify themselves and carefully explain what they are doing before it is done. Quickly moving the patient, starting an intravenous line, or starting oxygen will all increase anxiety if the actions are not understood. Movement from a bed to a stretcher may intensify pain. One must always listen carefully to the patient and show respect for the patient's values and opinions.

Because an elderly person may present with significant medical emergencies with apparently benign symptoms, one must be particularly cautious about downgrading pre-hospital transport from an advanced life support unit to a basic life support unit. Basic pre-hospital care procedures, including oxygen by nasal cannula, an intravenous line with normal saline, and rhythm electrocardiogram (ECG) monitoring, should be considered whenever emergent conditions are possible. Encouraging the patient to bring all medications to the hospital could facilitate ED workup. Elderly trauma victims have a particularly high morbidity and mortality.[32] These patients should be promptly transported to an ED capable of dealing with seriously ill trauma victims. Elderly trauma victims may not appear ill initially and then may deteriorate rapidly.[33,34] Because of their decreased cardiovascular reserve, it is most important that they receive definitive care as soon as possible.[33,34] Specific elements of the history and physical examination unique to elderly patients will be discussed later in this chapter. Pre-

PARAMEDIC REPORT FORM

Name			Priority	Hosp.	Run no. ☐☐ . ☐☐☐☐☐

No problem noted ☐   Could not eval. ☐

Date ☐☐ ☐☐ ☐☐

Age	Race	Sex	Contact	Home	Lives alone	Ong pt.	>1 pt.
	W B O	M F	Phone	Y N	Y N	Y N	Y N

Names of additional persons: _____

_____

_____

ENVIRONMENT
    Temperature _____
    Odor _____
    Sanitation _____
    Hazards _____

SOCIAL
    Support _____
    Trauma _____
    Food _____
    ADL _____

MEDICAL
    Hygiene _____
    Senses _____
    Medicines _____
    Conditions _____

MENTAL
    Confusion _____
    Affect _____
    ETOH _____

_____
Paramedic

FIGURE 6-3 Sample follow-up report. (Adapted from Gerson LW, Schelble DT, Wilson JE. Using paramedics to identify at-risk elderly. *Ann Emerg Med.* 1992;21:688–691.)

hospital personnel may begin the evaluation process by applying some of the recommended tools in the field such as a standardized mental status examination (see Chapters 7 and 8).

INITIAL EMERGENCY DEPARTMENT ASSESSMENT

The initial assessment of the patient will focus on presenting symptoms, vital signs, and a brief overview of the patient's condition. The initial assessment may be done by the emergency physician, nurse, or both. Its purposes are to (1) evaluate the acuity of the patient's condition and (2) determine the need for immediate interventions or monitoring, as described in Figure 6–1.

The initial assessment is an opportunity for emergency health care professionals to establish rapport with the patient and set the tone of the ED encounter. Shaking hands is a useful technique to touch the patient, note skin temperature, and initiate a positive relationship. Introductions and simple questions regarding the chief complaint give an impression of how the patient talks, understands, and responds to questions. An initial open-ended question allows the patient to express concerns. It is unfortunate that, in elderly patients, the chief complaint is frequently complex. Emergency health care professionals, because of time constraints and pressure to see multiple patients quickly, can find this frustrating. In the traditional emergency care model, chief complaints are boxed efficiently into simple categories that lead to a focused history, physical examination, and diagnostic tests. Elderly patients with complex complaints, multiple medications, and comorbid diseases do not fit easily into diagnostic categories. A fall with a Colles' fracture of the wrist may be symptomatic of a cardiac dysrhythmia or an acute gastrointestinal bleed.

VITAL SIGNS

The vital signs are an important component of the initial evaluation. Abnormal vital signs give a clue to a serious underlying condition. However, elderly patients may have serious diseases even with normal vital signs. An elderly patient with fever is more likely to have a life-threatening illness, and the rate of pathogenic isolates is higher than for younger febrile patients.[35] Hypothermia is also associated with many severe illnesses in the elderly population (e.g., hypothyroidism, stroke) but is easily missed. If the oral temperature is 35° C (95° F), which is as low as most thermometers register, take the temperature rectally with a low-register thermometer. If the temperature falls below 32° C (90° F), urgent treatment is required.

Criteria for the diagnosis of hypertension in elderly patients are a systolic pressure higher than 160 mmHg or a diastolic pressure higher than 95 mmHg. The cross-sectional prevalence of isolated systolic hypertension increases from 3% at 50 years of age to 22% of men and 34% of women at 65-74 years of age, with further increased prevalence for persons older than 75 years.[36] A series of at least three readings must be taken to establish an accurate baseline blood pressure (BP).

BP may be overestimated in elderly patients because of arterial stiffness. This "pseudohypertension" is suspected if the radial or brachial artery is still palpable after the BP cuff has been inflated to a pressure greater than the systolic pressure (Osler's sign).[37] The evaluation of orthostatic BP change may be useful in some older patients. Readings are obtained with the patient lying down, sitting, and/or standing. A decline of more than 20 mmHg in systolic pressure upon standing is seen in elderly patients who have symptomatic postural hypotension caused by dehydration or blood loss. When there is no increase in heart rate, an autonomic nervous system disorder or the ingestion of beta-blocking medications may be considered as possible causes.[38]

Pulse rates may vary between 60 and 100, regular and irregular, depending on the patient's past history of cardiac disease and current medications. Tachycardia may indicate a systemic problem with thyrotoxicosis, or it may suggest occult blood loss and may be the only significant abnormal finding on examination. When any pulse irregularity is noted, listening to the apical heartbeat with the stethoscope while palpating the radial pulse will determine the pulse deficit. Bradycardia (sinus bradycardia, sinoatrial exit block, second-degree or third-degree atrioventricular [AV] block) is rare in healthy elderly patients.[39] Irregular pulse rates often will indicate a need for cardiac monitoring.

Respiratory rate does not change with age; therefore, abnormal rates may be a subtle sign of a serious disease. Tachypnea may be due to hypoxia from infection, pulmonary embolus, or congestive heart failure or from nonhypoxic causes such as sepsis or hypovolemia. Medications such as aspirin in high doses can also cause tachypnea and a respiratory alkalosis.

A respiratory rate greater than 25 breaths/min suggests the possibility of a lower respiratory tract infection before the appearance of other clinical signs. It is not uncommon for the relatives of elderly invalids to report "attacks of breathlessness," which, in fact, are periodic episodes of Cheyne-Stokes respirations—a very common condition in the elderly age group, characterized by intervals of hyperpnea that alternate with intervals of apnea. Cheyne-Stokes breathing can come and go over a period of weeks or months without any noteworthy change in the patient's condition.

Weight is a useful measurement; unfortunately, it often is not recorded. It may be used both to monitor a patient's nutritional status and to judge the efficacy of diuretic therapy for congestive heart failure.

The initial evaluation alerts the physician or nurse to the potential acuity of the patient's condition. Patients with potentially life-threatening diseases have anticipatory monitoring or treatment started. This includes the establishment of an intravenous line, placement of ECG monitors, pulse oximetry, and oxygen supplementation. It also should trigger the need for a prompt, full history and physical examination. This may be done simultaneously with the performance of diagnostic testing. Cerebrovascular or cardiovascular insufficiency, abdominal catastrophe, and sepsis should be considered in the initial assessment and differential diagnosis of ill-appearing elderly patients with vague and nondescript symptoms.

Emergency Department
GERIATRIC MEDICAL RECORD - Part 1

NAME

ADDRESS

	CITY		STATE	ZIP CODE

DATE OF BIRTH	PLACE OF BIRTH		INFO. SOURCE

HOME PHONE	WORK PHONE	SOCIAL SECURITY NO.

EMPLOYER	USUAL PHYSICIAN / SERVICE	PHONE /PAGER	TRIAGE / ARRIVAL TIME

HEALTH INSURANCE COVERAGE	

AUTHORIZATION E.D. TREATMENT	REGISTRATION TIME

ADVANCE DIRECTIVES	NEXT OF KIN	PHONE	

TRIAGE LEVEL A B C	MODE OF ARRIVAL	ROOM NO.

INITIAL BP	TEMP	PULSE	RESP	AGE	SEX	CC	TIME IN ROOM

PAST MEDICAL HISTORY	LAST TETANUS	INFLUENZA	PNUEMOVAX	DISPOSITION COMPLETE

CURRENT MEDICATIONS	WEIGHT	

ALLERGIES	SOCIAL SUPPORT	CAREGIVER	DISCHARGE COMPLETE

ACTIVITIES OF DAILY LIVING

Ambulation _____   Transfer _____   Toileting _____

Bathing _____   Dressing _____   Feeding _____

MENTAL STATUS EVALUATION

Delirium/Confusion _____   CAM Score _____   Mini-Mental State Score _____

Orientation _____   Three-Item Recall _____

CASE SCREENING

Nutrition   Depression   Falls

Alcohol   Incontinence   Abuse

HISTORY

PHYSICAL EXAM

ED ASSESSMENT/PLAN

PHYSICIAN _____   NURSE _____

FIGURE 6-4   Geriatric medical record.

Emergency Department GERIATRIC MEDICAL RECORD - Part 2

ED COURSE / RESPONSE TO TREATMENT

TIME	MEDICATION / PROCEDURE	DOSE	ROUTE	RN	PURPOSE / SIDE EFFECTS REVIEWED	TIME / EVALUATION	TIME	B / P	HR	RESP.	TEMP. AND / OR OTHER
					YES NO						
					YES NO						
					YES NO						
					YES NO						
					YES NO						
					YES NO						

VITAL SIGNS

NURSING NOTES

CBC   LFTs ————————   ABG ————
             ————————   CXR ————
LYTES   ————————   C-SPINE ————
U / A ————————   ECG ————————   ABD SERIES ————
————————   CT ————

COGNITIVE STATUS

FUNCTIONAL STATUS

ADL (ambulation, transfer, toileting, bathing, dressing, feeding)

IADL (telephone, shopping, meals, laundry, medicines, finances)

"Get up and go" test

SOCIAL (CAREGIVER)

OTHER

DIAGNOSTICS (LAB AND X-RAY)

CASE FINDING

DISCHARGE PLAN

DISCHARGE DIAGNOSIS   TREATMENT   FOLLOW UP
1. ————   ————   ————
2. ————   ————   ————
3. ————   ————   ————
4. ————   ————   ————

PHYSICIAN ————————   NURSE ————————

FIGURE 6-4   CONTINUED

HISTORY

Adequate time must be devoted to obtaining accurate histories from elderly patients (Figure 6–4). As the proportion of elderly patients increases, physician and nurse staffing patterns need to reflect an increased time commitment. Data gathering for the history often will include interviews with the patient, family, or caregivers; review of past medical records; and a telephone interview with the primary care physician. Access to prior records and hospitalizations can provide invaluable data to emergency health care professionals. Fax machines in the ED can readily provide information from other health care facilities. Elderly patients may have non-specific ST-T wave abnormalities on ECG testing, and access to a previous ECG can provide crucial information on whether the ECG changes are new.

The history includes the following elements.

Presenting Symptom

In elderly patients, as discussed previously, the presenting symptom is often complex. There may be multiple concerns that may or may not be related to one disease process. Even a straightforward chief complaint such as a laceration following a fall should trigger questions regarding frequent falls, balance, gait, and possible etiologies including dysrhythmia, medication toxicity, and orthostasis. Questions about elder abuse should be asked even if this is not initially brought up by the patient.

Formal Mental Status Examination

Elderly patients should have a formal evaluation of cognitive function as part of the history. Abnormal cognitive function may play an important role in the patient's ability to relate the rest of the history accurately. Studies also have shown that up to one third of elderly ED patients may have an unrecognized, moderate cognitive deficit.[13] Instruments to assess cognitive status and ED work up when abnormalities are detected are presented in Chapters 7 and 8.

Functional Status Assessment

The functional status of the patient is an essential part of the history. Functional status includes an assessment of the patient's ability to perform ADLs such as bathing, dressing, toileting, transferring, and feeding as well as performing functions in the environment such as preparing meals, doing laundry, and managing money. Functional status can be assessed with one of the formal tools discussed in Chapters 7 and 9. Obtaining information about the patient's social and environmental resources will be essential in planning the disposition of the patient following ED workup.

Past Medical History

Elucidation of the past medical history with an emphasis on comorbid diseases is essential for all elderly ED patients. A knowledge of these conditions is crucial for assessment of the patient's complaint as well as for planning management strategies. Questions regarding patient treatment preferences and the presence of advance directives also should be considered in patients with significant medical diseases.

Medications

A medication history is essential that includes both over-the-counter and prescription medicines.

Review of Systems

A brief review of systems is important to help evaluate the chief complaint and put it in context. Inquiries regarding problems in the respiratory, cardiovascular, gastrointestinal, genitourinary, musculoskeletal, neurologic, and psychologic systems can provide important information.

Case Screening for Relevant Conditions

Questions to determine patients at risk for significant problems also should be part of the ED history. These include risks for abuse, suicide, nutritional deficiencies, and incontinence. The importance of finding these problems in the ED encounter is discussed in Chapters 7 and 9.

The physical examination of the elderly patient in the ED depends on the ED presentation. Since elderly patients frequently present atypically with serious diseases, a thorough physical examination is generally indicated, especially with regard to the heart, lungs, abdomen, and neurologic status. It is important to note that specific elements of the physical examination may be unique for the elderly.

PHYSICAL EXAMINATION

Skin

The elderly patients skin can be notably thin and dry, with a loss of elasticity. These changes make an evaluation of dehydration less reliable. The lateral aspect of the cheek is often the best site for evaluation of skin turgor. An increased capillary fragility may result in reddish purple spots that appear on the hands and forearms (senile purpura). Bruisability, however, also may reflect fragile skin, vitamin deficiency, coagulopathy, liver disease, or abuse. Patients who have been confined to a wheelchair or bed for long periods of time should be examined for pressure sores. Increased pressure over a bony prominence (e.g., heels or sacrum) leads to a cone-shaped pressure gradient with the base of the cone on the bone. For this reason the size of the ulceration seen on the skin surface underestimates the size of the soft-tissue lesion.

Neoplasia is associated with aging in virtually all organ systems but is especially common in the skin.

Neoplasia is associated with aging in virtually all organ systems but is especially common in the skin. One or more benign proliferative growths are present in nearly every adult over 65 years of age, and most individuals have dozens of lesions. Because emergency personnel are often the first to confront the myriad skin lesions seen in this population, it is important to recognize the various types and to know when to refer the patient for further evaluation.

Eyes

With aging, there is a loss of orbital fat, gradually displacing the eye backward into the orbit (enophthalmos). Thus sunken eyes are not a reliable indicator of dehydration in elderly patients. Wrinkling and loosening of skin around the eyelids produce an eversion, or ectropion, of the eyelids with exposure of the conjunctiva. Entropion, or inversion of the eyelids, may result in irritation of the conjunctiva by the eyelashes. Arcus senilis, often cited in the past as a marker of premature cardiovascular disease, loses its clinical significance with advancing age (generally over 50 years of age) and, in fact, for the elderly population is frequently a result of depigmentation within the iris associated with normal aging.

The optic disc may be scrutinized for pressure atrophy caused by glaucoma; the macula may be checked for evidence of macular degeneration; and the retinal field may be evaluated for diabetic or hypertensive angiopathy. Many elderly patients have had cataracts extracted, in which case, an ophthalmoscope with a positive diopter lens should be used. Measurement of normal intraocular pressure by tonometry may not exclude glaucoma because of the considerable diurnal variation in this pressure. Thus funduscopic examination and visual field testing are at least as important in screening, especially in persons at high risk.[40]

Ears, nose, and throat

Wax accumulation is a common cause of hearing loss. Patients reported as senile may simply be hard of hearing. Presbycusis (loss of auditory acuity from nerve degeneration) may cause loss of ability to hear high-pitched sounds, progressing to loss of ability to hear normal speech sounds. If a patient wears a hearing aid, it should be removed and examined; the ear mold and plastic tubing can become plugged with wax. If the battery is dead, a whistle (feedback) will not be heard when the volume is increased.

Patients reported as senile may simply be hard of hearing.

Women with osteoporosis may have florid periodontal disease caused by loss of alveolar bone that supports the teeth. If a person wears dentures, they should be removed before examining the mouth for bleeding or swollen gums, fungal infections, and signs of oral cancer (leukoplakia, erythroplasia, ulceration, and tumor mass).[37]

The neck, as usual, is examined for palpable lymph nodes, thyroid enlargement, and carotid bruits. The range of motion of the cervical spine should be evaluated. Cervical spondylosis is common in the elderly and may be responsible not only for neck pain but also for occipital headaches and pain in the upper extremities and chest area. A tortuous aorta may interfere with assessment of jugular venous pulse elevation, particularly on the left side of the neck.

Thorax

Breast cancer is a disease of the elderly as well as of middle-aged and younger women. Lesions that are 1 cm or larger can be palpated in otherwise normal breasts. Most tumors feel irregular and hard, whereas cysts usually are round, smooth, and almost elastic on palpation. Carcinomas also tend to be relatively fixed in the surrounding breast tissue and have indistinct edges (caused by local infiltration). However, normal changes in breast tissue that occur with aging may be misleading if diagnosis is based solely on clinical examination.[41] For example, the decrease in the glandular elements and fat envelope may cause some lesions (e.g., fibroadenomas) that have been present for years to become more prominent, giving the impression of a new or growing mass. In addition, shrinkage and fibrotic changes may cause nipple retraction, also mimicking cancer.

An examination of the lungs should determine the pattern of respiration and expansion of the chest, as well as the ability to cough. Rales at the lung bases may be normal in the elderly population. Elderly patients tend to have stasis of blood and lung secretions because of weakness of respiratory muscles, changes in lung mechanics, and a diminished cough reflex. Dullness at the base of the lung may be an early sign of consolidation in the toxic-appearing elderly patient without other signs of pneumonia, and wheezing may represent incipient pulmonary edema.

Chemoreceptors are less sensitive to hypoxia, and elderly patients with acute asthma produce less tachycardia and pulsus paradoxus for the same degree of hypoxia in a younger patient.[42] The insensitive chemoreceptor also may be partly responsible for an elderly subject's poor perception of dyspnea during bronchoconstriction.

Cardiovascular system

Systolic ejection murmurs are common in people over 70 years of age and generally are due to hemodynamically insignificant aortic valve sclerosis. These murmurs are crescendo-decrescendo and usually are no louder than grade 2/6. Grade 3/6 or louder murmurs or the presence of symptoms such as angina or exertional syncope warrants an echocardiogram. Diastolic murmurs are always significant.

A narrowing of the gap between the aortic and pulmonary components of the second heart sound during inspiration indicates strain or reduced function of the left ventricle, probably caused by a recent myocardial infarction (MI) or left bundle branch block. As in younger persons, a third heart sound indicates ventricular dilatation and failure. A chronic fourth heart sound is heard frequently enough to be considered consistent with the norm; this probably reflects a decreased compliance instead of failure of the left ventricle. However, an S_4 gallop that develops suddenly in a person with angina may indicate an acute change, such as a silent MI.[43]

Carotid and femoral pulses should be auscultated for bruits. A carotid bruit not accompanied by other symptoms serves to arouse suspicion of generalized atherosclerosis, rather than to predict the presence of a specific carotid lesion. The dynamics of the carotid pulse may indicate aortic valvular disease if it is rapidly collapsing (insufficiency)

Systolic ejection murmurs are common in people over 70 years of age and generally are due to hemodynamically insignificant aortic valve sclerosis.

or significantly slow in the upstroke stenosis. However, this sign may be obscured by the vessel stiffening seen in some elderly patients.[38]

Gastrointestinal system

With the abdominal wall often thin, examining the gastrointestinal area is simplified. A palpable abdominal aortic aneurysm should be distinguished carefully from a simple tortuous aorta, which is less than 3 cm wide and seldom has an associated bruit. Palpate for possible hernias, which often are more localized in the elderly. Acute abdominal emergencies may be difficult to discern because typical local and systemic signs may not be present. Perforation of a viscus and gangrene of the bowel may be marked by nothing more than sudden confusion.

The rectal examination provides invaluable information about the prostate gland in men and the cervix, uterus, rectal wall, and contents of the lower abdominal cavity in women.

Pelvis

A pelvic examination in an elderly woman and a rectal examination in an elderly man are important especially in light of the increased incidence of malignancy. When positioning an elderly woman for a pelvic examination, remember that degenerative changes in the lumbar spine and hips may make the classic lithotomy position painful. As an alternative, position the patient comfortably in the supine position with the knees flexed and the legs dropped to each side. With the patient in this position, the clinician may adequately examine the external genitalia. Begin with careful inspection and palpation of the vulvar area, which is often ignored on the pelvic examination. Note any abnormal changes in the skin, including erythema, leukoplakia, ulceration, or masses. Next, observe and palpate the urethra, Skene's glands, and Bartholin's glands. To perform the vaginal examination, guide the patient onto the left lateral position with the knees flexed. A small vaginal speculum (1- to 1.5-cm Pederson) is recommended for the patient with an atrophic vulva and vagina.[44] If the speculum cannot be inserted easily, explore the vagina carefully with a gloved fingertip. In older women who are not sexually active, the vaginal walls may have adhered, precluding a visual examination of the vagina. A Papanicolaou (Pap) smear should be obtained from any abnormal areas visualized in the vagina or in the cervix.

A patient receiving estrogen replacement may tolerate the usual bimanual examination without much difficulty. The atrophic vagina and vulva may, however, admit only one digit easily. Uterine size, shape, and mobility are all important factors to be evaluated. Any enlargement in the ovaries is abnormal and will require further evaluation. In women more than 5 years after menopause, a palpable ovary is suspicious for neoplasia.[45]

Pelvic prolapse refers to a group of anatomic, sometimes symptomatic, defects, including uterine prolapse (descensus), relaxation of the anterior vaginal wall (urethrocele and cystocele), relaxation of the posterior wall (rectocele), and herniation of the peritoneum of the cul-de-sac (enterocele). Some form of pelvic prolapse occurs in one fourth of patients over 60 years of age and may be symptomatic in 10%.[46] Pessaries remain a useful palliative strategy for patients who wish to avoid surgery or are otherwise at high risk for surgical repair. A recent review[47] describes the variety of major and minor complications that may be seen in patients who use pessaries.

Nervous system

Mental status testing by a reasonably sensitive, standard screening instrument is mandatory in assessing older individuals with or without complaints, both to establish baseline norms and to detect abnormalities requiring further workup (see Chapters 7 and 8). Symmetric diminution or disappearance of the gag reflex and vibratory sensation in the toes are common age-related changes and should not, in isolation, be attributed to disease. Frontal release signs (e.g., snout reflex), often touted as evidence of dementing disease, have been shown to occur with normal aging and are not correlated with cognitive impairment.[48] Cerebellar function is tested by watching the gait and noting fine movements of the extremities. A senile tremor, which occurs at a rate of 3-7 per second, is coarser than a parkinsonian tremor and involves the head, jaw, and hands. The tremor occurs with movement and does not involve limb rigidity.

Symmetric diminution or disappearance of the gag reflex and vibratory sensation in the toes are common age-related changes.

After the standard examination is completed, it is important to observe gait. Spastic weakness, if unilateral, is usually due to the effects of a stroke. The problem is stiffness of the affected leg combined with persisting plantar flexion. In peripheral neuropathy, flaccid weakness is combined with some loss of feeling. The result is a high-stepping gait caused by footdrop and a general incoordination of movement because weak muscles are always clumsy. Trauma or pressure neuropathy will frequently produce a unilateral gait problem with a limp and with dorsolumbar scoliosis if the sciatic or femoral nerves are involved. Parkinson's disease produces a characteristic gait disorder marked by rigidity of muscles, with slowness of response producing difficulty in starting any walking movement. Once begun, the gait is shuffling with a forward-stooping posture, causing patients to take small, rapid steps to avoid falling forward. Ataxic gait may be either motor or sensory. In motor ataxia the problem is one of muscle incoordination, and the patient walks on a wide base, wandering from side to side as if intoxicated. The acute onset of such an ataxia in an older individual is almost always of vascular origin. In sensory ataxia the problem is not knowing where the feet are in relation to the ground. The gait is slow with the head held down. In the elderly patient, this condition is caused by disorders that affect the posterior columns (e.g., vitamin B_{12} deficiency, cervical spondylosis).[49]

EMERGENCY DEPARTMENT DIAGNOSTIC WORKUP

The ED history and physical examination dictate a differential diagnosis as illustrated in Figure 6–1. Emphasis will be initially on life-threatening illnesses that may cause the presenting complaint. Sometimes, no clear differential diagnosis will emerge from the symptom complex. The priorities for the geriatric patient will, however, remain the same. Does this symptom complex represent myocardial ischemia? Does this represent acute cerebrovascular disease? Does this represent an infectious process? Does this represent an acute abdominal condition?

The secondary priority in developing the differential diagnosis is to assess the signs and symptoms with respect to urgent or common diseases. Are the symptoms related to patient medications? Are the symptoms an exacerbation of a pre-existing disease? Do the symptoms fit a new disease process?

Following the history and physical examination one must also decide whether more than one symptom needs to generate a differential diagnosis. For example, the elderly patient who falls warrants two questions:

1. What were the injuries from the fall?
2. What caused the fall (arrhythmia, medications, dehydration, etc.)?

Each of these questions will generate its own diagnostic workup. Diagnostic tests will help answer some of the questions and decrease the likelihood of missing catastrophic diseases. The results of diagnostic testing will help refine the differential diagnosis.

ED management will focus on (1) treatment for specific diseases diagnosed, (2) therapy for symptoms (pain, etc), and (3) addressing problems elicited in the ED workup (abnormal cognitive status, polypharmacy, etc.).

EMERGENCY DEPARTMENT DISCHARGE PLANNING

The concept of discharge planning is standard for hospitalized patients and can be applied to elderly patients being discharged from the ED.[26,50-58] Different aspects of the ED workup, including cognitive status, functional status, and case finding, will all dictate the plan and need for follow-up care. Involvement of social service agencies, primary care physicians, and home health care may be an important part of the discharge plan (Figure 6–5). For example, in patients in whom there is concern about elder abuse but for whom there is no immediate danger, a follow-up visit by the social service agency and involvement with the primary care physician would be appropriate. A knowledge of hospital and community resources is important to ensure adequate discharge planning.

Ideally, discharge planning should begin at the time of admission to the ED as part of the initial assessment. Elder patients require a comprehensive discharge plan to improve health outcomes and, subsequently, prevent readmission to the ED. A comprehensive discharge plan integrates an assessment of the patient's highest level of function and independence with the needs of the patient and family or primary caregiver. The patient's home environment and social support systems also must be considered to anticipate physical, emotional, and geographic constraints.

Traditionally the emergency nurse is responsible for coordinating a multidisciplinary discharge plan for the elderly patient. Social work

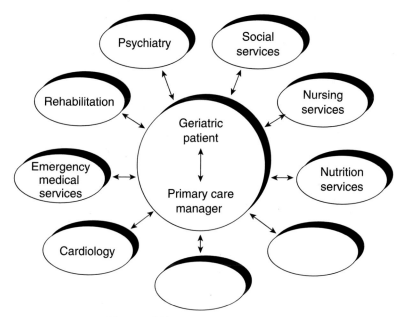

FIGURE 6-5   Geriatric care model.

services, whether assigned to the ED on a permanent or an on-call basis, are an additional resource.

A sample patient discharge form is provided in Figure 6–6. It includes elements elicited during the ED visit such as cognitive and functional assessments with plans for follow-up care. The discharge plan addresses psychosocial factors as well as the home environment. Functional assessment at discharge will include an evaluation of the patient's ability to perform necessary activities such as shopping and cooking. Does the patient have social resources to overcome problems?

A second test to be done at discharge is the "get up and go test." Does the patient have the ability to walk out of the room?[50] If not, resources must be available to support the patient in the home environment.

FAMILY AND CAREGIVER ASSESSMENT

Caregiving by family and friends can be provided at several levels, from emotional support to actual physical care and ADLs.[51] However, the caregiver also may be older and have multiple needs. Caregiving creates potential stressors at any level of support, and discharge assessment must include caregiver preparedness, needs of the caregiver, and signs of caregiver strain.

Assessment of caregiver preparedness is based on the subjective views of the caregiver combined with identified needs for support (e.g., supplies, transportation, mobility aids) in the caregiver role. Caregivers should feel capable of handling the physical and emotional needs of the patient while coping with the stress of providing care.[52]

Caregiver needs are specific to the situation and include awareness of the patient's capabilities and limitations or restrictions on discharge from the ED. Generally, caregivers require information, emotional support, financial assistance, and referral to community support services.

Emergency Department Discharge Plan

ED diagnosis _____

Treating physician _____   Nurse _____

Treatment plans

    Medications

    Follow-up

Special considerations

    Cognitive status

    Functional status

    ADLs (ambulation, transfer, toileting, bathing, dressing, feeding)

    IADLs (telephone, shopping, meals, laundry, medicines, finances)

    "Get up and go" test

    Social (caregiver)

    Case finding

    Other

FIGURE 6-6   Sample emergency department discharge form.

Signs of caregiver strain are often evidenced by dysfunctional behaviors that may not be readily identified in the ED setting. Caregiving that is motivated by a sense of guilt or financial necessity can create an unhealthy emotional situation for the elderly patient as well as for the caregiver. On the other hand, a history of open communication and problem solving without guilt or conflict indicates an effective elder–caregiver relationship.[53]

The caregiver's involvement must not detract from the autonomy and independence of the elderly patient. Many elderly patients fear a loss of control or being a burden to family. Health care providers should include the elderly patient in all aspects of discharge planning even when a primary caregiver is responsible for the patient.

Confidentiality can be an issue for those patients who live independently yet need assistance from a caregiver on discharge from the ED. ED personnel should receive permission from the patient before discussing details of his or her condition and plan of care with a family member or primary caregiver.

A history of abuse or neglect by any caregiver suggests a potential for current risk to the patient and should be taken into consideration in discharge planning. A social services referral is indicated in these cases or when there are signs of caregiver strain (Table 6-3).

HOME ENVIRONMENT ASSESSMENT

The elderly patient's daily routine and patterns of living are part of the home environment assessment (Table 6-4). The patient's environment may need temporary modifications to accommodate limited mobility. The elderly patient must be able to have basic needs met safely in the home environment. Ability to manage self-care activities such as eating,

Table 6–3 **Signs of Caregiver Strain**

Does the caregiver express feelings:
   of difficulty handling the role?
   of financial problems?
   of anger or resentment toward the patient?
   of guilt about the patient's condition?

Is the caregiver:
   complaining about the patient?
   arguing with the patient?
   blaming the patient?
   focusing conversation on self rather than the patient?

Does the caregiver appear tired or depressed?

Is the caregiver demanding that the patient be admitted when discharge is
   warranted?

Table 6–4 **Environmental Factors to Assess Before Discharge**

Will the patient have difficulty:
   Getting into the home? Are there stairs or ramp access to the home?
   Getting around the home? Are there stairs? Are the bathroom, bedroom,
     and kitchen on the same level?
   Preparing food? Are supplies and appliances in easy reach?
   Using bathroom facilities? Are there safety features, such as raised toilet
     seat and grab bars, in use?
   Using the telephone? Is there one in the home? Is it easy to reach and
     dial?

Does the patient have concerns about:
   Finances? Are there prescriptions to get filled? Are there medical supplies
     needed for home?
   Follow-up? Is there a physician appointment needed? Is there
     transportation to the office or clinic?
   Pet care? Is there one in the home? How much care does it need?

Safety is important when physical or cognitive function is impaired.

bathing, dressing, and toileting is most important for the patient's positive self-image. Safety issues need to be taken into consideration, especially when the elderly patient is not at his or her prior level of physical or cognitive function because of the emergency illness or injury.

Financial considerations need to be addressed as part of the patient's environment. The patient's financial status affects the practicality of both the discharge plan and expectations for follow-up care. Elderly patients on fixed incomes or with limited resources may not be able to afford discharge plans that include costly prescriptions and transportation to outpatient testing or physician office visits.

PATIENT AND FAMILY OR CAREGIVER TEACHING

Patient and family interaction and teaching are a focal part of the discharge planning procedure. Special considerations must be addressed in the process of patient teaching. Slower mental functions with short-term memory loss, diminished hearing and vision, and decreased physical capacities can affect the elderly patient's ability to absorb the necessary data.[54] The patient must be given enough information with which to make intelligent, informed choices while being allowed to maintain an appropriate level of autonomy and independence in self-care. This increases positive outcomes by promoting patient compliance with discharge planning goals and activities.

Most people experience sensory alterations with advancing age. Many aging individuals with sensory impairment ignore or attempt to hide the deficits and may be mistakenly considered confused or inattentive. ED personnel can use simple techniques in communicating with these elderly patients.[54]

Hearing-impaired patients should be spoken to slowly in even, low tones with short, simple sentences. If the patient has a "good" ear, that side should be addressed when speaking to the patient. Some hearing-impaired persons are able to read lips, so the discharge planner should face the patient and maintain direct eye contact during discussion of any instructions. Health care providers should wait for the patient to acknowledge each instruction before proceeding to the next topic. Whenever possible, the area used for discharge teaching should be situated away from the main treatment room and free from distracting noises.

Visually impaired patients need written instructions in large, bold print on matte-finish paper. If special large-print discharge forms are not available, magnifying hand lenses should be considered for use in the ED. Discharge teaching should take place in a well-lighted area without shadows or glare. Written and other visual diagrams should be held at eye level. Discharge personnel should encourage the patient who wears corrective lenses to use them when reviewing materials.

Patients with impaired cognition may not have the attention span and short-term memory ability to recall simple instructions in the discharge planning process. In these cases a caregiver must be involved in discharge planning and participate in instruction to help ensure a positive outcome for the patient.

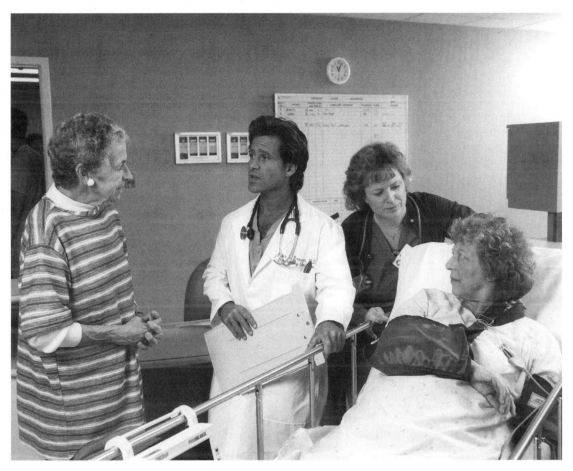

Patients who come in after a fall may be treated appropriately for their injury. However, a more comprehensive assessment and management of the patient through a fall-prevention program can be done using a geriatric assessment unit.

ROLES OF HEALTH CARE PROFESSIONALS

The role that each member of the health care team plays will be determined by resources in individual hospitals and communities. It is essential, however, that emergency health care professionals understand the training, function, and language of colleagues who interact with the elderly. For example, the problem of elder abuse is underrecognized by emergency health care professionals in most communities. Detection of elder abuse, however, is only a small part of the solution.[19] The issue of elder abuse can be addressed only by a comprehensive plan involving multidisciplinary teams. Each member of the team must understand his or her own role and contribution.[2,19]

Similarly in the emergency care model for elderly patients, it is essential that emergency health care workers develop collaborative relationships with geriatricians, primary care physicians who deal with the elderly, and with social service agencies. Emergency physicians will be directly responsible for the emergency medical care of elderly patients presenting to hospital emergency departments. Pre-hospital care providers including paramedics and basic emergency medical technicians need to work with their base station medical director to develop protocols to meet the needs of geriatric patients. Emergency nurses will be responsible for triaging patients, discharging patients, and coordinating ED discharge care. Emergency nurses also can perform many of the standardized tests evaluating cognitive status, functional status, and at-risk case finding. Nurses can give valuable insight into the relationship of caregivers to the patient and bridge the care to outside social service and nursing agencies, if necessary. Social services are provided in most hospital emergency departments, although consultation may not be available 24 hours per day at all hospitals. Social service workers will be able to work with emergency health care professionals in implementing discharge planning and involvement of home-visit follow-up to ensure that the patient is capable of functioning in the community. Geriatric physicians will be key resources in designing protocols for the ED evaluation of specific complaints (elder abuse, fall assessment, etc.) as well as for ensuring appropriate follow-up. Specific geriatric consultations in the ED may be useful in managing difficult cases.

Assessment by multidisciplinary geriatric clinical teams has been shown to be efficacious in preventing morbidity and decreasing mortality in many groups of geriatric patients, especially frail elderly persons who do not live in long-term care facilities. For example, patients who come in after a fall may be treated appropriately for their injury. However, a more comprehensive assessment and management of the patient through a fall-prevention program can be done using a geriatric assessment unit. The use of standardized assessment criteria for cognitive and functional assessments in the ED will provide a consistent baseline for comprehensive evaluation and management by other health care professionals who care for the patient.[59,60]

Finally, since most patients will require the use of emergency care systems, emergency health care providers must be considered part of the multidisciplinary planning and approach to the patient. Geriatricians and primary care managers need to understand the principles, environment, and role of emergency health care professionals in the care of the elderly.

NURSING HOME TRANSFER PROCESS

The transfer of patients from a long-term care facility to an ED for evaluation of a specific problem can be done efficiently and professionally with good communication between facilities as to what is needed. More commonly, however, there is a breakdown in communication as to the history, baseline cognitive and functional status, presence of advance directives, and extent of workup required. Many of the problems are the result of differences in mind-sets and models of care used in emergency medicine and long-term care facilities. The situation could be greatly improved by a mechanism providing necessary information to the ED on transfer of the patient.[61,62] Similarly, information should be provided to the long-term care facility on transfer of the patient back to the nursing home. Once again, this requires close coordination among ED personnel, geriatricians, and the staff of long-term care facilities. Standardized tests for cognitive and functional status will also help with information transfer. Figure 6–7 gives a transfer form that can be adapted for universal use in local communities.[62]

Nursing Home to Hospital Transfer Form

Name _____ Gender _____ DOB _____

Transferring facility _____ Religion _____

Address _____ Phone _____

Dates of stay _____

SS# _____ Medicare # _____ Insurance # _____

Responsible relative/guardian _____

Address _____ Phone _____

Physician _____ Phone _____ Nurse _____ Phone _____

Other physician _____

Date/time of transfer _____ Recent vital signs _____

Reason for transfer _____

Physician orders on transfer _____

Hospitals/facilities discharged within 60 days _____

Advance directives _____

Critical care plan _____

Allergies _____ Immunizations _____

Medications _____

Other treatments (PT, resp, diet, etc.) _____

Past medical history _____

Primary diagnosis _____

Secondary diagnosis _____

Surgical history _____

Tobacco/alcohol _____

BASELINE INFORMATION

Ambulation _____

Activities of Daily Living

Bathing _____   Transfer _____

Dressing _____   Continence _____

Toileting _____   Feeding _____

Disabilities

Amputation _____   Contracture _____

Paralysis _____   Decubitus ulcer _____

Impairments

Speech _____   Vision _____

Hearing _____   Sensation _____

Usual Mental Status

Alert _____   Oriented _____   Wanders _____

Combative _____   Confused _____   Withdrawn _____

Other _____

Mini-mental status _____

Appliances/supports (e.g., wheelchair, cane, walker, prosthesis) _____

Other information to emergency providers _____

FIGURE 6-7   Transfer form, nursing home to hospital.

DISCHARGE AND RETURN TO THE NURSING HOME

In the event that a nursing home resident is discharged for return to the long-term care facility after emergency treatment and evaluation, interfacility communication is essential. The discharge instructions should be documented along with a summary of the emergency care given. A verbal report by telephone should be given nurse to nurse. Discharge instructions should be reviewed with the patient at his or her level of comprehension and with next of kin if available. A copy of the discharge instructions should accompany the patient back to the nursing home.

The emergency physician should contact the primary care physician to review the discharge plan. Prescriptions for medication, recommendations for specific treatments, or any changes in diet and activity must be ordered by the patient's primary care physician after return to the facility.

ED staff need to be aware that most long-term care facilities must process requests for medications and other supplies from providers after verifying the orders from the primary care physician. The turnaround time may be several hours in some cases, depending on the time of day. It may be necessary to send medication or supplies with the resident to cover the transition period when such items are not immediately available in the long-term care facility.

FOLLOW-UP PROTOCOL

A system of postdischarge follow-up for elderly patients should be considered in the basic protocol for discharge planning. Telephone "call backs" to elderly patients or caregivers provide additional information or referral to community resources and may decrease unnecessary return visits to the ED. These also can be used as mechanisms with which an ED can evaluate discharge planning effectiveness for high-risk elderly persons. High-risk factors that may prompt telephone follow-up include the following:

- Musculoskeletal injury limiting mobility
- Pain medication that may decrease responsiveness level
- Upper respiratory infection
- Gastrointestinal infection
- Genitourinary infection
- Mental health disorder

Questions to ask the patient or caregiver during telephone follow-up may include the following:

- Have you been able to have your prescriptions filled?
- Do you have any questions about how to take your medication?
- Do you have all of the supplies you need to complete _____? (as appropriate)
- Who is helping you with your meals?
- How will you get to _____ for your follow-up appointment? (as appropriate)
- How have you changed your daily routine or home setting because of your illness or injury?

Telephone follow-up may occur within 24 hours for high-risk elderly patients, even if they are transferring back to a nursing home facility. The telephone call provides the ED staff with data that can be used in quality improvement audits, in developing or revising discharge protocols, and in promoting the public relations mission of the hospital.

Discharge planning for the elderly patient requires more time and assessment data than for a younger patient. Data collection begins in triage when information about transportation, treatment before arrival, current medications, and prior medical history is obtained. While interacting with the patient, the health care provider is assessing the patient's sensory and cognitive abilities. If a caregiver accompanies the patient, additional information can be elicited concerning caregiving responsibilities and functional abilities of the patient.

Throughout the ED visit, additional data are integrated. By the time of discharge, the health care provider should have an appreciation of what impact this illness or injury may have on the patient or family resources. Social service and community resource agency referrals should be contacted if elder neglect or abuse is suspected, and the patient should not be discharged to the same home situation.

A list of community resources relating to elderly care services should be developed for the ED's geographic locale. The hospital's social services department can be instrumental in the development of a thorough listing of available resources. Such a listing saves time for ED personnel and should be posted near all telephones in the department.

Numerous services for the elderly are available through local departments on aging. The National Eldercare Locator Service (1-800-677-1116) will identify the local aging office. Some typical community services are home health care, homemaker, friendly visitor, meals on wheels, telephone reassurance, personal emergency response system, dental services, nutrition site, and senior center. Support groups and respite care for caregivers also may be available.

SUMMARY

The elderly have a unique physiology, pattern of disease presentation, and psychosocial needs. Optimal care in EDs will require a new model of care. The new model will take into account the elderly patient's functional, cognitive, emotional, and social status when evaluating the patient's complaint as well as in discharge planning. Principles of geriatric emergency medicine have been defined. Issues such as the complexity of the chief complaint, atypical disease presentation, confounding effects of comorbid diseases, polypharmacy, cognitive impairment, altered normal values in some diagnostic tests, decreased functional reserve, psychosocial support, and functional status will all influence ED care.

SUMMARY POINTS

- There is a great deal of heterogeneity among the elderly; therefore physiologic rather than biologic age should guide use of the geriatric emergency care model.

- The high-stress environment of most EDs makes many patients very uncomfortable; the elderly are generally frightened by and do not cope well with the rapid pace of most EDs. Interpersonal interactions with emergency health care personnel as well as simple physical changes in the environment can help reduce stress and provide a more therapeutic environment.
- Communication barriers can be addressed through the use of interpersonal skills and respect.
- Pre-hospital care professionals can provide an important assessment of the elderly patient's home environment.
- The elderly patient should have a formal evaluation of cognitive status.
- An assessment of the elderly patient's functional status will give context to historical information.
- The differential diagnosis should assess whether the chief complaint represents, for example, myocardial ischemia, acute cerebrovascular disease, an occult infectious process, or an acute abdominal condition.
- Discharge planning for elderly patient's can be formally done with an evaluation of their functional status in the context of the home environment.
- Health care for elderly patients is often optimized through the use of multidisciplinary teams coordinated by a primary care physician.
- Transfer of patients from the nursing home to the ED can be greatly facilitated through the use of a universal transfer form communicating the patient's baseline status and the extent of ED workup needed.

CHAPTER AUTHORS

Arthur B. Sanders, MD, FACEP, FACP
Donald B. Witzke, PhD
Jeffrey S. Jones, MD
Kathleen Richmond, RN, BS
Pamela Kidd, RN, PhD, CEN

REFERENCES

1. Hamilton GC. Orientation to emergency medicine. In: Hamilton GC, Sanders AB, Strange GR, Trott AT, Eds. *Emergency medicine: an approach to clinical problem solving.* Philadelphia, PA: WB Saunders; 1991:1–18.
2. Sanders AB. Emergency care. In: Schrier RW, Jahnigan D, eds. *Geriatric medicine.* 3rd ed. Cambridge, MA: Blackwell Scientific Publications; 1995. In press.
3. Horattas MC, Guyton DP, Wu D. A reappraisal of appendicitis in the elderly. *Am J Surg.* 1990;160:291–293.
4. Freund HR, Rubinstein E. Appendicitis in the aged: is it really different? *Am Surg.* 1984;50:573–576.
5. Bayer AJ, Chadha JS, Farag RR, et al. Changing presentation of myocardial infarction with increasing old age. *J Am Geriatr Soc.* 1986;34:263–266.
6. Cocchi A, Franceschini G, Incalzi RA, et al. Clinico-pathological correlations in the diagnosis of acute myocardial infarction in the elderly. *Age Ageing.* 1988;17:87–93.
7. Beck JC, Ed. *Geriatric review syllabus: a core curriculum in geriatric medicine.* New York, NY: American Geriatrics Society, 1991.

8. Eliastam M. Elderly patients in the emergency department. *Ann Emerg Med.* 1989;18:1222–1229.

9. American Medical Association Council on Scientific Affairs. American Medical Association white paper on elderly health. *Arch Intern Med.* 1990;150:2459–2472.

10. Cassel CK, Riesenberg DE, Sorensen LB, et al. *Geriatric medicine.* New York, NY: Springer-Verlag; 1990.

11. Singal BM, Hedges JR, Rousseau EW, et al. Geriatric patient emergency visits: part I. Comparison of visits by geriatric and younger patients. *Ann Emerg Med.* 1992;21:802–807.

12. Singal BM, Hedges JR, Rousseau EW, et al. Geriatric emergency visits: part II. Perceptions of visits by geriatric and younger patients. *Ann Emerg Med.* 1992;21:808–813.

13. Gerson LW, Counsell SR, Fontanarosa PB, Smucker WD. Case finding for cognitive impairment in elderly emergency department patients. *Ann Emerg Med.* 1994;23:813–817.

14. Lewis LM, Miller DK, Morley JE, et al. Unrecognized delirium in ED geriatric patients *Am J Emerg Med.* 1995;13:142–145.

15. Gerson LW, Rousseau E, Hogan T, Bernstein E, Kalbfleisch N. A multi-center study of case findings in elderly emergency department patients. *Acad Emerg Med.* 1994;1:A16.

16. Fulop G, Reinhardt J, Strain JJ, et al. Identification of alcoholism and depression in a geriatric medicine outpatient clinic. *J Am Geriatr Soc.* 1993;41:737–741.

17. Koenig HG, Meador KG, Cohen, et al. Depression in elderly hospitalized patients with medical illness. *Arch Intern Med.* 1989;148:1929–1936.

18. Gerson LW, Schelble DT, Wilson JE. Using paramedics to identify at-risk elderly. *Ann Emerg Med.* 1992;21:688–691.

19. Jones J, Dougherty J, Schelble D. Emergency department protocol for the diagnosis and evaluation of geriatric abuse. *Ann Emerg Med.* 1988;17:1006–1015.

20. Rousseau EW, Sanders AB, Perkins T. Attitudes of emergency health care professionals towards elderly patients. *Acad Emerg Med.* 1994;1:A16.

21. Katch MP. A negentropic view of the aged. *J Gerontol Nurs.* 1983;9:656–660.

22. Topol EJ, Califf RM. Thrombolytic therapy for elderly patients. *N Engl J Med.* 1992;327:45–47.

23. Krumholz HM, Pasternak RC, Weinstein MC, Friesingen GC, Ridken PM, Tosteson AN, Goldman L. Cost effectiveness of thrombolytic therapy with streptokinase in elderly patients with suspected acute myocardial infarction. *N Engl J Med.* 1992;327:7–13.

24. Doorey AJ, Michelson EL, Topol EJ. Thrombolytic therapy of acute myocardial infarction. *JAMA.* 1992;268:3108–3114.

25. Baraff LJ, Bernstein E, Bradley K, et al. Perceptions of emergency care by the elderly: results of multicenter focus group interviews. *Ann Emerg Med.* 1992;21:814–818.

26. Sanders AB. Care of the elderly in emergency departments: conclusions and recommendations. *Ann Emerg Med.* 1992;21:830–834.

27. McNamara RM, Rousseau E, Sanders AB. Geriatric emergency medicine: a survey of practicing emergency physicians. *Ann Emerg Med.* 1992;21:796–801.

28. Strange GR, Chen EH, Sanders AB. The use of emergency departments by elderly patients: projections from a multicenter data base. *Ann Emerg Med.* 1992;21:819–824.

29. Marston WA, Ahlquist R, Johnson G Jr, et al. Misdiagnosis of ruptured abdominal aortic aneurysms. *J Vasc Surg.* 1992;16:17–22.

30. Phillips SL, Burns GP. Acute abdominal disease in the aged. *Med Clin North Am.* 1988;72:1213–1224.

31. Balsano N, Cayten CG. Surgical emergencies of the abdomen. *Emerg Med Clin North Am.* 1990;8:399–410.

32. Finelli FC, Jonsson J, Champion HR, Morelli S, Fouty WJ. A case control study for major trauma in geriatric patients. *J Trauma.* 1989;29: 541–547.

33. Scalea TM, Simon HM, Duncan AO, Atweh NA, Sclafani SJ, Phillips TF, Shaftan GW. Geriatric blunt multiple trauma: Improved survival with early invasive monitoring. *J Trauma.* 1990;30:129–136.

34. Pellicane JV, Byrne K, DeMaria EJ. Preventable complications and death from trauma victims. *J Trauma.* 1992;33:440–444.

35. Keating HJ III, Klimek JJ, Levine DS, et al. Effect of aging on the clinical significance of fever in ambulatory adult patients. *J Am Geriatr Soc.* 1984;32:282–287.

36. Schoenberger JA. Epidemiology of systolic and diastolic systemic blood pressure elevation in the elderly. *Am J Cardiol.* 1986;57:45C–52C.

37. Starer PJ, Libow LS. History and physical examination. In: Abrams WB, Berkow R, Eds. *The Merck manual of geriatrics.* Rahway, NJ: Merck & Co; 1990:153–169.

38. Cassel CK, Walsh JR, Shepard M, et al. Clinical evaluation of the patient. In: Cassell CK, Riesenberg DE, Sorensen LB, et al., Eds. *Geriatric medicine.* 2nd ed. New York, NY: Springer-Verlag; 1990:102–110.

39. Jones J, Srodulski Z. The aging electrocardiogram. *Am J Emerg Med.* 1990;8:240–245.

40. Eddy DM. The value of screening for glaucoma with tonometry. *Surv Ophthalmol.* 1983;28:194–199.

41. Rybolt AH, Waterburgh L. Breast cancer in older women: trends in diagnosis. *Geriatrics.* 1989;44:69–82.

42. Connolly MJ, Crowley JJ, Vestal RE. Clinical significance of bronchoconstriction provoked by metacholine in elderly asthmatic and normal subjects as measured on a simple awareness scale. *Thorax.* 1992;47:410–413.

43. Cannon LA. Valvular cardiac emergencies. In: Bosker G, Schwartz GR, Jones JS, et al., Eds. *Geriatric emergency medicine.* St Louis, MO: Mosby–Year Book; 1990:188–201.

44. Leiblum S, Bachmann G, Kemmann E, et al. Vaginal atrophy in the postmenopausal woman. *JAMA.* 1983;249:2195–2198.

45. Harwood-Nuss AL, Benrubi GI, Nuss RC. Management of gynecologic oncology emergencies. *Emerg Med Clin North Am.* 1987;5577–5599.

46. Ranney B. Enterocele, vaginal prolapse, pelvic hernia: recognition and treatment. *Am J Obstet Gynecol.* 1981;140:53–61.

47. Zeitlin MP, Lebherz TB. Pessaries in the geriatric patient. *J Am Geriatr Soc.* 1992;40:635–639.

48. Basavaraju NG. Primitive reflexes and perceptual sensory tests in the elderly: their usefulness in dementia. *J Chronic Dis.* 1981;34:367–370.

49. Kay AD, Tideiksaar R. Falls and gait disorders. In: Abrams WB, Berkow R, Eds. *The Merck manual of geriatrics.* Rahway, NJ: Merck & Co; 1990:52–68.

50. Mathias S, Nayak US, Issacs B. Balance in elderly patients: the get up and go test. *Arch Phys Med Rehabil.* 1986;67:387–389.

51. Phillips L. Social support of the older client. In: Chenitz W, Stone J, Salisbury S, Eds. *Clinical gerontological nursing: a guide to advanced practice.* Philadelphia, PA: WB Saunders; 1991:535–545.

52. Archbold P, Stewart B, Greenlick M, Harvath T. The clinical assessment of mutuality and preparedness in family caregivers to older frail people. In: Funk S, Tornquist E, Champagne M, Wiese R, Eds. *Key aspects of elder care.* New York, NY: Springer Publishing; 1992:328–339.

53. Henderson M, McConnell E. Gerontological care in community care settings. In: Matteson M, McConnell E, Eds. *Gerontological nursing: concepts*

and practice. Philadelphia, PA: WB Saunders; 1988:763–791.

54. Needham J. *Gerontological nursing: a restorative approach.* Albany, NY: Delmar Publishers; 1993.

55. Naylor M. The implications of discharge planning for hospitalized elders. In: Fulmer T, Walker M, Eds. *Critical care nursing of the elderly.* New York, NY: Springer Publishing; 1992:331–347.

56. Eagle D, Rideout E, Price P, McCann C, Wonnacott E. Misuse of the emergency department by the elderly population: myth or reality? *J Emerg Nurs.* 1993;19(3):212–218.

57. Heckheimer E. *Health promotion of the elderly in the community.* Philadelphia, PA: WB Saunders; 1989.

58. Zeman S. Nurses and family systems. In: Corr D, Corr C, Eds. *Nursing care in an aging society.* New York, NY: Springer; 1990:301–319.

59. Tinetti ME, Speechley M, Ginter SF. Risk factors for falls among elderly persons living in the community. *N Engl J Med.* 1988;319:1701–1707.

60. Rubenstein LZ, Robbins AS, Josephson KB, Schulman BL, Osterweil D. The value of assessing falls in an elderly population—a randomized clinical trial. *Ann Intern Med.* 1990;113:308–316.

61. Rubenstein LZ, Ouslander JG, Wieland D. Dynamics and clinical implications of the nursing home-hospital interface. *Clin Geriatr Med.* 1988;4:471–491.

62. Jones JS, Dwyer P, Firman R, Dougherty J, White LJ. Patient transfer from nursing home to emergency department: outcome and policy implications. *Acad Emerg Med.* 1994;1:A16.

Specific Instruments for the ED Assessment

7 *Functional Assessment, Mental Status and Case Finding*

LEARNING OBJECTIVES

1. Demonstrate the ability to perform a delirium and cognitive status examination and interpret the results in the ED environment.
2. Define the hierarchy of functional status and explain how changes in functional status may lead to unusual presentations of disease.
3. Recognize that the evaluation of elderly persons must adopt a comprehensive approach, assessing physical, mental, and social function and the patient's environment, including social support system.
4. Demonstrate an ability to elicit information for functional assessment, activities of daily living (ADLs), and instrumental activities of daily living (IADLs), and apply results to appropriate disposition and discharge planning.
5. Understand the importance of and demonstrate case findings for the following conditions:
   a. Depression and risk of suicide
   b. Alcohol and other drug abuse (including cigarette smoking)
   c. Malnutrition
   d. Incontinence

The emergency care model for elderly patients emphasizes the importance of a comprehensive assessment. This includes assessment of cognitive as well as functional status, with case finding as indicated in selected patients. The National Institutes of Health (NIH) Consensus Development Conference Statement on Geriatric Assessment of 1987 recommends that assessment target those persons who are most likely to benefit, who have acute changes in health status, or who are in the transitional period from home to nursing home or hospital to home, and who are frail but not terminally ill. In addition, the statement emphasizes the need to link the detection of disabilities with management, referral, and close follow-up of any positive findings.[1] This chapter addresses the ED assessment of mental status, functional status, social, environmental, and economic supports, depression, alcohol abuse, malnutrition, and incontinence (Figure 7–1). It also describes and recommends a number of highly sensitive, specific, reliable and validated assessment instruments that are appropriate for use in the ED.

ED Assessment of Elderly Persons

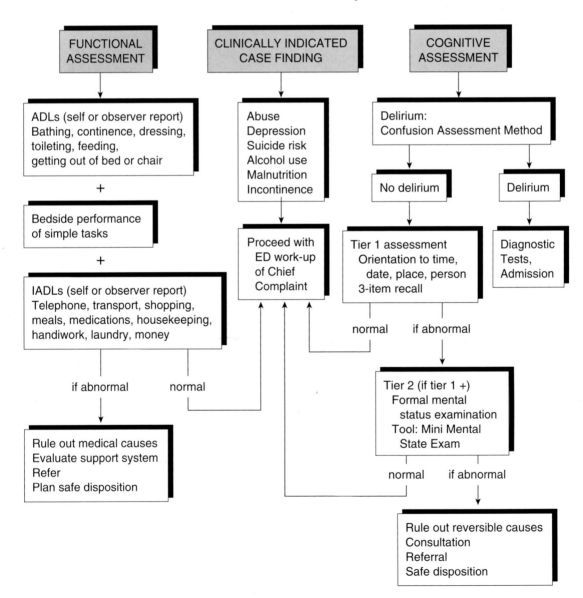

FIGURE 7-1   Sample algorithm for a comprehensive ED assessment of elderly patients.

ASSESSMENT OF MENTAL STATUS

Cognitive status in elderly patients (patients 70 years or older or patients 60 years or older who are frail) should be evaluated for the following reasons:

1. There is a high incidence of impaired cognition in patients older than 69 years; among 85-year-olds, the fastest growing geriatric age group, the rate of dementia is 50%.
2. Abnormalities are often subtle and easily missed unless a formal mental status evaluation is undertaken.
3. Reliability of the history depends on normal cognitive function.
4. An acute confusional state or subtle change in mental status may be the only indicator of a serious disease process such as an acute myocardial infarction (MI), congestive heart failure (CHF), sepsis, metabolic or electrolyte abnormalities, hypothermia, or hypoxia.
5. Eleven percent of cognitive impairment is thought to be reversible, and even patients with progressive, irreversible dementia benefit from early detection, support services, and monitoring.[2]
6. The mental status evaluation provides information needed for clinical practice, including assessment of patient compliance, and decisions about disposition.[3]

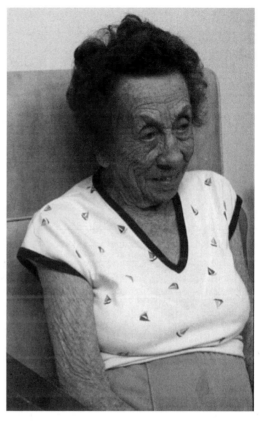

Delirium is often missed in the ED setting, or is misdiagnosed as depression, dementia, or aging.

Altered mental status is a challenge for the clinician because of the difficulty in distinguishing acute confusional states (delirium) from chronic cognitive conditions (dementia). Acute conditions also may be complicated by underlying chronic conditions. Screening every patient 70 years of age and older for delirium is recommended, because an acceptable assessment of cognitive function such as orientation and memory cannot be obtained in the presence of delirium. Also, signs of delirium can be subtle and easily missed without a systematic assessment. Screening instruments can increase accuracy and comprehensiveness and save time. Acute confusional states (delirium) must be identified promptly in order to evaluate differential diagnoses, address causes, and admit patients to the appropriate hospital setting.

And yet, delirium is often missed in the ED setting, or is misdiagnosed as depression, dementia, or aging. If the underlying cause is not addressed in the early stage, the prognosis is considerably worse. Approximately 10% of elderly ED patients meet the criteria for a diagnosis of delirium when formally tested. In recent studies, this abnormality was not recognized by ED providers in most patients.[4,5] Among elderly hospitalized patients, the incidence of confusional states is 25-60%. Hospital stays are longer, and the patient is less likely to be discharged home. The case fatality rate is between 25% and 33%.[6]

ASSESSMENT OF DELIRIUM (ACUTE CONFUSIONAL STATE)

The Confusion Assessment Method (CAM) is recommended as a brief, sensitive, specific, reliable and easy-to-use instrument for differentiating delirium from dementia[6] (Figure 7–2). The four criteria used to make the diagnosis of acute confusional states are as follows:

1. Acute onset or fluctuating course
2. Inattention
3. Disorganized thinking
4. Altered level of consciousness

Confusion Assessment Method (CAM) Worksheet

I. ACUTE ONSET OR FLUCTUATING COURSE

BOX 1

Is there evidence of an acute change in mental status from the patient's baseline?

or

Did the (abnormal) behavior fluctuate during the day (i.e., tend to come and go or increase and decrease in severity)?   No   Yes

II. INATTENTION

Did the patient have difficulty focusing attention (e.g., being easily distractible or having difficulty keeping track of what was being said)?   No   Yes

III. DISORGANIZED THINKING

Was the patient's thinking disorganized or incoherent (e.g., rambling or irrelevant conversation, unclear or illogical flow of ideas, or unpredictable switching from subject to subject)?   No   Yes

BOX 2

IV. ALTERED LEVEL OF CONSCIOUSNESS

Overall, how would you rate the patient's level of consciousness?

—Alert (normal)

—Vigilant (hyperalert)
—Lethargic (drowsy, easily aroused)
—Stupor (difficult to arouse)
—Coma (unarousable)

Do any checks appear in this box?   No   Yes

FIGURE 7-2   The diagnosis of delirium is suggested with the presence of the first two criteria and either the third or fourth criteria. Reproduced with permission from Inouye SK, van Dyck CH, Alessi CA, et al. Clarifying confusion: the confusion assessment method—a new method for detection of delirium. *Ann Intern Med* 1990;113:941–948.

Making an assessment regarding many of the key criteria of the CAM scale may involve observation of th the patient over time. An accurate and consistent history from the patient with confirmation from the family, caregiver and the medical record is key. Observation of patient behavior over time during the prehospital and emergency department stay is important in assessing a fluctuating course. It may be useful to supplement these observations with several structured questions, such as the following:

> Orientation to person, place, day, date, time
> Three-item recall
> State the days of the week backward
> State the months of the year backward

Using the CAM Worksheet, the key criteria can be assessed as follows:

- Acute onset - history
- Fluctuating course - history
  > ED observation
- Inattention - history
  > ED observation
  > structured questions
- Disorganized thinking - history
  > ED observation
  > structured questions
- Altered level of conciousness - history
  > ED observation

There is some variation with the use of the CAM Scale in emergency department settings. Some researchers are evaluating modifications of the CAM Scale with the addition of classifications for "probable" and "possible" delirium for patients who meet some but not all criteria.[5] Further research in this area will continue because of the importance of recognizing delirium.

When the CAM Scale was applied by trained observers in both inpatient and clinic settings, its sensitivity (detection of disease when present) was greater than 91%. The specificity (negative in health) is the test's ability to rule out disease and has been found to be above 90%. The positive predictive accuracy, the ability to identify a positive patient in the entire population sampled, was greater than 91%.[6]

ASSESSMENT OF DEMENTIA (CHRONIC CONFUSIONAL STATE)

If the patient fails to meet the criteria for delirium, a cognitive assessment is performed using a two-tier approach. In *tier one*, the patient is assessed for orientation to time/date or year, place, and person. This is followed by testing the patient's ability to recall three items after a 1-minute interval. Short-term memory is a sensitive test of cognitive impairment.[7] The instructions are as follows:

1. The patient is told by the ED provider, "I shall say three words for you to remember. Repeat them after I have said all three words ... shirt ... brown ... honesty."
2. After 1 minute the patient is asked, "What are the three words that I asked you to remember?"

3. For each word failed, a cue is provided, for example, "something to wear." If there is no recall, three choices are offered for each word, such as "shoes, pants, and shirt."[8]
4. If the patient fails to recall the three items, even after prompting, a formal mental status examination should be performed (*tier two*).

A number of screening tests are available, including Folstein's Mini-Mental State Examination (MMSE),[9] Blessed's BIMC and BOMC,[10,11] Pfeiffer's Short MSE,[12] and Jacobs.[13] The MMSE, however, is the most widely used and is available in many languages, although these versions have not all been validated (Figure 7–3). It can be administered in less than 5 minutes. The MMSE has been evaluated the most extensively in the literature.[14] It has been used as a brief screen for cognitive problems with different examiners in both community settings and institutions, as well as in clinical trials in order to observe changes in mental status over time. This instrument is recommended by the National Institute of Neurological and Communicative Disorders and Stroke and the Alzheimer's Disease and Related Disorders Association (NINCDS-ADRDA).[15]

The MMSE has a high level of sensitivity for moderate to severe deficits and a satisfactory reliability and construct validity compared to the DSM-III-R, clinical diagnosis, and NINCDS-ADRDA criteria. At a cutoff of 23/30 or less, sensitivity and specificity are 87% and 82% respectively, in hospitalized patients.[16] A score of 18/30 to 23/30 indicates mild impairment, and 0-17 indicates moderate to severe impairment. Crum et al, administered the MMSE to 18,000 adults to develop reference standards by age and educational level. Clinicians can compare their patients to the reference age and education groups.[17]

The MMSE screening instrument is recognized to be affected by age, education level, culture, and race *but not by gender.* Caution should be exercised in interpreting scores in the mild impairment range. This is especially true for patients who are 85 years old or older, who have very little education, and who score between 20 and 24. If the patient is highly educated then more sensitive neuropsychiatric testing may be required. Another caveat is that if a family member or caregiver says there is a problem despite scores in the normal range, ED personnel need to *listen* and pursue the workup with a more formal evaluation.

Some of the chronic but possibly reversible causes of altered mental status include depression, medication side effects, chronic subdural hematoma, hypothyroid disease, B_{12} and thiamine deficiency, and malnutrition. Any findings of chronic dementia warrant a search for reversible causes and a plan for further cognitive assessments to rule out Alzheimer's disease, multi-infarct dementia, Huntington's chorea, or other currently irreversible and progressive dementias. Appropriate consultation, referrals, and a safe discharge plan should be made before the patient leaves the ED.

FUNCTIONAL ASSESSMENT

Assessment of the elderly patient's activities of daily living (ADL) can provide subtle indicators of illness as well as important data for discharge decision making. ADLs measure the abilities needed for independent self-maintenance and are more important than biologic age in predicting morbidity and mortality. As in mental status changes, a

Mini-Mental State Exam (MMSE)

Add points for each correct response.   Score   Points

Orientation

		Score	Points
1. What is the:	Year?	____	1
	Season?	____	1
	Date?	____	1
	Day?	____	1
	Month?	____	1
2. Where are we?	State?	____	1
	County?	____	1
	Town or city?	____	1
	Hospital?	____	1
	Floor?	____	1

Registration

3. Name three objects, taking one second to say each. Then ask the   ____   3
   patient to repeat all three after you have said them.

   Give one point for each correct answer. Repeat the answers until
   patient learns all three.

Attention and calculation

4. Serial sevens. Give one point for each correct answer. Stop after five   ____   5
   answers. Alternate: Spell WORLD backwards.

Recall

5. Ask for names of three objects learned in question 3. Give one point   ____   3
   for each correct answer.

Language

6. Point to a pencil and a watch. Have the patient name them as you   ____   2
   point.
7. Have the patient repeat "No ifs, ands, or buts."   ____   1
8. Have the patient follow a three-stage command: "Take a paper in your   ____   3
   right hand. Fold the paper in half. Put the paper on the floor."
9. Have the patient read and obey the following: 'CLOSE YOUR EYES."   ____   1
   (Write it in large letters.)
10. Have the patient write a sentence of his or her choice. (The sentence   ____   1
    should contain a subject and an object and should make sense. Ignore
    spelling errors when scoring.)
11. Have the patient copy the design. (Give one point if all sides and   ____   1
    angles are preserved and if the intersecting sides form
    a quadrangle.)

____ = Total   30

In validation studies using a cutoff score of 23 or below, the MMSE has a sensitivity of 87%, a specificity of 82%, a false-positive ratio of 39.4%, and a false-negative ratio of 4.7%. These ratios refer to the MMSE's capacity to accurately distinguish patients with clinically diagnosed dementia or delirium from patients without these syndromes.

FIGURE 7-3   Mini-Mental State Examination (MMSE). Courtesy Marshall Folstein, MD. Reprinted with permission from Folstein MF, Folstein S, McHugh PR. Mini-Mental State: a practical method for grading the cognitive state of patients for the clinician. *J Psych Res.* 1975;12:189–198. Elsevier Science Ltd., Pergamon Imprint, Oxford, England.

For additional information on administration and scoring refer to the following references:
1. Anthony JC, LeResche L, Niaz U, et al. Limits of "Mini-Mental State" as a screening test for dementia and delirium among hospital patients. *Psych Med.* 1982;12:397–408.
2. Folstein MF, Anthony JC, et al. Meaning of cognitive impairment in the elderly. *J Am Geriatr Soc.* 1985;33(4):228–235.
3. Spenser MP, Folstein MF. The Mini-Mental State Examination. In: Keller PA, Ritt LG. *Innovations in clinical practice: a source/book.* 1985;4:305–310.

The change in activity rather than an absolute test score is most critical, and it is important to ascertain the onset, acute or gradual, the duration and the severity as one would do with any important symptom.

decline in ADLs can be the only symptom of serious diseases such as urosepsis, CHF, or MI (see Chapter 9). Functional assessment is a useful tool for the detection of disease and its severity, and it is an essential element for guiding and evaluating treatment, planning disposition, observing deterioration or improvement over time, and matching socioeconomic and community resources with patient needs.

Functional assessment can be derived from self-report or observer-report data. Patients, as a rule, tend to rate self-function higher than do family members or nurses. Therefore, performance measures are more reliable than reports, and it is recommended that, when possible and safe, ED personnel observe the patient getting off the stretcher, walking, and using hands to perform simple tasks such as combing hair, writing, or drawing.

The Katz functional assessment of ADLs is routinely used in primary care and is recommended for ED screening as well[18] (Figure 7–4). The ADL screening includes questions related to activities necessary for independent living and can be administered in less than 5 minutes.

The items are rated on a scale of 1-3, with 3 = performing activities without assistance, 2 = some assistance, and 1 = considerable assistance required. These questions should be incorporated routinely into the medical interview of the elderly patient. The following questions can be asked: "Do you need any assistance with bathing, dressing, toileting, getting out of bed into a chair, controlling your urine or bowel movements or feeding yourself?" A change in any one of these ADL functions should raise the index of suspicion for a serious, underlying acute illness (see Chapter 9). The *change* in activity rather than an absolute score is most critical, and it is important to ascertain the following:

1. Onset (acute or gradual)
2. Duration
3. Severity

Treat these changes as one would treat any important symptom. The patient's self-report should be confirmed by caregivers. Caregivers can provide a wealth of information about recent impairment. The level of social support should be assessed concurrently to determine the advisability of patient discharge.

The physical examination will reveal information about personal hygiene, dress, and nutritional status to corroborate the patient's self-reported ADLs. In addition, when safe, the physical examination should include a demonstration by the patient of his or her ability to "get up and go"—for example, observe the patient's ability to:

1. Get off the stretcher.
2. Walk (to assess gait, balance, and stability).

A patient's failure to perform ADLs and "get up and go" in the absence of a home social support system suggests the need for admission. If social services are available in the ED it may be possible in some cases to refer the patient directly to a rehabilitation center or intermediate-level care facility for further assessment.

At the time of discharge planning, an ED staff member needs also to assess higher functions that are more likely to deteriorate before

Activities of Daily Living (ADL) Scale: Evaluation Form

Name _____   Day of evaluation _____

For each area of functioning listed below, check description that applies. (The word "assistance" means supervision, direction, or personal assistance.)

Bathing—either sponge bath, tub bath, or shower

☐ Receives no assistance (gets in and out of tub by self, if tub is usual means of bathing)

☐ Receives assistance in bathing only one part of the body (such as back or a leg)

☐ Receives assistance in bathing more than one part of the body (or not bathed)

Dressing—gets clothes from closets and drawers, including underclothes and outer garments, and uses fasteners (including braces, if worn)

☐ Gets clothes and gets completely dressed without assistance.

☐ Gets clothes and gets dressed without assistance, except for assistance in tying shoes

☐ Receives assistance in getting clothes or in getting dressed or stays partly or completely undressed

Toileting—going to the "toilet room" for bowel and urine elimination, cleaning self after elimination and arranging clothes

☐ Goes to "bathroom," cleans self, and arranges clothes without assistance (may use object for support such as cane, walker, or wheelchair and may manage night bedpan or commode, emptying same in morning)

☐ Receives assistance in going to "bathroom" or in cleansing self or in arranging clothes after elimination or in use of night bedpan or commode

☐ Does not go to bathroom for the elimination process

Transfer

☐ Moves in and out of bed as well as in and out of chair without assistance (may be using object for support, such as cane or walker)

☐ Moves in and out of bed or chair with assistance

☐ Does not get out of bed

Continence

☐ Controls urination and bowel movements completely by self

☐ Has occasional "accidents"

☐ Supervision helps keep urine or bowel control; catheter is used or person is incontinent

Feeding

☐ Feeds self without assistance

☐ Feeds self except for getting assistance in cutting meat or buttering bread

☐ Receives assistance in feeding or is fed partly or completely by using tubes or intravenous fluids

FIGURE 7-4   Reprinted with permission Katz S, Ford AB, Moskowitz RW, et al. Studies in illness in the aged. The index of ADL: Standardized measure of biologic and psychosocial function. *JAMA.* 1962; 185:914-919. Copyright 1962, American Medical Association.

For additional information on administration and scoring refer to the following references:
1. Katz S. Assessing self-maintenance: activities of daily living, mobility, and instrumental activities of daily living. *J Am Geriatr Soc.* 1983;31:721–727.
2. Katz S, Akpom CA. A measure of primary sociobiologic functions. *Int J Health Services.* 1976;6:493–508.
3. Katz S, Downs TD, Cash HR, et al. Progress in development of the index of ADL. *J Gerontol.* 1970;10(1):20–30.

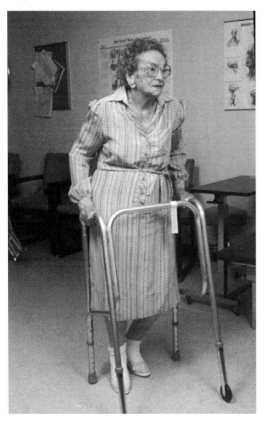

When possible, the physical examination includes a demonstration of the ability to "get up and go."

ADLs reveal functional decline and impairment. The instrumental activities of daily living (IADLs) assessment, developed by Lawton and Brody, is the instrument commonly used and recommended[19] (Figure 7–5). This instrument can be administered in less than 5 minutes and includes the patient's ability to perform routine tasks.

Deficiencies in these areas need to be evaluated and acted on before discharge. Referral to a social service agency and back to the primary care physician or a geriatric assessment unit should be arranged. It is critical to provide long-term follow-up and address positive findings. The patient can be asked if there is a need for such services as the following:

1. A homemaker
2. Food stamps
3. Meals on wheels
4. Transportation
5. Public transportation discounts
6. A Medicaid card
7. Home health care services
8. Senior citizen center activities
9. Friendly visitors

CASE FINDING: A MULTIDISCIPLINARY APPROACH

Case finding is defined as the search for problems in patients who are being treated for unrelated symptoms.

The system of ED care for the elderly patient needs to expand beyond the limits of the patient-physician relationship. A multidisciplinary team approach is essential. Nonphysician clinic personnel such as physicians' assistants (PAs), registered nurses (RNs), emergency medical technicians (EMTs), and medical students have successfully administered formal geriatric assessment tools in clinical settings. Miller et al, published a study in which PAs and RNs did case finding and used formal instruments for elderly medical outpatients. The MMSE took less than 4 minutes. In addition, they assessed depression, gait and balance, and nutritional status.[20] Gerson et al, described an important pre-hospital screening program for elderly persons. Those elderly persons identified with potential problems such as neglect, abuse, or a hazardous home environment were referred to the area agency on aging for more extensive home evaluation and referral to services by an experienced social worker.[21]

A recent multicenter ED-based pilot study by Gerson and colleagues, adapting Lachs and colleagues[7] outpatient screening instrument to the ED, showed the feasibility and efficacy of a brief comprehensive case-finding program among elderly patients (Table 7–1).[22] In one center, referrals were made to the area agency on aging and at an-

Instrumental Activities of Daily Living (IADL)Scale

1. Can you use the telephone:
   without help | 3
   with some help, or | 2
   are you completely unable to use the telephone? | 1

2. Can you get to places out of walking distance:
   without help | 3
   with some help, or | 2
   are you completely unable to travel unless special arrangements are made? | 1

3. Can you go shopping for groceries:
   without help | 3
   with some help, or | 2
   are you completely unable to do any shopping? | 1

4. Can you prepare your own meals:
   without help | 3
   with some help, or | 2
   are you completely unable to prepare any meals? | 1

5. Can you do your own housework:
   without help | 3
   with some help, or | 2
   are you completely unable to do any housework? | 1

6. Can you do your own handyman work:
   without help | 3
   with some help, or | 2
   are you completely unable to do any handyman work? | 1

7. Can you do your own laundry:
   without help | 3
   with some help, or | 2
   are you completely unable to do any laundry at all? | 1

8a. Do you take medicines or use any medications?
   (If yes, answer Question 8b) Yes | 1
   (If no, answer Questions 8c) No | 2

8b. Do you take your own medicine:
   without help (in the right doses at the right time), | 3
   with some help (take medicine if someone prepares it for you and/or reminds you to take it), or | 2
   (are you/would you be) completely unable to take your own medicine? | 1

8c. If you had to take medicine, can you do it:
   without help (in the right doses at the right time, | 3
   with some help (take medicine if someone prepares it for you and/or reminds you to take it), or | 2
   (are you/would you be) completely unable to take your own medicine? | 1

9. Can you manage your own money:
   without help | 3
   with some help, or | 2
   are you completely unable to handle money? | 1

FIGURE 7-5 Instrumental Activities of Daily Living (IADL) scale: self-rated version extracted from Multilevel Assessment Instrument (MAI). Adapted from Lawton MP, Brody EM. Assessment of older people: self-maintaining & instrumental activities of daily living. *Gerontologist.*1969;9:179–185. Copyright © The Gerontological Society of America. Reprinted with Permission.

For additional information on administration and scoring refer to the following references:
1. Lawton MP, Scales to measure competence in everyday activities. *Psychopharm Bull.* 1988;24(4):609–614.
2. Lawton MP, Moss M, Fulcomer M, et al. A research and service-oriented Multilevel Assessment Instrument. *J Gerontol.* 1982;37:91–99.

Table 7–1 **Results of Outpatient Screening of 242 Persons
(281 Conditions Identified)**

Patients (%)	Condition
79	Limitations in ADLs or IADLs
55	Vision problems
54	Lacked flu vaccination
49	Hazards in home environment
46	Some cognitive impairment
40	Fall in past year
36	Felt depressed
32	Potential inadequate nutrition
26	Incontinence
6.6	Potential drinking problem
2.5	Potential abuse case

other site to an outpatient geriatric assessment unit. Of the 76 patients evaluated at a follow-up visit, 47 newly identified problems were confirmed, and a treatment plan was developed for 53% of the problems. These studies provide encouraging evidence that in the near future ED providers can incorporate a brief mental status, functional, and psychosocial assessment into their clinical practice.

The ED brief assessment and case finding for elderly patients are recommended when clinically indicated, especially in situations in which the problems of depression and suicide risk, alcohol and drug abuse, malnutrition, and incontinence are prevalent. Case finding is defined as the search for problems in patients who are being treated for unrelated symptoms. A computerized data base can be established so that changes in baseline status can be monitored on subsequent ED visits. Early detection also decreases costly future testing and treatment.

DEPRESSION AND SUICIDE RISK

Thirty-two percent of elderly patients in a cross-sectional study of an outpatient clinic population tested positive for mild depression, and 6% tested positive for severe depression; however, only one third of these problems had been previously identified by a geriatric team.[23] Depression and medications account for the majority of cases of reversible dementia. Among older inpatients, 12% had major depression and 23% had depressive syndromes.[24] Therefore, all elderly ED patients should be questioned about whether they have recently felt depressed, sad, or hopeless or whether they have had thoughts of self-harm. If there is an immediate suicide risk, emergency psychiatric consultation is required. Elderly divorced or single males have the highest suicide risk of any group. A positive response to these questions warrants administration of the abbreviated Geriatric Depression Scale (GDS)[25] (Figure 7–6).

The GDS takes less than 4 minutes to administer. It is a 15-item, forced choice, yes or no questionnaire. The cutoff score (higher than 5) suggests depression that requires referral and further evaluation. Depression in the eldelry patient is responsive to medications and psychotherapy in many instances. When depression is detected and treated early, the patient's quality of life and that of the caregiver are both improved, and a decreased utilization of emergency services is possible.

ALCOHOL ABUSE

The absolute number of elderly persons with alcohol problems is at least 0.5 million and may exceed 2.5 million (a population rate of 2-10%).[26] Women make up two thirds of all older, late-onset alcoholics.

Geriatric Depression Scale

Choose the best answer for how you felt over the past week.

1. Are you basically satisfied with your life?   yes/no
2. Have you dropped many of your activities and interests?   yes/no
3. Do you feel that your life is empty?   yes/no
4. Do you often get bored?   yes/no
5. Are you in good spirits most of the time?   yes/no
6. Are you afraid that something bad is going to happen to you?   yes/no
7. Do you feel happy most of the time?   yes/no
8. Do you often feel helpless?   yes/no
9. Do you prefer to stay at home, rather than going out and doing   yes/no
   new things?
10. Do you feel you have more problems with memory than most?   yes/no
11. Do you think it is wonderful to be alive now?   yes/no
12. Do you feel pretty worthless the way you are now?   yes/no
13. Do you feel full of energy?   yes/no
14. Do you feel that your situation is hopeless?   yes/no
15. Do you think that most people are better off than you are?   yes/no

This is the scoring for the scale. One point for each of these answers. Cutoff: normal (0-5), above 5 suggests depression.

1. no	6. yes	11. no
2. yes	7. no	12. yes
3. yes	8. yes	13. no
4. yes	9. yes	14. yes
5. no	10. yes	15. yes

FIGURE 7-6   Geriatric Depression Scale: short form. Reprinted with Permission. Copyright 1986. The Haworth Press, Inc. Binghamton, NY. Sheikh JI, Yesavage JA. Geriatric Depression Scale: recent evidence and development of a shorter version. *Clin Gerontol.* 1986;5:165–172.

For additional information on administration and scoring refer to the following references:
1. Yesavage JA, Brink TL, Rose TI., et al. Development and validation of a geriatric depression rating scale: a preliminary report. *J Psych Res.* 1983;17:27.

General hospital rates have been reported between 15% and 50%.[27] Four patterns of use have been identified among elderly persons:

1. Chronic
2. Intermittent
3. Reactive (following significant psychosocial stresses)
4. Late onset

One third of elderly persons with alcohol dependency are in the reactive or late onset group.[26,28] Late-life alcohol abuse is underdiagnosed and underestimated, because the older person does not offer the typical presentation, such as problems on the job or with family members, motor vehicle crashes, or other trauma, as in the case of the younger person with alcohol dependence. By contrast, they present more frequently with medical illness, particularly gastrointestinal disease. The elderly persons' physiologic response is greater at lower levels of intake and frequency of drinking because of reduced total body fluid volume.[28]

The validity of self-report is affected by memory problems and patient denial. Patients' attempts to hide drinking problems reflect the shame, fear of social stereotypes, and the moral and legal ethos surrounding alcoholism in this generation. Drinking problems may commonly be misdiagnosed as depression, problems with memory or sleep, or the effects of aging.[29-31] Despite difficulty in diagnosing alcohol-related problems, treatment is very effective in the older person. The high prevalence and rate of successful treatment emphasize the importance of detection and referral by the ED staff.

A recent study showed that, among elderly persons presenting to the ED, 24% had lifetime alcohol problems and 14% had current alcohol problems.[32] The CAGE questions given below are recommended for detection of alcohol problems in EDs with high prevalence rates or when clinical indicators such as the following are present:

1. Gastrointestinal complaints
2. Hypertension
3. Insomnia
4. Depression
5. Falls
6. Pedestrian injuries
7. Motor vehicle trauma

CAGE is a mnemonic for the following:

C = Cutting down: "Have you ever felt you ought to cut down on your drinking?"
A = Annoyed: "Have you ever been annoyed (upset or concerned may be a more acceptable choice of words) by being questioned about your alcohol use?"
G = Guilty: "Have you ever felt guilty about your drinking?"
E = Early morning drinking/Eye-opener: "Have you ever felt the need for an eye opener?"

A positive response to one CAGE question for the elderly patient has a sensitivity of 86% and a specificity of 78%. A cutoff of one positive response is most appropriate when in communities with a high prevalence.[33] A cutoff for two questions has a sensitivity of 70% and a specificity of 91%. Sensitivity increases to 90% and specificity to 85% for current drinking if, in addition to two positive CAGE questions, a patient has consumed alcohol in the past 24 hours and admits to having or having had a drinking problem. Therefore also ask: when was your last drink? Have you ever had a drinking problem?[34]

It is important to ask the time of the patient's last drink to help distinguish between lifetime and current problem drinking. Once the problem is detected, a brief intervention involving respectful, active, empathic listening and a review of how the patient interprets the problem, consequences, and readiness to change has been shown to encourage a change in behavior. The goal of case finding is to motivate patients to seek further assessment and to match patients with appropriate treatment modalities.[35,36]

PROTEIN ENERGY UNDERNUTRITION

Eighteen percent of elderly persons presenting to the ED are undernourished. About one third of outpatients will be undernourished because of depression. A number of other treatable causes of undernutrition have been identified (Table 7–2). A simple screening test for patients at risk for undernutrition has been developed (Table 7–3). Undernutrition is associated with recurrent infections and poor response to treatment because of such factors as an impaired immune system, decubitus ulcers, and weakness. Aggressive identification of the cause of undernutrition and appropriate treatment should decrease hospital admissions. Elderly patients with undernutrition should be referred to a geriatrician or primary care physician for further workup.

Table 7–2 **Common Causes of Malnutrition in Elderly Persons***+

Medications (e.g., digoxin, psychotropic drugs)

Emotional (depression)

Anorexia (nervosa or tardive) or alcoholism

Late-life paranoia

Swallowing disorders

Oral factors (e.g., loss of teeth)

No money (absolute or relative poverty)

Wandering (dementia)

Hyperthyroidism or hyparparathyroidism

Entry problems (malabsorption)

Eating problems

Low-salt or low-cholesterol diet

Shopping and food-preparation problems

From Morley, John E. Why do Physicians Fail to Recognize and Treat Malnutrition in Older Persons. *JAGS.* 1991;39:1139–1140.
*organized by the acronym MEALS ON WHEELS.
+In addition, consider infection (tuberculosis), gallstones, and chronic obstructive pulmonary disease (COPD).

Table 7–3 **SCALES Protocol for Evaluating Risk of Malnutrition in Elderly Persons***

Item Evaluated	Criterion for Assigning 1 Point	Criterion for Assigning 2 Points
Sadness (as measured on Yesavage Geriatric Depression scale)	10–14	≥15
Cholesterol	≤160 mg/dl	—
Albumin	3.5–4 g/dl	<3.5 g/dl
Loss of weight	1 kg (or 1/4 inch in mid-arm circumference) in 1 mo	3 kg (or 1/2 inch in mid-arm circumference) in 6 mo
Eating problems	Patient needs assistance	—
Shopping and food preparation problems	Patient needs assistance	—

From Morley, John E. Why do Physicians Fail to Recognize and Treat Malnutrition in Older Persons. *JAGS.* 1991;39:1139–1140.
* Total scores ≥ 3 indicate patients at clear risk.

INCONTINENCE

Incontinence, a common problem in the elderly ED patient, is present in up to 26% of this population.[22] Incontinence is defined as the involuntary loss of urine, and is one of the precipitating factors in admission to a nursing home. It also can result in social isolation and depression. The causes of acute incontinence are best remembered by the mnemonic DRIP:

D = **D**rugs, **d**elirium
R = **R**etention of urine, **r**estricted mobility
I = **I**nfection, **i**mpaction of feces
P = **P**olyuria, **p**rostatism

All patients with incontinence should have a urine analysis and culture and a rectal examination to rule out an enlarged prostate or fecal impaction. Chronic incontinence has multiple causes, which are summarized in Table 7–4. In most cases incontinence is a treatable or curable condition, and referral to a geriatrician or urologist should be initiated from the ED.

PREVENTATIVE CONSIDERATIONS

The following screening and case-finding recommendations are consistent with the Year 2000 National Health Objectives[37] and the findings of the US Preventive Services Task Force for older adults.[38] The year 2000 objectives target opportunities for improvement of health status among the elderly by accomplishing the following goals.

1. Reducing to "no more than 90 per 1000 people the proportion of all people age 65 and older who have difficulty in performing two

Table 7–4 **Types and Common Treatments of Chronic Incontinence**

Type	Treatment
Overflow	
Obstruction	Transurethral prostatectomy (TURP)
	Proscar
Neurogenic	Bethanechol
	Catheter
Stress (i.e., loss of urine with maneuvers that increase intraabdominal pressure [e.g., cough, sneeze])	Kegel exercises
	Estrogen
	Surgery
Urge (i.e., inability to control urine following first urge to void)	Oxybutynin
Reflex (as in paraplegia)	Intermittent catheterization
Functional (e.g., dementia)	Frequent toileting

or more personal care activities, thereby preserving independence (baseline: 111 per 1000 in 1984-85)";

2. Reducing "suicides among white men aged 65 and older to no more than 39.2 per 100,000 (age-adjusted baseline: 46.1 per 100,000 in 1987)";

3. Increasing "to at least 60% the proportion of providers of primary care for older adults who routinely evaluate people aged 65 and older for urinary incontinence, impairment of vision, hearing, cognition, and functional status (baseline data available 1992)."

Health promotion issues discussed in other chapters, such as reducing the risk of morbidity and mortality of motor vehicle accidents, falls, fires, and intentional injuries, are also health status objectives targeted by *Healthy People 2000*. ED providers can incorporate into the discharge plan patient education on the use of safety restraints, smoke detectors, and home and pedestrian safety and assess the risk for elder abuse. There are also opportunities, when appropriate, to make referrals for alcohol, drug, and smoking cessation counseling, immunizations, Pap smears, and mammograms.

With the growing emphasis on primary and secondary prevention in health care policy, the ED provides an opportune setting for identifying elderly patients with these impairments and linking them with appropriate diagnostic, treatment, and psychosocial support services. Emergency medical personnel are in a unique position to develop a comprehensive and collaborative approach to the care of our elderly patients and, together with them and other providers (public health and social services personnel), contribute to improving the quality of their lives.

SUMMARY POINTS

- Abnormalities in cognitive status are easily missed unless formal assessment is performed in the ED. Cognitive status is evaluated through a two-step process: (1) orientation to person, place, and time and (2) three-item recall after 1 minute. If these are abnormal, a formal mental status instrument, the Mini-Mental State Examination, can be used to assess the patient's cognitive abilities.
- Delirium or acute confusional states can easily be missed in elderly patients in the ED unless a formal evaluation is done. The Confusion Assessment Method (CAM) Scale can be used to evaluate delirium with regard to the following:
  1. Acute onset or fluctuating course
  2. Inattention
  3. Disorganized thinking
  4. Altered level of consciousness.
- Changes in the elderly patient's functional ability can be important indicators of serious illness. It is recommended that the elderly patient have an assessment of activities of daily living (ADLs), including questions with regard to bathing, dressing, toileting, continence, transferring, and feeding.
- Patients who are to be discharged from the ED can be further evaluated by the instrumental activities of daily living (IADL) assessment to evaluate the patient's ability to perform routine tasks of daily living such as use of the telephone, preparing meals, shopping, housekeeping, and laundry.
- Elderly patients are at a significant risk for depression and suicide. A screening question regarding feelings of depression or hopelessness can help evaluate the patient for depression. The Geriatric Depression Scale (GDS) can be used to screen patients with positive responses.
- Alcohol abuse is a significant problem in the elderly population. Patients suspected of alcohol abuse can be screened using the CAGE scale.
- Undernutrition and incontinence are treatable and significant problems among elderly persons. Screening tests in high-risk populations can be part of the ED evaluation.
- Significant numbers of older patients do not have appropriate or preventive care such as immunizations. The ED encounter provides an opportunity for elderly patients to be evaluated for preventive health measures and health promotion issues.

CHAPTER AUTHOR

Edward Bernstein, MD, FACEP

REFERENCES

1. National Institute of Health, Consensus Development Conference Statement. Geriatric assessment methods for clinical decision making. *J Am Geriatr Soc.* 1988;36:342.
2. Clarfield AM. The reversible dementias: do they reverse? *Ann Intern Med.* 1988;109:479–486.
3. Rubenstein LV, Calkins DR, Greenfield S, et al. Health status assessment for the elderly patients. *J Am Geriatr Soc.* 1988;37:562–569.

4. Naughton BJ, Moran MB, Kadah H, Heman-Ackah Y, Longanu J: Delirium and other cognitive impairment in older adults in an emergency department. *Ann Emerg Med* 1995;25:751–755.
5. Lewis LM, Miller DK, Morley JE, et al. Unrecognized delirium in ED geriatric patients. *Am J Emerg Med* 1995;13:142–145.
6. Inouye SK, van Dyck CH, Alessi CA, et al. Clarifying confusion; the confusion assessment method—a new method for detection of delirium. *Ann Intern Med* 1990;113:941–948.
7. Lachs MS, Feinstein AR, Cooney LM, et al. A simple procedure for general screening for functional disability in elderly patients. *Ann Intern Med* 1990;112:699–706.
8. Teng EL, Chui HC. The Modified Mini-Mental State (MMSE) Examination. *J Clin Psychiatry.* 1987;48:314–318.
9. Folstein MF, Folstein SE, McHugh PR. 'Mini-Mental State.' A practical method for grading the cognitive state of patients for the clinician. *J Psychiatr Res.* 1975;12:189–198.
10. Blessed G, Tomilison BE, Roth M. The association between quantitative measures of dementia and of senile changes in the cerebral grey matter of elderly subjects. *Br J Psychiatry.* 1983;114:610–612.
11. Katzman R, Brown T, Fuld P, et al. Validation of a short orientation-memory-concentration test of cognitive impairment. *Am J Psychiatry.* 1983;140:734–739.
12. Pfeiffer E. A short portable mental status questionnaire for the assessment of organic brain deficit in elderly patients. *J Am Geriatr Soc.* 1975;23:433–441.
13. Jacobs JW, Bernhard MR, Delgado A, Strain JJ. Screening for organic mental syndromes in the medically ill. *Ann Intern Med* 1977;86:40–46.
14. Tombaugh TN, McIntyre NJ. The Mini-Mental State Examination: a comprehensive review. *J Am Geriatr Soc.* 1992;40:922–935.
15. McKhann G, Drachman D, Folstein M, et al: Clinical diagnosis of Alzheimer's disease: report of the NINCDS-ADRDA Work Group under the auspices of Department of Health and Human Services Task Force on Alzheimer's disease. *Neurology.* 1984;34:939–944.
16. Anthony JC, LaResche L, Niaz U, et al. Limits of the 'Mini-Mental State' as a screening test for dementia among hospital patients. *Psychol Med.* 1982;12:397–408.
17. Crum RM, Anthony JC, Bassett SS, Folstein MF. Population-based norms for the Mini-Mental State examination by age and educational level. *JAMA.* 1993;269:2386–2391.
18. Katz S. Assessing self maintenance; activities of daily living, mobility, and instrumental activities of daily living. *J Am Geriatr Soc.* 1983;31:721–727.
19. Lawton MP, Moss M, Fulcomer M, et al. A research and service-oriented multilevel assessment instrument. *J Gerontol.* 1982;37:91–99.
20. Miller DK, Morley JE, Rubinstein LZ, et al. Formal geriatric assessment instruments and the care of older general medical outpatients. *J Am Geriatr Soc.* 1990;38:645–651.
21. Gerson LW, Schelble DT, Wilson JE. Using paramedics to identify at-risk elderly. *Ann Emerg Med.* 1992;21:688–691.
22. Gerson LW, Rousseau E, Hogan T, Bernstein E, Klabfleisch N. A multicenter study of case finding in elderly emergency department patients. *Acad Emerg Med.* 1995. [In press.]
23. Fulop G, Reinhardt J, Strain JJ, et al. Identification of alcoholism and depression in a geriatric medicine outpatient clinic. *J Am Geriatr Soc.* 1993;41:737–741.
24. Koenig HG, Meader KG, Cohen HJ, et al. Depression in elderly hospitalized patients with medical illness. *Arch Intern Med.* 1989;148:1929–1936.
25. Sheikh JL, Yesavage JA. Geriatric depression scale: recent evidence and development of a shorter version. In: Brink TL, ed. *Clinical Gerontology.* New York, NY: Haworth Press;1986:165–173.

26. Gomberg ES. Alcohol use and alcohol problems among the elderly. In: *Special population issues* (alcohol and health monograph no. 4); DHHS publication no. (ADM) 82-1193. Rockville, MD: National Institute on Alcohol and Alcohol Abuse, 1982;263–290.

27. Bristow MF, Clare AW. Prevalence and characteristics of at-risk drinkers among elderly medical inpatients. *Br J Addict.* 1992;87:291–294.

28. Scott R, Mitchell M. Aging, alcohol and the liver. *J Am Geriatr Soc.* 1988;36:255–265.

29. Schuckit MA. Geriatric alcoholism and drug abuse. *Gerontologist.* 1977;17:168–174.

30. Stinson FS, Dufour MC, Bertolucci D. Epidemiologic bulletin #20: alcohol related morbidity in the aging population. *Alcohol Health Research World.* 1989;13:80–87.

31. Beresford T, Blow FC, Brower KJ, Adams KM, Hall RC. Alcoholism and aging in the general hospital. *Psychosomatics.* 1988;29:61–72.

32. Adams WL, Magruder-Habib K, Trued S, Broome HL. Alcohol abuse in the elderly emergency department patients. *J Am Geriatr Soc.* 1992;40:1236–1240.

33. Buchsbaum DG, Buchanan BA, Welsh MA, Centor RM, Schnoll SH. Screening for drinking in the elderly using the CAGE questionnaire. *J Am Geriatr Soc.* 1992;40:662–665.

34. Cy M, Wartman S, The effectiveness of routine screening questions in the detection of alcoholism. *JAMA.* 1988;259:51.

35. Rollnick S, Kinnersley P, Scott N. Methods of helping patients with behavior change. *Br Med J.* 1993;307:188–190.

36. Miller WR, Rollnick S. *Motivational interviewing: preparing people to change addictive behavior.* New York, NY: Guilford; 1991.

37. Department Of Health And Human Services. *Healthy people 2000; national health promotion and disease prevention objectives: full report, with commentary.* Boston, MA: Jones & Bartlett, 1992. (Originally published: USDHHS, PHS, Publication No. [PHS] 91-50212. Washington, DC: US Government Printing Office; 1991.)

38. U.S. Preventive Services Task Force. *Guide to clinical preventive services: an assessment of the effectiveness of 169 interventions; report of the U.S. Preventive Services Task Force.* Baltimore, MD: Williams & Wilkens; 1989.

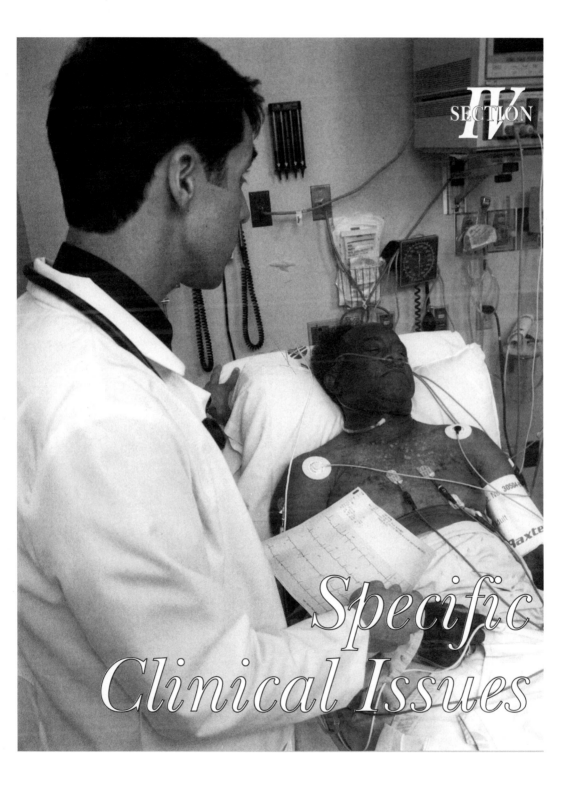

Specific
Clinical Issues

8 *Altered Mental Status*

LEARNING OBJECTIVES

1. Define delirium and dementia, and identify distinguishing characteristics.
2. Explain the potential impact of a missed diagnosis of deliruim on morbidity and mortality.
3. Apply the Mini-Mental State Examination (MMSE) and Confusion Assessment Method (CAM) to the ED evaluation of patients with altered mental status.
4. Identify factors unique to elderly persons that predispose to delirium.

Acute mental confusion as a presenting symptom holds a central position in the medicine of old age. Its importance cannot be overemphasized, for acute confusion is a far more common herald of the onset of physical illness in an older person than are, for example, fever, pain, or tachycardia.

H.M. Hodkinson[1]

An elderly patient with altered mental status may be among the most challenging patients the emergency physician sees to effectively and accurately diagnose and treat. The spectrum of the clinical presentation is diverse—violent to withdrawn, agitated to comatose, subtle to dramatic. In most circumstances a complex interplay of predisposing and precipitating factors denies the emergency care provider a simple, single, readily apparent cause. Etiologies to an altered mental status are protean, are often multifactorial, and cover the spectrum of medical, surgical, neurologic, and psychiatric illnesses seen in the elderly population (Table 8–1). Medications are often contributory (Table 8-2).

The nature of the signs and symptoms often precludes a valid history from the patient. Collaborative information is often not readily available. An accurate medical history including current problem or a medication list may be of pivotal importance but may not be readily accessible. The cause or causes of altered mental status, even when found, may not be readily treatable or reversible and are often associated with morbidity and mortality. Frequently, significant diagnostic uncertainty remains even after meticulous and directed evaluation in the ED.

Table 8–1 **Causes of Altered Mental Status in the Elder Person**

Causes Affecting the Central Nervous System Indirectly

Cardiovascular
Congestive heart failure
Myocardial infarction
Arrhythmias
Other disease states producing hypoperfusion

Pulmonary
Pulmonary embolism
Other disease states producing hypoxia

Fluid, Electrolyte and Metabolic Distrubances
Dehydration/Water intoxication
Electrolyte imbalance
Acid/Base Imbalance
Hypoglycemia/Hyperglycemia
Vitamin deficiency
Renal insufficienty
Hepatic insufficiency
Endrocrinopathies
Inborn errors of metabolism

Infections
Pneumonia
Urinary tract infections
Sepsis
Cellulitis
AIDS
Any infection with systemic effect

Other
Neoplasm
Para neoplastic syndrome
Reye's syndrome

Other (continued)
Thrombotic thrombocytopenic purpura
Anesthesia
Trauma
Surgery
Shock
Burns

Environmental/Sensory
Hypothermia/Heat stroke
Pain
Vision/hearing impairment
Sensory deprivation/overload
Immobilization
Sleep deprivation

Intoxication/Withdrawal/Poisoning
Intoxication by/withdrawal of presceiption and over-the-counter medications (See Table 8-2)
Intoxication by drugs of abuse including ethanol
Withdrawal of drugs of abuse syndromes
Carbon monoxide
Poisoning

Primary Central Nervous System Disorders
Head Trauma
Subdural/epidural
Intracerebral hematoma
Post Concussive Syndrome

Cerebrovascular Disease
Subarachnoid hemorrhage
CVA/TIA

Cerebrovascular Disease (continued)
Temporal arteritis
Complex migraine headache
Hypertensive encephalopathy

Infection
Cerebral abscess/meningitis
Encephalitis
Neurosyphilis

Other
Epilepsy and post-ictal states
Multiple sclerosis
Huntington's Chorea
Lupus cerebritis

Space-Occupying Masses
Benign intra-cerebral tumors
Primary and metastatic malignancy

Psychiatric Disorders
Organic withdrawal syndromes
Organic intoxication syndromes
Bipolar Disorder
Agitated Depression
Paranoid Delusional Disorders
Anxiety Disorders
Schizophrenia
Schizophreniform psychosis
Brief reactive psychosis
Psychogenic unresponsiveness
Catatonia
Some forms of malingering
Pseudoseizure
Conversion reaction

Dementia
Alzheimer's
Vascular (formerly multi-infarct)

Table 8–2 **Medications Associated with Altered Mental Status in the Elderly**

Sedative-hypnotics
Antidepressants
Steroids
Barbiturates
Anticonvulsants
Neuroleptics
Antihistamines
Diuretics
Antiparkinson agents
Antihypertensive agents
Theophylline
Antiemetics
Antispasmodics
Cardiac (digitalis, lidocaine); other antiarrhythmics
Antibiotics including anti-virals, antifungals
Lithium
Nonsteroidal anti-inflammatory drugs including salicylates
Ocular cycloplegics and mydriatics
H_2 blockers
Psychotropics

SPECTRUM OF ALTERED MENTAL STATUS

Coma, stupor, obtundation, lethargy, somnolence, and agitation in the patient with an altered mental status are best described as a disturbed *level* of consciousness (i.e., wakefulness/awareness). Delirium, confusional state, reversible dementia, organic brain syndrome, encephalopathy, and psychosis in the patient with an altered mental status are best characterized as a disturbed *content* of consciousness. Thus disturbed level of consciousness and disturbed content of consciousness represent two different ways of describing mental status alterations. Clinically, patients with altered mental status invariably present with compromise to a certain extent of both (Table 8-3).

A disturbed level of consciousness or a disturbed content of consciousness are two ways of describing an altered mental status.

This chapter focuses on important features of transient altered mental status in elderly persons and discusses emergency management of the patient from pre-hospital transport through disposition from the ED.

DEFINITIONS

COMA

Coma is a condition in which the patient appears to be asleep and is at the same time incapable of being aroused by external stimuli or inner physiologic needs.[2]

DEMENTIA

The essential feature of dementia is impaired short- and long-term memory associated with impaired abstract thinking, impaired judg-

Table 8–3 **Clinical Features of Coma, Delirium, Dementia, and Psychosis**

Characteristic	Coma	Delirium	Dementia	Psychosis
Onset	Variable	Variable	Insidious, progressive	Variable
Course over days	Variable	Fluctuating with lucid intervals and nocturnal exacerbation	Stable	Stable
Consciousness	Decreased	Reduced	Clear	Variable
Attention	Absent	Globally disordered	Normal except in severe cases	May be disordered
Alertness	Decreased	Abnormally low or high	Normal	Abnormally low or high
Cognition	Absent	Globally disordered	Impoverished	May be selectively impaired
Hallucinations	Absent	Usually visual or visual and auditory	Often absent	Predominantly auditory
Delusions	Absent	Fleeting, poorly systematized	Often absent	Sustained, complex, systematized
Orientation	Nonverbal	Usually impaired	Often impaired	Variable
Psychomotor activity	Variable, often markedly reduced or absent	Increased, reduced, or shifting; unpredictable	Often normal	Variable
GCS	8 or less	11 or greater	11 or greater	11 or greater
Speech	Incoherent if present	Often incoherent; slow or rapid	Patient has difficulty finding words; perseveration	Normal, slow, or rapid; coherent
Involuntary movements	Variable; often markedly reduced	Often asterixis, coarse tremor, or myoclonus	Often absent	Usually absent
Vital signs	Typically abnormal	Typically abnormal; sympathetic hyperactivity	Normal	Usually afebrile (tachypneic, tachycardic)
Prior psychiatric history	No causal relationship	Psychiatric history predisposed	No causal relationship	Frequent
Age at onset	Variable	Very young or elderly	Elderly	Usually before 40 yr
Agitation	Variable	Frequent	Variable	Frequent
Electroencephalogram	Usually normal	Characteristic changes persist	Often normal	Normal
Duration	Variable	Limited	Nonfluctuating, progressive	Limited, recurrent
Evidence of physical illness or drug effect	Yes	Yes	Variable	Variable

Adapted from Beresin EV. Delirium in the elderly. *J Geriatr Psychiatry Neurol.* 1988;1:127–143; Francis J, Delirium in older patients. *J Am Geriatr Soc.* 1992;40:829–838; and Lipowski ZJ. Delirium in the elderly patient. *N Engl J Med.* 1989;320:578–582.

ment, other disturbances of higher cortical function, or personality change (Table 8-4).

DELIRIUM

Delirium is defined as an organic mental syndrome characterized by a global disorder of cognition and attention, a reduced level of consciousness, a disturbed sleep-wake cycle, and either abnormally increased or decreased psychomotor activity. The attention deficit is the cornerstone of delirium and is particularly helpful in distinguishing dementia from delirium.

Any elderly patient with an acutely disturbed content of consciousness should be assumed to have delirium until it is ruled out.

ACUTE PSYCHOSIS

Acute psychosis is a general term for any major mental disorder of psychiatric or emotional origin characterized by personality derangement and loss of contact with reality.

The more common functional psychiatric causes of altered mental status in the elderly population include some types of depression, such as agitated depression, paranoid delusional disorders, anxiety disorders, schizophrenia, and bipolar disorder. Unless the patient has a history of one of the latter two illnesses, it is unlikely that a new-onset altered mental status can be accounted for by these psychiatric disorders.[3]

Mood disorders, including anxiety and depression, are common, particularly among frail and institutionalized elderly persons. These mood disorders may have psychotic features.

Table 8–4 **Diagnostic Criteria for Dementia**

A. The development of multiple cognitive deficits manifested by both
  (1) memory impairment (impaired ability to learn new information or to recall previously learned information
  (2) one (or more) of the following cognitive disturbances:
    (a) aphasia (language disturbance)
    (b) apraxia (impaired ability to carry out motor activities despite intact motor function)
    (c) agnosta (failure to recognize or identify objects despite intact sensory function)
    (d) disturbance in executive functioning (i.e., planning, organizing, sequencing, abstracting)
B. The cognitive deficits in Criteria A1 and A2 each cause significant impairment in social or occupational functioning and represent a significant decline from a previous level of functioning.
C. The course is characterized by gradual onset and continuing cognitive decline.
D. The cognitive deficits in Criteria A1 and A2 are not due to any other disease entity.

Adapted from American Psychiatric Association: *Diagnostic and Statistical Manual of Mental Disorders,* Fourth edition. Washington DC, American Psychiatric Association, 1994

DELIRIUM

Any elderly patient with an acutely disturbed content of consciousness should be assumed to have delirium until it is ruled out and another diagnosis that may account for the patient's altered mental status is established. It is imperative that the emergency provider consider superimposed delirium within the differential diagnosis of patients presenting with worsened altered mental status who have a history of dementia or psychiatric illness, because elderly patients who have a psychiatric history or a diagnosis of dementia are very susceptible to developing delirium. Failure to recognize delirium is most likely to happen in the case of a patient with underlying dementia, psychiatric illness, or significant functional impairment, whose delirium may be misinterpreted as merely an exacerbation of dementia or worsening functional decline. Dementia is probably the greatest single risk factor for development of delirium, and up to two thirds of presentations in elderly patients have delirium superimposed on a pre-existing dementia.[4,5] Forty percent of demented elderly patients develop delirium sometime during their hospitalization.[6]

Elderly patients who have a psychiatric history or a diagnosis of dementia are very susceptible to developing delirium.

Although delirium has been recognized as a clinical syndrome since antiquity, it was not until 1980 when the third edition of the *Diagnostic and Statistical Manual (DSM)* was published that standardized diagnostic criteria were established. Minor revisions occurred in 1987 as *DSM-IIIR*.[7]

Inouye et al.[8] operationalized the diagnostic criteria for delirium based on *DSM-IIIR* standards. Their instrument, called the confusion assessment method (see CAM in Chapter 7), takes less than 5 minutes to complete and is a validated and reliable assessment tool to diagnose delirium in hospitalized elderly patients. Although other operational instruments are available[9] the CAM has growing acceptance as a research tool. Validation of this instrument in an ED setting is an active area of research at several EDs throughout the United States.

DSM-IV,[10] published in 1994, further defines, for research and clinical purposes, four broad categories of delirium: (1) delirium caused by a general medical condition, (2) substance-induced delirium, including intoxication and withdrawal syndromes. (3) delirium from multiple etiologies, and (4) delirium not otherwise specified. Table 8–5 details criteria for clinical application. For example, criteria A, B, and C are always present in a patient diagnosed with delirium, however, diagnostic specificity, and therefore appropriate management, is enhanced by consideration of etiology, as defined in criteria D through G. Delirium due to a general medical condition, therefore, would meet criteria A, B, C, and D, meaning there is evidence from the history, physical examination, or laboratory findings that the disturbance is caused by the direct physiologic consequences of a general medical condition. Delirium due to substance withdrawal would mean the patient exhibits criteria A, B, C, and F. Inouye recently published a review of controversial issues in the diagnosis of delirium,[11] observing that the diagnostic criteria for delirium continue to evolve, that diagnostic criteria remain somewhat difficult to apply clinically, and that current instruments lose sensitivity and specificity when delirium is superimposed on dementia.

Table 8–5 **General Diagnostic Criteria for Delirium**

A. Disturbance of consciousness (i.e., reduced clarity of awareness of environment) with reduced ability to focus, sustain, or shift attention.
B. A change in cognition (such as memory deficit, disorientation, language disturbance) or the development of a perceptual disturbance that is not better accounted for by a preexisting, established, or evolving dementia.
C. The disturbance develops over a short period of time (usually hours to days) and tends to fluctuate during the course of the day.

Additional criteria aid in establishing an etiologic diagnosis. These are used when there is evidence from the history, physical examination, or laboratory findings that the disturbance is caused by one of the following:

D. Direct physiologic consequences of a *general medical condition.*
E. *Substance abuse*
　1. The symptoms in Criteria A and B developed during *Substance Intoxication.* (This diagnosis should be made instead of a diagnosis of Substance Intoxication only when the cognitive symptoms are in excess of those usually associated with the intoxication syndrome and when the symptoms are sufficiently severe to warrant independent clinical attention.)
　2. *Substance-induced delirium* should be recorded as the diagnosis when medication use is etiologically related to the disturbance.
F. *Substance-withdrawal* delirium.
G. *Multiple etiologies* (e.g., more than one etiologic general medical condition, or a general medical condition plus substance intoxication or medication side effect.)

Adapted from American Psychiatric Association: *Diagnostic and Statistical Manual of Mental Disorders,* Fourth edition. Washigton DC, American Psychiatric Association, 1994

PREDISPOSING FACTORS AMONG THE ELDERLY

The elderly patient, particularly the oldest individuals and frail elderly, is uniquely prone to delirium because of anatomic, physiologic, psychiatric, cognitive, and metabolic senescent changes.[6,12–17] As a consequence, any condition that impairs cerebral metabolism and promotes neurotransmitter disequilibrium even modestly may precipitate a delirium. Such circumstances include conditions such as hypotension or uncontrolled hypertension, hypoglycemia, hypothermia or hyperthermia, hypoxia, electrolyte imbalance, dehydration, sensory deprivation, and medications at otherwise therapeutic doses.[18] In addition, almost any physical illness, no matter how minor, may precipitate delirium.

Recognized *risk factors* for delirium, in addition to age, cognitive impairment, functional impairment, severity of medical illness, and medications, include trauma, particularly hip fracture and closed head injury, surgery, and substance abuse.[19] Medications, both prescription and over-the-counter, remain the most common reversible cause of delirium[18] (Table 8-2). Nearly all classes of drugs have been associated with delirium in the elderly, even at therapeutic dosages. Diuretics, antidepressants, antipsychotics, anti-Parkinson agents, antihypertensives, antidysrhythmics including beta-antagonists and digitalis compounds, pain medications including narcotics, steroids, and H_2 receptor blockers are frequently associated with delirium. Over-the-

Failure to recognize delirium is most likely to happen when the patient has co-morbid conditions, such as dementia, psychiatric illness or significant functional impairment.

counter medications commonly implicated include antihistamines, cold remedies, sleep aids, and non-steroidal antiinflammatory drugs. The relative risk of altered mental status increases dramatically when the elderly patient takes multiple medications, because the effect is not additive but synergistic.[24]

Benzodiazepine-induced and alcohol withdrawal-induced altered mental status is common. Delirium tremens (DT), a syndrome seen with alcohol withdrawal, perhaps is the classic teaching model. DT is associated with significant mortality, up to 27% in one series.

GERIATRIC CASCADE

Infection of the urinary tract (UTI) is the most common infectious cause of delirium and illustrates a concept called the *geriatric cascade*. This concept represents the complex interplay of compromised host defense mechanisms, decreased physiologic reserve, pre-existing morbid conditions, atypical or subclinical symptom presentation, and perhaps decreased cognitive ability or aphasia.

Ten to 22% of elderly delirious patients died during their index hospitalization; 20% to 25% died in the first month; 39% died in 3 months; and 50% died within 2 years.

Uncomplicated UTI in younger patients is often easily diagnosed by presenting symptoms, readily confirmed by urinalysis, and effectively treated with oral medications. Often there are no compromised host defense mechanisms, comorbid diseases, or impediments to communication. Diagnosis is straightforward, and treatment is straightforward. In this setting, UTI is rarely associated with long-term morbidity or mortality.

In contrast, in the elderly population, particularly frail elderly persons, failure to diagnose UTI may lead to urosepsis, which has an extremely high morbidity and mortality. Roughly 50% of institutionalized elderly patients and virtually all elderly patients with long-term indwelling Foley catheters have bacteriuria, which often is asymptomatic. Frail elderly persons may have functional or cognitive impairment that affects effective clinical evaluation and detection. The patient may become agitated, necessitating treatment with medications or restraints, or perhaps may suffer a fall leading to hip fracture or closed head injury. Thus a relatively benign condition such as a UTI may be life threatening, and acute confusion or delirium may be the only sign of the underlying infection.

PREVALENCE AND INCIDENCE

With few exceptions, published studies based on *DSM-III* or *DSM-IIIR* criteria of the prevalence and incidence of delirium in the elderly population are based solely on hospitalized patients. A clue to the *prevalence* rate of delirium in the ED setting may be in research studies designed to screen elderly patients for delirium within 48 hours of hospital admission. These studies report a prevalence rate in this subgroup of 10% to 16% for medical patients, 10% to 15% for general surgery patients, 20% to 30% for patients with hip fracture, and 10% to 30% for psychiatric patients.[4,14,15,20–22]

The prevalence of delirium in the emergency department is not adequately known.

The *incidence* of delirium diagnosed during the course of hospitalization varies from 24% to over 50%, particularly in patients requiring intensive care and surgery.[13–15,23] Delirium that manifests after admission to the hospital is so common that Beresin believes it may be the most common adverse outcome for hospitalized elderly patients.[14]

The prevalence of delirium in older patients being evaluated in an ED setting is an area of active research and is not adequately known. Lewis and colleagues[24] were the first to report their research on the prevalence of delirium in an urban teaching hospital ED. They found 10% of elderly (65 years or older) patients evaluated met *DSM-IIIR* criteria of probable delirium using the CAM. In another study Naughton and colleagues found a 10% incidence of delirium in ED patients 70 years and older.[25]

PROGNOSIS

Delirium is a clinical marker signaling an underlying profound organic process that is associated with increased morbidity and mortality, lengthened hospitalization, and increased risk of institutionalization for those patients who survive. Delirium is a potential medical emergency.

An acute change in mental status that meets criteria for delirium may be the sole presenting feature among elderly patients subsequently diagnosed with a life-threatening condition such as myocardial infarction, cerebrovascular accident, pneumonia, gastrointestinal hemorrhage, meningitis, sepsis, or pulmonary embolism.

Review of several studies of elderly patients admitted to medical, surgical including orthopaedic, or psychiatric floors and subsequently diagnosed with delirium noted high mortality.[14] Ten to 30% of elderly delirious patients die during their index hospitalization. These earlier studies did not control for the effect of delirium independent of underlying comorbid disease or severity of illness. Recently published studies[5,19,26] controlled for severity of illness in the presence of delirium, and their analysis challenged whether or not delirium is an independent risk factor for increased mortality in the hospitalized elderly. The literature remains consistent that delirium is associated with significantly longer and more costly hospital stays, and with increased risk of long-term institutionalization[26,27]

Clinically, delirium by definition is a transient disorder. The supposition is that if delirium is accurately and rapidly diagnosed, and the underlying cause of the delirium is a condition that can be effectively treated, a majority of surviving patients will recover to or near their premorbid baseline. Francis[15] correctly notes, however, that reversibility is not part of the criteria for defining delirium—a point that Levkoff et al.[26] dramatically illustrated in a recent study that found only 4% of hospitalized patients diagnosed with delirium returned to their pre-delirium cognitive status before hospital discharge and only 20% of delirious patients returned to their cognitive baseline at 6 months.

In-hospital psychiatry services report that up to 50% of in-hospital patients for whom psychiatric consultation was obtained had unrecognized delirium.

MISDIAGNOSIS

Delirium in the elderly population is poorly documented, unrecognized, and misdiagnosed. Lewis et al.[24] reported only 13% of patients who met CAM criteria for delirium or probable delirium in an ED were diagnosed with delirium or equivalent terminology. A significant portion of patients who met criteria for delirium using the CAM instrument were subsequently discharged from the ED. Discharging a patient from the ED without recognizing delirium appears to place the patient at significant risk for morbidity and mortality. Preliminary results showed an increase in mortality in these patients sent home with delirium at 3-month follow-up, but the findings did not reach statistical significance ($P = .20$), in part because of the small number of patients in this subgroup.

PRE-HOSPITAL CONSIDERATIONS

Initial assessment and stabilization should focus on airway, breathing, and circulation, since delirious or comatose patients are critically ill. The patient may require airway adjuncts, intubation, or respiratory support. Administer supplemental oxygen and monitor oxygen saturation via pulse oximetry if available. Vital signs must be taken frequently. A cardiac monitor is essential to assess cardiac stability. Emergency medical services (EMS) personnel should be vigilant, because patients with an alteration in mental status may deteriorate rapidly during transport. The potential for cervical spine injury should always be considered in the overall management of the patient, particularly in those older patients with a history of trauma or evidence of trauma on physical examination.

Vital signs including temperature must be taken promptly as a guide to initial supportive or resuscitative efforts. As intravenous (IV) access is established, determine the blood glucose level in the field, if feasible. Retain a blood sample for subsequent confirmation in the ED. Even if EMS personnel are unable to obtain a blood sample, empiric treatment with one ampule of D50 intravenously is indicated as rapidly as possible. When IV access is unobtainable, buccal administration of concentrated glucose is a useful alternative. However, the emergency care provider should administer the buccal glucose with the patient in a side-lying position if feasible to prevent possible aspiration of the glucose solution.

Elderly patients with altered mental status with a recent or proximate history of trauma, or with evidence of trauma on physical examination, should be considered for entrance into a trauma system even when lateralizing neurologic findings are not present.

An acute change in mental status may be the sole presenting feature of myocardial infarction, pneumonia, gastrointestinal hemorrhage, sepsis, or pulmonary embolism.

For the elderly patient with a clinical presentation consistent with Wernicke-Korsakoff syndrome, IV or intramuscular (IM) administration of 100 mg of thiamine before the glucose infusion may help prevent an exacerbation of symptoms. The syndrome is most common among elderly patients with malabsorption, malnourishment, and chronic alcohol use. Wernicke's encephalopathy may manifest as oculomotor dysfunction, confusion, or ataxia. Korsakoff's psychosis consists of apathy, amnesia, and logorrheic confabulation.

The frail elderly patient may be unusually susceptible to narcotic medications, even at "therapeutic" doses, presenting with somnolence and unresponsiveness. Paradoxically, the elderly patient may present with hallucinations, agitation, and confusion when he or she is prescribed narcotics.[15] Narcotic withdrawal syndromes are associated with delirium, and the administration of naloxone may worsen the clinical presentation. Routine utilization of naloxone is reserved for the elderly patient who presents with decreased respiratory drive, somnolence, and unresponsiveness. The confused and agitated patient should not be given naloxone.

Patients with access to benzodiazepines may present a similar clinical spectrum to that associated with narcotics. A benzodiazepine withdrawal syndrome almost always includes confusion and agitation. Administration of the benzodiazepine antagonist flumazinil may dramatically worsen the clinical presentation, including status epilepticus, particularly if the patient is taking tricyclic medications. Therefore flumazinil in the pre-hospital setting should rarely if ever be administered.

Safety of the patient and EMS personnel is paramount. Delirious, agitated patients may be dangerous to themselves and to personnel helping them. The delirious patient may need to be restrained to prevent removal of an endotracheal tube or IV line or becoming assaultive. This is particularly important in aeromedical transport. When appropriate, physical restraint is preferred, although chemical restraint may be used in unusual circumstances. Regardless of the methodology of the restraint, pre-hospital personnel must be familiar with state and local laws and follow existing protocols. The restrained patient is directly observed at all times and monitored closely for respiratory effort and level of consciousness.

The ideal therapeutic agent for chemical restraint does not exist. Ideally the agent should be able to be administered without an IV line if necessary, have a rapid onset and a short half-life, be reversible, and have no side effects such as hypotension or a reduction in respiratory drive. Droperidol and haloperidol are phenothiazines commonly used for chemical restraint. Initial doses should be lower for elderly persons than for younger adults (i.e., 1-2 mg haloperidol intramuscularly or intravenously, 0.75 mg droperidol intramuscularly or intravenously). When closed head injury, alcohol, or benzodiazepine withdrawal delirium is present, or if the agitated or violent patient is post-ictal, the tranquilizing agent of choice is a benzodiazepine with the same characteristics described above. Lorazepam at initial IV or IM doses of 1 mg is often useful in this circumstance.

INITIAL EMERGENCY DEPARTMENT ASSESSMENT AND STABILIZATION

Patients with altered mental status may be critically ill and need immediate intervention. Again, initial methods for assessment and stabilization are determined by the status of the patient's airway, breathing, and circulation. If glucose was not administered in the field, the emergency physician may immediately check blood glucose and treat if indicated. Thiamine and naloxone are also considered, depending on the history and presentation.

Once the patient has been resuscitated and stabilized, the ED physician must search for the underlying cause of the delirium using a directed history, physical examination, and diagnostic tests. The patient with altered mental status does not, by definition of the condition, have decision-making capacity; therefore, emergency assessment and management are governed by implied consent and the emergency

Myoclonus and asterixis when present are pathognomonic for delirium.

rule, unless contravening requests exist by a legitimate health care proxy or guardian.

HISTORY

An attempt to get information directly from the awake patient yields important information even if the ED physician suspects the patient has a disturbed content of consciousness. Should the patient's speech be disorganized, rambling, nonsensical, or incoherent, little reliable information would be obtained from further history taking from the patient alone. Thus the physician's time is most efficiently spent obtaining information from others.

The patient with a more subtle derangement in content of consciousness is more difficult to accurately diagnose. Simple assessments such as determining orientation to person, place, day of the week, reciting days of the week backward, or correctly identifying loved ones who accompanied the patient to the ED may help identify an impediment. The ED clinician subsequently could ask the patient to repeat and then recall at one-minute 3 items as a screening tool. If the patient is unable to repeat the 3 items, even with prompting, formal mental status testing, with the Folstein Mini-Mental State Exam (MMSE) and the Confusion Assessment Method (CAM) should be undertaken.

Information is gathered from as many sources as feasible, including family members, companions, caregivers, EMS personnel, and the patient's primary physician. Information about the patient's baseline functional and cognitive status, as well as the onset, progression, and temporal course of symptoms and signs, is obtained. Closed head injury precipitated by a ground-level fall may be overlooked as a cause of the patient's condition, particularly if the fall occurred days to weeks prior to the ED presentation.

Review of the patient's ADLs and IADLs (Chapter 7) may reveal a recent worsening of functional status such as inability to feed oneself or incontinence and may reflect an accurate temporal course of the altered mental state. New-onset incontinence is the most common presentation of delirium.

Medication history is critical not only for identifying all current prescription and over-the-counter drugs, but also for learning if any medications have recently been started or stopped, or if doses have been increased, decreased.[10,15,18] Medications remain the most common single cause of reversible delirium.

PHYSICAL EXAMINATION

A thorough physical examination is warranted to look for medical or surgical causes for the patient's condition. The general appearance of the patient may give important and subtle clues to the patient's underlying condition and acuity. Take the time to observe the patient not only while the patient is interacting with other staff or family, but also when the patient is not conversing. The patient may appear lethargic, agitated, confused, or attending to irrelevant internal or external stimuli.

A patient's responses to your questions may be perseverant; alternatively, the patient may stop mid-task or mid-sentence, as though he or she has forgottten what is supposed to be done. Classically, a delirious patient may fall asleep mid-sentence or when physical or verbal stimulation is absent. Remember, physical evidence of proximate trauma may be subtle. The underlying cause often may be found efficiently by this approach, confirmed as necessary by selected laboratory and ancillary tests.

Tachycardia, diaphoresis, fever, and relative hypertension or hypotension secondary to autonomic instability should be sought, as well as evidence of dehydration. A structured and meticulous neurologic examination to look for focal neurologic signs should be undertaken. The neurologic examination is the most critical aspect of the physical examination in patients with altered mental status after the patient has been stabilized. The neurologic examination should include an assessment of pupillary and cranial nerve function as well as a meticulous examination for sensory and motor (including reflex) lateralizing signs. Oculocephalogyric (caloric) tests may be helpful with unusual clinical presentations for the ED clinician and are beyond the scope of this discussion. Focal neurologic deficits are considered new unless evidence to the contrary is available from the caregiver, primary physician, or medical record. Myoclonus and asterixis when present are pathognomonic for delirium.

DIAGNOSTIC TESTS

Knowing what diagnostic tests to order is problematic since the causes of altered mental status are numerous and the diseases within the differential diagnosis cover the widest spectrum, from UTI to myocardial infarction (see Table 8–1).

An incomplete or inadequate examination is not likely to shed light on the underlying etiology, causing the clinician to rely on a shotgun approach to laboratory tests and imaging modalities.

INSTRUMENTS TO EVALUATE LEVEL OF CONSCIOUSNESS

Instruments to evaluate and objectify altered mental status have been developed. Clinicians often are familiar with the instruments and tests that are utilized to evaluate a decreased level of consciousness. The mnemonic AVPU subjectively and hierarchically characterizes the patient's level of consciousness from alert (A) to unresponsive (U) (Figure 8–1).

A   Alert
V   Responds to Vocal stimuli
P   Responds only to Painful stimuli
U   Unresponsive

The primary practical and clinical limitation to AVPU is that it has not been predictive of patient outcome. The Glasgow Coma Scale (GCS) (Table 8–6) is an instrument that provides a quantitative and

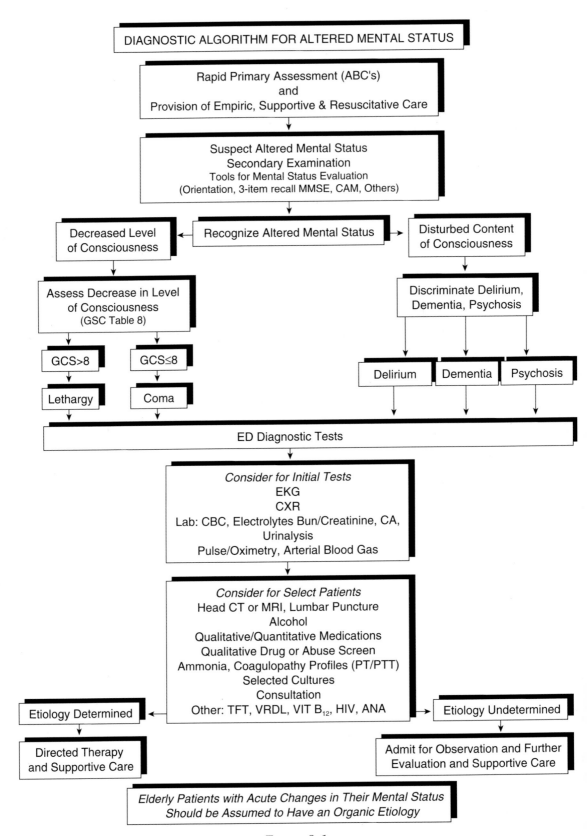

FIGURE 8–1

Table 8–6 **Glasgow Coma Scale (GCS)**

1. Eye-opening response (E)
   a. Spontaneous (already open with blinking): E = (4)
   b. To speech (not necessarily to a request for eye opening): E = (3)
   c. To pain: E = (2)
   d. None: E = (1)
2. Verbal response (V)
   a. Oriented (knows name, age, etc.): V = (5)
   b. Confused conversation (still answers questions): V = (4)
   c. Inappropriate words (speech is either exclamatory or random, but recognizable words are produced): V = (3)
   d. Incomprehensible sounds (grunts and groans are produced, but no actual words are uttered; do not confuse with partial respiratory obstruction) V = (2)
   e. None: V = (1)
3. Best motor response (M)
   a. Obeys (moves limb to command and pain is not required): M = (6)
   b. Localizes (changing the location of the pain stimulus causes purposeful motion toward the stimulus): M = (5)
   c. Withdraws (pulls away from painful stimulus): M - (4)
   d. Abnormal flexion (decorticate posture): M = (3)
   e. Extensor response (decerebrate posture): M = (2)
   f. No movement: M = (1)

Coma defined as no eye opening (E = 1), no word verbalization (V = 1-2), no ability to follow commands (M = 1-5). All patients with a GCS below 8 are comatose, most patients with GCS of 8 are comatose as well.

Adapted with permission from *Resources for Optimal Care of the Injured Patient: 1993,* Committee on Trauma, American College of Surgeons, p. 20.

objective measure of level of consciousness, developed as a field assessment for trauma. The patient is assessed in three particular areas: eye opening (E), verbal responsiveness (V), and best motor response (M). Each area has a maximum score (E = 4, V = 5, and M = 6). The GCS score is summative. The maximum score, 15, is representative of a normal level and content of consciousness. For purposes of outcomes research, coma as a descriptor of decreased level of consciousness, has been set at a GCS of 8 or less. Scores greater than 8 and less than 15 indicate an altered mental status but are not representative of coma (Figure 8-1).

Clinically, the value of using either the AVPU or the GCS tool is that it forces the clinician to look at the patient's level of consciousness. Neither the AVPU nor the CGS tool was designed to evaluate content of consciousness, and both are most useful when the decreased level of consciousness is due to a mass lesion or head injury.

INSTRUMENTS TO EVALUATE CONTENT OF CONSCIOUSNESS

A formal evaluation of the patient's current mental status is necessary, addressing cognition, mood, and behavior. Two instruments are valuable to perform in the setting of altered content of consciousness. The

Folstein Mini-Mental State Examination (MMSE) (Figure 7–1) is a valid and reliable 30-point instrument to measure cognitive status of the patient but is not designed specifically to discriminate delirium from dementia or affective disorders.[28] Scores of 23 or less are considered abnormal. However, Folstein and Folstein reported 30% of patients diagnosed with delirium had scores of 23 or higher, indicating this instrument is not sensitive to diagnosing delirium.[16]

The CAM, or confusion assessment method,[8] (Figure 7–2) is based on *DSM-IIIR* criteria for delirium and is currently being revised to reflect *DSM-IV*. The instrument may stand alone when its four features are specifically sought by the emergency care provider:

1. acute onset or fluctuating course,
2. inattention,
3. disorganized thinking, and
4. altered level of consciousness

However, information obtained in concert with the Folstein MMSE and the history and physical examination may also be utilized. The diagnosis of delirium requires the presence of features 1 *and* 2, and either 3 *or* 4. After the physician has made the diagnosis, attention should focus on finding the underlying cause of the delirium.

LABORATORY TESTS AND IMAGING MODALITIES

Tests that should be routinely considered in most elderly patients with altered mental status include chest roentgenogram, electrocardiogram (ECG), complete blood count, urinalysis, and admission panel with electrolytes, including calcium and liver function tests.

An *electrocardiogram* can be helpful in elderly patients, since 60% of persons older than 80 years do not have chest pain in association with acute myocardial infarction, and altered mental status may be the sole presenting feature.

A *chest roentgenogram* and pulse oximetry or arterial blood gases are indicated in patients with a possible acute pulmonary process or congestive heart failure.

An *arterial blood gas* (ABG) should be obtained with the initial battery of laboratory and ancillary tests, but usually does not reveal an etiology.

In the elderly patient with hypothermia or fever in whom an occult infectious cause of the delirium is suspected, selected cultures will help guide inpatient management. The erythrocyte sedimentation rate (ESR) plays little role in the ED evaluation of the elderly patient with altered mental status, because the ESR is neither sensitive nor specific and is often elevated in the healthy older person.

If the emergency provider has not found a specific etiology to account for the patient's altered mental status, further laboratory tests may be considered for selected patients. Patients taking certain medications associated with altered mental status that may be quantified such as digoxin, theophylline, lithium, tricyclic antidepressants, or aspirin may have drug levels assessed in the ED. Often the patient's history and physical examination will give additional clues to a suspicion of medication toxicity. Screens for drugs of abuse rarely play a role except in very selected circumstances. Acute alcohol intoxication may be the underlying cause of the delirium and of other forms of altered mental status. If alcohol intoxication is suspected, quantification of serum alcohol should be obtained.

The elderly patient with gastrointestinal bleeding and abnormal hepatic metabolism may have hepatic encephalopathy, a well-recognized and common cause of delirium. Serum ammonia levels may support the diagnosis.

Those individuals who present with a history or signs and symptoms of suspected head trauma and an altered mental status, even in the absence of focal neurologic deficits, should have a non-contrast head computed tomography (CT) scan performed.

Elderly patients presenting with altered mental status and new focal neurologic deficits should have a CT scan performed without contrast, although fewer than 10% of cases of delirium are associated with acute central nervous system (CNS) lesions.[29]

For patients with evidence of infection as the underlying cause but in whom no source of infection is found after thorough physical examination and screening laboratory tests, a spinal tap should be performed. For those patients with a focal neurologic examination and evidence of CNS infection, a head CT scan with and without contrast is obtained before the spinal tap.

Thyroid function tests, vitamin B_{12}, VDRL, and HIV antibody tests may yield important information; however, the results routinely are not available soon enough to impact medical decision making in the ED.

EMERGENCY DEPARTMENT MANAGEMENT AND DISPOSITION

As with any type of potential medical emergency, many diagnostic and therapeutic steps are undertaken simultaneously and not sequentially (Figure 8-1). Management of the elderly patient with altered mental status is based on the following principles:

1. Rapid primary assessment and subsequent provision of empiric, supportive, or resuscitative care before confirmation of cause (for example, empiric glucose administration in a patient with altered mental status)
2. Recognition of altered (or worsened) mental status, assuming a significant organic cause
3. Broad categorization of the patient with altered mental status as having either (a) a decreased level of consciousness or (b) a disturbed content of consciousness
4. In patients with primarily a disturbed content of consciousness, differentiation of delirium from dementia and psychosis
5. Diagnosis of the underlying cause (or causes) with reevaluation as data base evolves
6. Frequent reassessment and monitoring as directed treatment and supportive care are given

Altered mental status manifests as either a decreased level of consciousness, an altered content of consciousness, or a combination of disorders and can be categorized broadly into five groups.

1. Disease states affecting the central nervous system indirectly and diffusely
2. Primary central nervous system disease
3. Psychiatric disorders
4. Dementias
5. Multifactorial or no clearly defined etiology

Most elderly patients with acute changes in mental status are admitted to hospital for further work-up and observation. Some patients who have subacute or chronic cognitive impairment (dementia) may be discharged providing (a) prompt medical follow up and (b) safe home environment with reliable caregiver are assured.

The management and disposition of patients with altered mental status will depend upon the dignostic category that best fits the diagnostic tests and patient presentation. The causes of altered mental status may be categorized into four groups, adapted from *DSM-IV* discussed below. A fifth category (no clearly identified etiology) is also discussed.

CAUSES AFFECTING THE CENTRAL NERVOUS SYSTEM DIFFUSELY

The most common etiology of altered mental status in the elderly is not primary central nervous system disease, but rather is a systemic effect of metabolic or physiologic derangements, such as hypoxia, hypoglycemia, electrolyte disturbance, or non-CNS infection. Management should be directed at finding the underlying etiology, treating those reversible causes and providing supportive care to correct any metabolic or physiologic derangements.

Patients with delirium or decreased mental status should be hospitalized.

Disease processes with systemic effects associated with altered mental status in the elderly population are protean. Each disease process has a characteristic history, physical examination, and laboratory findings. It is unfortunate that many diseases present subclinically, subtly, or atypically in elderly persons, making the initial diagnosis more challenging. In systemic illness, focal signs may not be found (Table 8–1). Assume that the elderly patient who presents with altered mental status has a treatable, reversible organic cause. Patients with delirium or decreased mental status should be hospitalized. Patient stability, cause of the altered mental status, and level of acuity determine admission status (intensive care or observation ward).

Elderly patients who present with altered mental status in which the cause is traditionally treated as an outpatient (such as UTI) still should generally be hospitalized. They remain at significant risk for falls, dehydration, or wandering away. Even if the cause is readily and rapidly treatable, as in the above circumstance, the altered mental status often remains far longer than the precipitating cause. If the patient is discharged, it must be to a safe and structured environment where the patient will be constantly monitored. Most nursing homes, foster homes, and families do not have the resources to provide such an environment.

The role of *medication* in inducing altered mental status in the elderly population should not be understated and deserves elaboration. It remains the most common cause of altered mental status in this age group. Importantly, an altered mental status caused by therapeutic agents is likely to be reversed if the drug is stopped.

> *Medications are the most common cause of altered mental status in the elderly.*

PRIMARY CENTRAL NERVOUS SYSTEM DISEASE

Primary central nervous system disease, unless manifest with acute onset of focal neurological deficit such as seen in certain CVA syndromes or with clinically relevant clinical findings such as meningismus in the febrile patient with altered mental status, may present quite subtly. As mentioned earlier, often there are objective neurological findings when the neurological examination is thorough.

Primary CNS disease should always be entertained if the initial laboratory and ancillary tests do not identify the etiology. Neurological consultation after initial ED evaluation may be warranted. If the etiology of the patient's decreased LOC or altered content of consciousness is not found, a brian-imaging study such as CT or MRI is indicated, often followed by a lumbar puncture. The timing of such imaging is dependent on the presentation of the patient. For instance, if a patient presents with a significantly reduced level of consciousness, with meningeal signs and headache, emergent CT and subsequent LP are standard of care. If, however, the patient presents to the ED with behavioral changes and aggressiveness without lateralizing neurological signs, the patient would likely get an urgent or routine brain imaging study, followed by the LP.

Brain tumors, mass lesions such as subdural and epidural hemorrhages, and strokes that manifest as altered mental status in the elderly patient *without* focal neurologic findings are exceedingly rare. The primary CNS infections of meningitis, encephalitis, and abscess typically present with fever, an elevation in the white blood cell (WBC) count, and meningismus. However, the elderly patient may present without fever, abnormal WBC count, or meningeal signs, particularly if the patient has severe cognitive and functional impairment, is malnourished, or is taking immunosuppressive medications.

Seizures in elderly persons may have a very prolonged post-ictal state with altered mental status. Non-convulsive status epilepticus and partial complex status epilepticus are recognized neurologic diseases that may be very difficult to diagnose. An electroencephalogram may be helpful in this setting.

PSYCHIATRIC DISORDER

Elderly patients with a history of psychiatric disease or dementia represent a significant challenge to the ED clinician. A history of either dementia or psychiatric disease not only is a well-recognized risk factor for developing delirium, but both conditions are notorious for masking superimposed delirium.

It is possible for elderly patients to present with altered mental status caused by a new-onset functional psychiatric disorder, but this is very rare without a history of previous schizophrenia or bipolar disorder. Again, the emergency care provider should assume a non-psychiatric precipitation of the patient's altered mental status until a thorough workup is completed. Delirium superimposed on psychiatric illness may be particularly hard to determine in the ED setting. Psychiatric consultation after ED evaluation may be warranted. The patient should be admitted to the hospital for observation and further evaluation. Psychiatric disposition before a thorough evaluation for medical or neurologic causes should be discouraged.

DEMENTIA

Critical Question: Is presentation caused by a natural progression of the patient's underlying dementia or by a superimposed delirium?

Two scenarios may confront the emergency care provider evaluating elderly patients with dementia. In the first case an elderly patient with a well-documented diagnosis of dementia is brought to the ED for evaluation of agitation, aggressive behavior, new incontinence, inability to get out of bed, or other issues relating to activities of daily living. The critical question is as follows: Is this presentation caused by a natural progression of the patient's underlying dementia or by a superimposed delirium? A superficial approach to evaluation is unlikely to reveal any superimposed delirium or allow diagnosis of the underlying cause of the delirium. The charge to the emergency care provider is to consider the patient to have an altered (here worsened) mental status and aggressively investigate the patient's condition. Only after a thorough evaluation and negative workup is it appropriate to discharge the patient from the ED.

Critical Question: Does patient have unrecognized dementia or is some behavior or cognitive trait manifesting that requires ED evaluation?

In the second scenario the elderly patient is brought to the ED for similar complaints but without a suspicion or diagnosis of dementia. From the history obtained from the patient and caregivers, abnormal mental status is evident. Here the question is as follows: has this person had an unrecognized dementia and is this patient now manifesting some behavior or cognitive trait that is sufficiently disconcerting to the patient or caregiver to warrant ED evaluation? Again, a thorough workup is warranted to look for reversible causes of altered mental status. It is unfortunate that the CAM is less sensitive and specific in this scenario for detecting delirium than it is in other scenarios. The MMSE can detect cognitive deficits but is unable to discriminate whether the deficits are new or old. Thus the emergency care provider may not be able to determine in the ED the nature of the altered mental status. If the patient's workup is negative, the patient should be admitted for observation and further assessment. Under unusual circumstances the patient may be discharged to a responsible caregiver for prompt outpatient workup of the dementia if a safe environment in the interim is ensured.

COMA AND DECREASED LEVEL OF CONSCIOUSNESS

Decreased level of consciousness represents a wide spectrum of clinical presentations from the comatose patient unable to protect his or her airway, breathe spontaneously, or respond to stimuli to a sleep-deprived house staff unable to keep his or her eyes open or talk without some external stimulation. Dozens of terms have been utilized to describe this continuum of decreased level of consciousness, including stupor, lethargy, and obtundation. These terms lack precision of definition and clinical applicability. What one clinician generalizes to represent lethargy may fit another clinician's description of obtundation. Emergency clinicians should instead describe the patient's responses to various stimuli. Both the mnemonic AVPU and the GCS utilize a more objective and structured assessment of the patient's level of consciousness and are particularly valuable for accurate communication between emergency care providers as well as for serial examinations of the patient.

Patients with altered mental status invariably present with compromise to a certain extent of both their level of consciousness and their content of consciousness. Those patients with a GCS of 8 or below are particularly vulnerable and require immediate assessment (ABCs) and resuscitation. As with any type of altered mental status, the underlying etiology or etiologies of the patient's comatose state or protean and include a broad spectrum of medical, surgical, neurological, and psychiatric illness as illustrated by Table 8–7.

Table 8–7 **Final Diagnosis in 500 Patients Admitted to Hospital with "Coma of Unknown etiology"**

Supratentorial mass lesions	101
Intracerebral hematoma	44
Subdural hematoma	26
Epidural hematoma	4
Cerebral infarct	9
Thalamic infarct	2
Brain tumor	7
Pituitary apoplexy	2
Brain abscess	6
Closed-head injury	1
Subtentorial lesions	65
Brainstem infarct	40
Pontine hemorrhage	11
Brainstem demyelination	1
Cerebellar hemorrhage	5
Cerebellar tumor	3
Cerebellar infarct	2
Cerebellar abscess	1
Posterior fossa subdural hemorrhage	1
Basilar migraine	1
Metabolic and other diffuse disorders	326
Anoxia or ischemia	87
Hepatc encephalopathy	17
Uremic encephalopathy	8
Pulmonary disease	3
Endocrine disorders (including diabetes)	12
Acid-base disorders	12
Temperature regulation	9
Nutritional	1
Nonspecific metabolic coma	1
Encephalomyelitis and encephalitis	14
Subasrachnoid hemorrhage	13
Drug poisoning	149
Psychiatric disorders	8

From Adams RD, Ed. Principles of neurology. 5th ed. New York: McGraw-Hill;1993:308

Initial assessment should focus on patency and adequacy of the airway, including gag response, and adequacy of breathing. Intubation should be considered to protect the airway and ensure adequate oxygenation. Empirical therapy with glucose, naloxone, or thiamin must be considered. Naloxone use should be selective. When clinically indicated in coma of unknown etiology, naloxone may prevent a patient from undergoing intubation by reversing the effect of narcotic medication.

Patients with a GCS of 9 or greater are not comatose clinically but may rapidly deteriorate, thus requiring serial neurological assessment. This group of patients also presents unique challenges to the emergency provider. They almost always are uncooperative, and often are aggressive, even combative. Chemical tranquilization or sedation may make the patient less combative and the ED environment less chaotic, but at the potential cost of further decreasing the patient's level of consciousness and ability to safely maintain and protect his or her airway. Conversely, physical restraint may worsen the patient's agitation and physically injure the patient. Physical restraint must be designed to protect the airway from aspiration. Patients who are chemically or physically restrained must have continuous one-on-one observation.

NO CLEARLY IDENTIFIED ETIOLOGY

Often the cause of the altered mental status is multifactorial, but in a significant minority of cases, the cause is never found, despite detailed evaluation in the ED. These patients should be hospitalized for observation and further evaluation. Even if the cause remains cryptic, mortality, morbidity, length of hospitalization, and risk of institutionalization are all increased.

SUMMARY POINTS

- Delirium in the elderly is associated with significant mortality and increased morbidity, length of hospitalization, and risk of institutionalization.
- Delirium is commonly misdiagnosed and not recognized.
- Assume every elderly patient with acute mental status changes to be delirious until proven otherwise.
- The elderly patient with delirium should be admitted to the hospital for further work up and treatment.

CHAPTER AUTHOR

Norm Kalbfleisch, MD, FACEP

REFERENCES

1. Hodkinson HM. Mental impairment in the elderly. *J R Coll Physicians.* 1973;7:305–317.
2. Adams RD, Ed. *Principles of neurology.* 5th ed. New York: McGraw-Hill; 1993:300.
3. Tueth MJ, Cheong JA. Delirium: diagnosis and treatment in the older patient. *Geriatrics.* 1993;48:75–80

4. Levkoff SE. Acute confusional states (delirium) in the hospitalized elderly. *Ann Rev Gerontol Geriatr.* 1986;6:1–26.
5. Francis J, Kapoor WN. Delirium in the hospitalized elderly. *J Gen Intern Med.* 1990;5:65–79.
6. Pousada L. Common neurologic emergencies in the elderly population, geriatric emergency care. *Clin Geriatr Med.* 1993;9(3):577–580.
7. American Psychiatric Association. *Diagnostic and statistical manual of mental disorders: DSM-III.* 3rd ed., revised. Washington, DC: American Psychiatric Press;1987.
8. Inouye SK et al. Clarifying confusion: the confusion assessment method. *Ann Intern Med.* 1990;113:941–948.
9. Levkoff S, Leptzin B, Cleary P, et al. Review of research instruments and techniques used to detect delirium. *Int Psychogeriatrics.* 1991;3(2):253–271.
10. American Psychiatric Association. Delirium, dementia, and amnestic and other cognitive disorders. In: *Diagnostic and statistical methodology: DSM-IV.* Washington, DC: American Psychiatric Press;1994.
11. Inouye SK. The dilemma of delirium: clinical and research controversies regarding diagnosis and evaluation of delirium in hospitalized elderly patients. *Am J Med.* 1994;97:278–288.
12. Johnson JC. Delirium in the elderly. *Emerg Med Clin North Am.* 1990;18(2): 255–265.
13. Lipowski ZJ. Delirium in the elderly patient. *N Engl J Med.* 1989;320: 578–582.
14. Beresin EV. Delirium in the elderly. *J Geriatr Psychiatry Neurol.* 1988;1:127–143.
15. Francis J. Delirium in older patients. *J Am Geriatr Soc.* 1992;40:829–838.
16. Folstein MF, Folstein SE. Syndromes of altered mental state. In: *Principles of geriatric medicine and gerontology.* Hazzard & Andres. 2nd ed. New York: McGraw-Hill, 1990; 1089–1101.
17. Tueth MJ, Cheong JA. Delirium: diagnosis and treatment in the older patient. *Geriatrics.* 1993;48:75–80.
18. Stewart RB. Acute confusional states in older adults and the role of polypharmacy. *Annual Rev Health.* 1992;13:415–430.
19. Shor JD et al. Risk factors for delirium in hospitalized elderly. *JAMA.* 1992; 267(6):827–831.
20. Johnson JC et al. Prospective versus retrospective methods of identifying patients with delirium. *J Am Geriatr Soc.* 1992;40:316–319.
21. Gustafson Y et al. Underdiagnosis and poor documentation of acute confusional states in elderly hip fracture patients. *J Am Geriatr Soc.* 1991;39: 760–765.
22. Francis J et al. A prospective study of delirium in hospitalized elderly. *JAMA.* 1990;263(8):1097–1101.
23. Inouye SK. A predictive model for delirium in hospitalized elderly medical patients based on admission characteristics. *Ann Intern Med.* 1993;119: 474–481.
24. Lewis LM, Miller DK, Morley JE et al. Unrecognized delirium in ED geriatric patients. *Am J Emerg Med.* 1995;13:142–145.
25. Naughton BJ, Moran MB, Kadah H, Heman-Ackah Y, Longano J. Delirium and other cognitive impairment in older adults in an emergency department. *Ann Emerg Med.* 1995;25:751–755.
26. Levkoff SE et al. Delirium: the occurrence and persistence of symptoms among elderly hospitalized patients. *Arch Intern Med.* 1992;152:334–340.
27. Francis J, Kapoor WN. Prognosis after hospital discharge of older patients with delirium. *J Am Geriatr Soc.* 1992;40:601–606.
28. Folstein SE, Folstein MF, et al. The Folstein mini-mental state examination: a practical method for grading the cognitive state of patients for the clinician. *J Psychiatr Res.* 1975;12:189–198.

29. Francis J, Hilko EM. Acute mental changes, when are head scans needed. *Clin Res.* 1991;39:103. (Abstract.)

SELECTED READINGS

Levkoff S. Epidemiology of delirium: an overview of research issues and findings. *Int Psychogeriatrics.* 1991;3(2):149–167.

Sanders AB. Recognition of cognitive problems in older adults by emergency medicine personnel. *Ann Emerg Med.* 1995;25:831–833.

9 *Functional Decline*

LEARNING OBJECTIVES

1. Explain the diagnostic and prognostic importance of functional decline in the ED evaluation and management.
2. Demonstrate appropriate application of instruments commonly used to assess functional disability.
3. Identify functional decline by applying specific instruments in combination with a medical history that emphasizes time landmarks.
4. Provide a differential diagnosis for functional decline.
5. Demonstrate proper evaluation of functional decline and determine when it can be safely ascribed to "physiologic" aging.
6. Identify methods for management or referral of patients with functional decline not referable to intercurrent medical illness.

Functional decline may be defined as recent or progressive difficulty or inability in performing various tasks that are necessary or highly desirable for independent living. The qualifier "recent" is intended to reinforce that the impairments are relatively new and that the tasks were at one time within the capabilities of the elderly patient. Thus, by definition, the recognition of functional decline requires some appreciation of premorbid functioning with regard to these tasks.

These personal or self-care tasks have been defined in a variety of ways, but they are most frequently measured using the activities of daily living (ADLs) scale[1] (see Figure 7–4). ADLs are feeding, toileting, grooming, dressing, bathing, and transferring (e.g., from bed to chair). If an elderly patient cannot perform these without assistance, then safe, independent living is highly unlikely. In fact, ADL impairment usually means that the patient requires a caregiver, paid or unpaid, to provide assistance. Thus the appearance of one or more new ADL impairments is of concern and may either be the chief complaint in an ED presentation or, alternatively, be discovered as an incidental finding when the patient presents with a more traditional chief complaint.

A second and higher level of function is linked more closely with the ability to maintain and manage a household. The IADL (instrumental activities of daily living) scale (see Figure 7–5) includes more sophisticated abilities, such as shopping, using the telephone, doing housework, and handling finances.[2] These are likely to become impaired before ADLs as underlying chronic disorders advance, but IADL impairments are of themselves probably less likely to result in an ED visit.

There are two errors that the ED physician can make with regard to functional decline. The first is to miss it. The second is to recognize it and to perfunctorily dismiss it as "normal aging."

The emergency health care professional can make two errors in the care of elderly patients with regard to functional decline. The first is to miss it. The second is to recognize it and to perfunctorily dismiss it as normal aging without an appropriate evaluation. Much of this chapter is dedicated to minimizing these two errors.

Functional decline is typically missed when it is not ascertained in a formal or structured way, such as with the use of instruments (validated questionnaires or assessments intended to cover the appropriate domains). Whatever comprises the tasks to be considered when assessing for functional decline, they should be determined in a standardized manner.

Functional decline is typically dismissed because it is often attributed to "normal aging." However, medical illness in elderly persons often presents with functional decline instead of with signs and symptoms traditionally referable to specific diseases. The appropriate posture in the ED is to assume that functional decline is a symptom of new underlying medical illness or established chronic diseases that are decompensating. Some examples include the following:

1. Coronary ischemia presenting as immobility instead of chest pain
2. Pneumonia presenting as confusion or a decline in self-care instead of dyspnea
3. Uncontrolled diabetes presenting as incontinence instead of polyuria

Thus the ED physician should be skilled in the recognition and evaluation of functional decline.

ASSESSING FUNCTIONAL DECLINE

The most valuable tool in assessing functional decline is the patient history and, whenever possible, corroborating or additional history from a caregiver or family member who is in a position to comment objectively on functional impairments that are new or have worsened. Two of the most commonly used instruments (standardized evaluations) for evaluating functional decline are the Katz ADL and Lawton

IADL scales (see Figure 7–4 and Figure 7–5). Although ADL impairment is a more common reason for an elderly person to be brought to the ED, the presence of any functional impairment should prompt the examiner to inquire about all these domains. Whereas some authorities have suggested obtaining this information in a dichotomous fashion (i.e., able vs. unable), others have suggested that a third response (able with assistance) provides a finer gradation with which to evaluate the overall picture of decline. Several aspects of the history are crucial in evaluating functional decline:

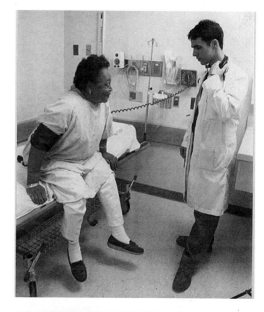

1. Landmarks should be used whenever possible to determine the trajectory of the decline. For example, if family members cannot reach a consensus to the question "when was your father last able to dress himself without your assistance?", offer time landmarks. For example, "Could your father dress himself without assistance last Christmas?"
2. When a functional impairment is present the clinician should determine how long it has been present.
3. The acute onset of a functional impairment suggests an acute underlying process (e.g., stroke) as opposed to a gradually progressive one (e.g., dementia).
4. The complete inability to reach consensus among family members as to the precise onset of ADL impairment suggests the unfolding natural history of chronic diseases as opposed to acute decompensations or new events.
5. When multiple ADL impairments are present, attempt to determine their chronology of onset. In the absence of specific disease processes that impact on a single ADL (e.g., a spinal cord lesion causing fecal incontinence), ADL impairments usually appear in a characteristic chronology: bathing, dressing, toileting, transferring, and feeding. Thus difficulty in feeding with other ADLs

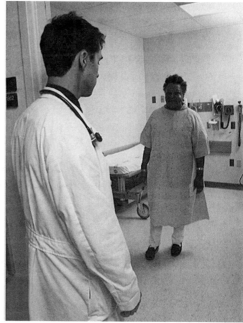

Functional status must be ascertained in a systematic assessment.

unimpaired suggests something about the underlying processes responsible. ADL impairment (e.g., incontinence) in the setting of preserved higher functions (i.e., IADLs) also suggests specific derangements (e.g., detrusor instability) as opposed to general frailty as the basis for functional decline.
6. Distinguish capability from ability. Is the functional decline caused by the legitimate inability to perform these tasks because of physical or cognitive impairments, or is the problem unwillingness

on the part of the patient? Patients capable of independent ADLs may not undertake them because of social withdrawal or depression. When possible, formal or informal performance-oriented measures wherein the patient is observed actually walking, transferring, feeding, or dressing (perhaps into a lab coat) will provide corroborative evidence of the ability or inability to perform the task. Figure 9–1, the physical performance test (PPT), is a useful instrument for this purpose when there is ample time available.[3]

The PPT is an objective performance-based measure of physical function that can be completed within 5 minutes by one examiner using a few easily obtainable props. Dimensions assessed by the PPT include: upper fine motor function, upper coarse motor function, balance, mobility, coordination, and endurance. The 9 items can be categorized by degree of difficulty, realizing that some variability is to be expected depending upon patients' physical or emotional handicaps. Items of perceived minimal difficulty are writing a sentence, simulated eating, and turning 360 degrees. Items of moderate difficulty are lifting a book (the Physician's Desk Reference), putting on and removing a jacket, picking up a penny from the floor, and walking 50 feet. The most difficult item is climbing stairs. By including items that extend across a broad range of difficulty, the test provides measures of physical function for a diverse group of elderly patients, ranging from those who are dependent in ADLs to those who are fully independent in IADLs but may demonstrate impairment on an item such as stair climbing. For each item, a five point scale (0–4) is used with 4 being most capable or fastest to 0 being "unable to do." Thus, scores could range from 0 to 36 (Figure 9–2).

7. Consider environmental factors as the basis for the functional decline. The traditional history and physical focus on patient-specific factors as the basis for chief complaints, but in elderly patients, the following environmental factors may be as important and must be considered. For example,

   A. Have new functional obstacles in the home environment produced functional disability?
   B. Is the patient in a new dwelling where the bathroom or kitchen is less accessible?
   C. Is a previously available caregiver now unavailable or less available?
   D. Have formal home care services been withdrawn?

8. Review the status of all chronic diseases the patient is known to harbor. Inability to transfer may be the cardinal feature of angina pectoris in a frail elderly patient. Exacerbation of chronic obstructive pulmonary disease (COPD) may cause dyspnea severe enough to limit mobility and result in incontinence. In these situations, attributing the functional decline to old age is a misdiagnosis that can have grave consequences.

9. If no single underlying process can be found, consider two or more interacting processes. Prostatism in itself might produce polyuria but not full-fledged incontinence until an exacerbation of arthritis

---

Physical Performance Test

Administer the physical performance test (PPT) outlined below. Subjects are told to perform each task at their usual speed and are given up to two chances to complete each item. Assistive devices are permitted for tasks 6 through 8.

1. Ask the subject, when given the command "go," to write the sentence "whales live in the blue ocean." Time from the word "go" until the pen is lifted from the page at the end of the sentence. All words must be included and legible. Period need not be included for task to be considered complete.

2. Five kidney beans are placed in a bowl, 5 inches from the edge of the desk in front of the patient. An empty coffee can is placed on the table at the patient's nondominant side. A teaspoon is placed in the patient's dominant hand. Ask the subject, on the command "go," to pick up the beans, one at a time, and place each in the coffee can. Time from the command "go" until the last bean is heard hitting the bottom of the can.

3. Place a *Physician's Desk Reference* or other heavy book on a table in front of the patient. Ask the patient, when given the command "go," to place the book on a shelf above shoulder level. Time from the command "go" to the time the book is resting on the shelf.

4. If the subject has a jacket or cardigan sweater, ask him or her to remove it. If not, give the subject a lab coat. Ask the subject, on the command "go," to put the coat on completely such that it is straight on his or her shoulders and then to remove the garment completely. Time from the command "go" until the garment has been completely removed.

5. Place a penny approximately 1 foot from the patient's foot on the dominant side. Ask the patient, on the command "go," to pick up the penny from the floor and stand up. Time from the command "go" until the subject is standing erect with the penny in hand.

6. With subject in a corridor or in an open room, ask the subject to turn 360°. Evaluate using scale on PPT scoring sheet.

7. Bring subject to start on 50-foot walk test course (25 feet out and 25 feet back) and ask the subject, on the command "go," to walk to 25-foot mark and back. Time from the command "go" until the starting line is crossed on the way back.

8. Bring subject to foot of stairs (9 to 12 steps) and ask subject, on the command "go," to begin climbing stairs until he or she feels tired and wishes to stop. Before beginning this task, alert the subject to possibility of developing chest pain or shortness of breath and inform the subject to tell you if any of these symptoms occur. Escort the subject up the stairs. Time from the command "go" until the subject's first foot reaches the top of the first flight of stairs. Record the number of flights (maximum is four) climbed (up and down is one flight).

The appropriate posture in the ED is to assume that functional decline is a symptom of new, underlying medical illness or established chronic diseases that are decompensating.

FIGURE 9-1   Reprinted with permission. Reuben DB, Siu AL. An objective measure of physical function of elderly outpatients. *J Am Geriatr Soc.* 1990;38:1105–1112.

limits mobility enough to lengthen a trip to the bathroom. A mild stroke might leave enough residual strength in the upper extremities for a patient to brush teeth or comb hair until a new rotator cuff tear is superimposed on this delicate balance.

Physical Performance Test Scoring Sheet

Physical Performance Test

	Time	Scoring	Score
1. Write a sentence (whales live in the blue ocean)	_____ sec*	≤10 sec = 4 10.5–15 sec = 3 15.5–20 sec = 2 >20 sec = 1 unable = 0	_____
2. Simulated eating	_____ sec	≤10 sec = 4 10.5–15 sec = 3 15.5–20 sec = 2 >20 sec = 1 unable = 0	_____
3. Lift a book and put it on a shelf	_____ sec	≤2 sec = 4 2.5–4 sec = 3 4.5–6 sec = 2 >6 sec = 1 unable = 0	_____
4. Put on and remove a jacket	_____ sec	≤10 sec = 4 10.5–15 sec = 3 15.5–20 sec = 2 >20 sec = 1 unable = 0	_____
5. Pick up penny from floor	_____ sec	≤2 sec = 4 2.5–4 sec = 3 4.5–6 sec = 2 >6 sec = 1 unable = 0	_____
6. Turn 360 degrees	discontinuous steps continuous steps unsteady (grabs, staggers) steady	0 2 0 2	_____
7. 50-foot walk test	_____ sec	≤15 sec = 4 15.5–20 sec = 3 20.5–25 sec = 2 >25 sec = 1 unable = 0	_____
8. Climb one flight of stairs	_____ sec	≤5 sec = 4 5.5–10 sec = 3 10.5–15 sec = 2 >15 sec = 1 unable = 0	_____
9. Climb stairs	Number of flights of stairs up and down (maximum 4)		_____
TOTAL SCORE (maximum 36 for 9-item, 28 for 7-item)			_____ 9-item _____ 7-item

*For timed measurements, round up to the nearest 0.5 second.

FIGURE 9-2   Reprinted with permission. Ruben DB, Siu, AL. An objective measure of physical function of elderly outpatients. *J Am Geriatr Soc.* 1990;38:1105–1112.

10. Consider pain as the basis for functional decline. Rather than complain of pain after a bony or soft tissue injury, elderly patients may not localize the discomfort and, instead, may limit their activity. Cognitive impairment increases this tendency. A history of recent injuries, especially falls, should prompt the clinician to palpate all bony structures likely to be affected by the injury, and joints should be examined through full active and passive range of motion. Observation of the gait is important in this setting. Several sites that are common sources of pain can be overlooked in a rapid examination: the mouth (e.g., dental abscess), the perineum (e.g., perirectal abscess, epididymitis), and the feet (e.g., bunions, ulcers, plantar fasciitis). These areas should be examined routinely.

11. Always consider the role of cognitive impairment in functional decline. Delirium and dementia are common problems whose prevalence rises with age. Both ADLs and IADLs require not only physical capability, but also cognitive coordination of these capabilities, including elements of praxis, visual memory, visuospatial skills, and orientation. Thus the presenting manifestation of acute or chronic cognitive impairment may be functional decline, well before it is appreciated that cognitive impairment is the underlying process. All patients with functional decline should therefore have formal mental status testing.

12. Consider psychiatric diagnoses, especially depression. The presentation may be atypical, and psychomotor retardation can produce significant functional decline that can be erroneously ascribed to physical frailty or dementia. Screening instruments for depression (described in Chapter 7) are appropriate once functional decline has been discovered.

13. Consider medications as a cause of functional decline. In some cases medications may impair cognitive ability such that functional impairments result. Alternatively, medications may affect specific functional abilities. For example, angiotensin converting enzyme (ACE) inhibitors may cause dysgeusia and secondary anorexia.

MANAGING FUNCTIONAL DECLINE

When a single underlying cause is the basis for functional decline (i.e., a new active process or an exacerbation of chronic disease), interventions should be directed at the underlying process. When multiple processes are the underlying problem, some will be potentially remediable, and some will not. The goal is to address all potentially remediable factors in the hope of improving the overall functional picture (Figure 9–3).

Functional decline attributed to frailty or failure to thrive is a diagnosis of exclusion after all the above possibilities have been considered. Patients who will be discharged home with this diagnosis (in the company of a caregiver) should have a formal, more comprehensive geriatric assessment on an outpatient basis.

In addition to the clinical importance of functional decline as a presenting manifestation of underlying illness, functional decline has direct relevance with regard to ED disposition. A patient with a new unresolved

Algorithm for Evaluation and Management of Functional Decline in the Elderly Patient

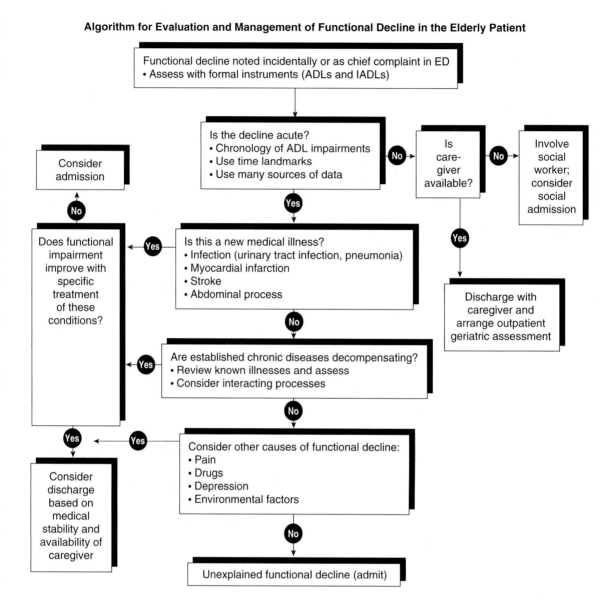

FIGURE 9-3

ADL impairment cannot return home unless someone is available to provide assistance with these activities. In the absence of such a caregiver, a patient cannot be discharged without other arrangements. In general, patients with an acute, unexplained change in functional status will require admission. If the impairment is chronic or subacute and a caregiver is available, ED discharge may be reasonable. If no caregiver is available, social services should be involved as soon as possible.

SUMMARY POINTS

- Functional decline may be defined as a *recent* or progressive difficulty or inability in performing various tasks that are necessary or highly desirable for independent living.
- The appearance of one or more new ADL impairments is of concern

and may either be the chief complaint in an ED presentation or, alternatively, may be discovered as an incidental finding when an elderly patient presents with a more traditional chief complaint.

- Medical illness in the elderly often presents with functional decline instead of with signs and symptoms traditionally referable to specific diseases.
- The most valuable tool in assessing functional decline is the patient history and, whenever possible, corroborating or additional history from a caregiver or family member who is in a position to comment objectively on new or worsening functional impairments.

CHAPTER AUTHOR

Mark S. Lachs, MD, MPH

Dr. Lachs is recipient of Academic Award #K0800580-01 from the National Institutes on Aging, an American College of Physicians Research Scholar, and a Paul Beeson Physician Faculty Scholar in Aging.

REFERENCES

1. Katz S, Ford AB, Moskowitz RW, et al. Studies of illness in the aged. The index of ADL: standardized measure of biologic and psychosocial function. *JAMA.* 1962;185:914–919.
2. Lawton MP, Brody EM. Assessment of older people—self-maintaining and instrumental activities of daily living. *Gerontologist.* 1969;9:179–185.
3. Reuben DB, Siu AL. An objective measure of physical function of elderly outpatients. *J Am Geriatr Soc.* 1990;38:1105–1112.

SUGGESTED READING

Cooperating Clinics Committee of the American Rheumatism Association: A seven day variability study of 499 patients with peripheral rheumatoid arthritis. *Arthritis Rheum.* 1965;8:302–334.
Jebsen RH, Taylor N, Trieschmann RB, et al. An objective and standardized test of hand function. *Arch Phys Med Rehabil.* June, 1969;311–319.
Kuriansky J, Gurland B. The performance test of activities of daily living. *Int'l J Aging and Human Development.* 1976;7(4):343–352.
Reuben DB, Siu AL. An objective measure of physical function of elderly persons: The physical performance test. *J Am Geriat Soc.* 1990;38:1105–1112.
Reuben DB, Siu A, Kimpau S. The predictive validity of self-report and performance-based measures of function and health. *J Gerontology: Medical Sciences.* 1992;47M106-110.

10 *Trauma and Falls*

LEARNING OBJECTIVES

1. Identify types of injuries most likely in the elderly.
2. Correlate physiologic changes associated with aging with principles of trauma resuscitation.
3. Explain the significance of determining the etiology of a fall as well as assessing injuries from a fall.
4. Demonstrate the appropriate history and physical examination of an elderly patient presenting to the ED with trauma.

Trauma is an important cause of morbidity and mortality in the elderly. For Americans aged 65 years and older trauma is the fifth leading cause of death. Elderly patients comprise 12-20% of all trauma patients and 28% of all trauma fatalities; they account for approximately one third of each dollar spent on trauma care. Although elderly persons are less likely to be injured than younger persons, when injured they are hospitalized more frequently and for longer periods. They are more likely to die from their injuries or related complications, and if they survive they will more often require long-term care.[1-3]

Falls account for the majority of traumatic injuries in the elderly population (Figure 10–1), followed by motor vehicle accidents, pedestrian accidents, violence (stab and gunshot wounds), and burns (Tables 10–1 and 10–2). The problem of falls is somewhat unique to the elderly population and is addressed separately in this chapter.

Persons over 65 years of age account for approximately 13% of all motor vehicle accidents. In contrast to younger drivers, older drivers are more often involved in collisions between two vehicles, at intersec-

The elderly comprise 12% to 20% of all trauma patients and consume approximately 1/3 of all dollars spent on trauma care.

153

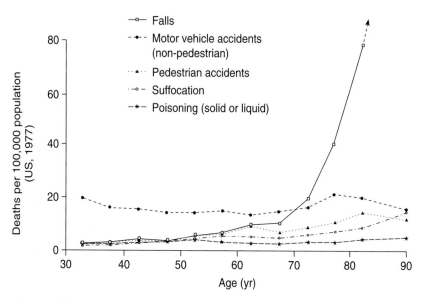

Figure 10–1   Deaths per 100,000 resulting from traumatic injury. From Baker SP, Harvey AM. Fall injuries in the elderly. *Clin Geriatr Med.*,1985;1:502.

Table 10–1 **Mechanism of Injury for Persons Under Age 65**

Cause	Cases (%)
Motor vehicle accidents	33.5
Stab and gunshot wounds	24.9
Falls	11.0
Pedestrian accidents	7.9

Adapted from Champion HR, Copes WS, Buyer D, et al. Major trauma in geriatric patients. *Am J Pub Health.* 1989;79:1278–1282. Reprinted with permission. Copyright 1989 American Public Health Association.

Table 10–2 **Mechanism of Injury for Persons Over Age 65**

Cause	Cases (%)
Falls	40.6
Motor vehicle accidents	28.2
Pedestrian accidents	10.0
Stab and gunshot wounds	8.1

Adapted from Champion HR, Copes WS, Buyer D, et al. Major trauma in geriatric patients. *Am J Pub Health.* 1989;79:1278–1282. Reprinted with permission. Copyright 1989 American Public Health Association.

tions, in good weather, during daylight hours, and closer to home. Persons over 65 years have the highest rate of pedestrian–motor vehicle accidents and a disproportionately high subsequent mortality (Table 10–3). The elderly tend to live in urban areas, making them increasingly subject to violent crimes. Elder abuse and neglect have only in re-

Table 10–3 **Accident Fatalities of Persons Aged 65 Years or Older by Cause**

Cause	No. of accident fatalities
Falls	10900 (38%)
Motor vehicle	7300 (25%)
Driver-passenger	5750
Pedestrian	1550
Suffocation: ingested objects	2050
Fire, burns	1350 (5%)
Drowning	500
Poisoning (solid, liquid)	750
Poisoning by gas	180
Firearms	170
Other	5500
Total	28700

From National Safety Council, *Accident facts.* Itasca, IL: The Council; 1994.

cent years become recognized as important health issues. Despite major advances in management of burn injuries the elderly have a much higher mortality from burns than younger adults. For example, full-thickness burns involving 50% of the total body surface area carry a 50% mortality in younger individuals, but the elderly patient faces nearly 100% mortality from a similar burn.[4]

PRE-HOSPITAL CONSIDERATIONS

Pre-hospital personnel need to be aware of the high morbidity and mortality experienced by elder trauma victims. Priorities in pre-hospital care include the basic ABCs (airway, breathing, and circulation) with the knowledge that the elderly tolerate shock very poorly and that prevention of cardiovascular collapse is very important. Fluids should be administered in discrete boluses rather than at "wide-open" rates, keeping in mind that fluid overload and congestive heart failure are potential complications. Prevention of further injury is a major priority. Immobilization with stiff cervical collars and spine boards may compromise the airway and impair the ability to ventilate adequately. The elderly often are unable to achieve thermoregulation efficiently, and provisions for maintaining normal body temperature should be made. These patients may have hearing and vision defects that make communication difficult and increase their fear and anxiety. Confusion should not be assumed to be a baseline condition but may result from inadequate oxygenation, ventilation, or impending shock.

The elderly patient is often unable to provide a complete and accurate history. Pre-hospital personnel should carefully survey the accident scene, looking for clues to the cause, with special attention to evidence of abuse or neglect. Witnesses are questioned about the patient's condition and behavior at the time of the accident. In addition to a general evaluation of living conditions, significant environmental hazards are noted, such as inadequate lighting, loose rugs, or dangerous stair-

The occasional need for a "social admission" runs against the trend to avoid hospitalization whenever possible and places great responsibility on the emergency physician to act as patient advocate.

ways. The presence of medications and potential intoxicants at the scene may be especially important.

Any elderly patient with a significant injury or multiple trauma should be transported to the nearest facility with resources for and experience in the specific management of elderly trauma victims.

TRAUMA RESUSCITATION

Fluids should be administered in discrete boluses rather than at a wide open rate, keeping in mind the potential complications of fluid overload and congestive heart failure.

Mortality from trauma begins to increase in the over-55-year age group and continues to increase with age. Basic principles of trauma resuscitation are unchanged when dealing with elderly persons. The priorities of establishing and protecting the airway, ensuring adequate oxygen delivery and ventilation, controlling hemorrhage, and supporting circulation, followed by primary and secondary injury surveys, should be observed. However, a number of basic principles that relate specifically to the elderly should be kept in mind. Most of these principles are based on the physiologic decline in major organ system reserve function and the disordered homeostasis that accompany aging.

In the elderly, mortality increases dramatically in the presence of shock (Figure 10–2). Along with multi-organ failure, shock represents the primary cause of death in the injured elderly. It is of utmost importance to recognize the potential for shock early on and to take steps to hemodynamically monitor and optimize cardiovascular function. Cardiovascular status is often difficult to assess in elderly patients. For example, the patient may not manifest tachycardia with loss of blood volume secondary to physiologic changes in intrinsic pacemaker activity or the presence of beta-adrenergic or calcium channel blocking drugs. A blood pressure in the low normal range may represent significant hypotension in the patient who is normally hypertensive. Persistent metabolic acidosis generally indicates underresuscitation but can also be a manifestation of overresuscitation in the patient with congestive heart failure. Urine output may not be a reliable indicator of cardiac output and organ perfusion because the elderly are less able to produce a concentrated urine, and decreased urine output may result from both underhydration and fluid overload. Some authorities in trauma care emphasize the value of invasive monitoring of hemodynamic parameters early in the management of multiply injured elderly patients. Data exists suggesting more favorable outcomes in elderly patients who receive early hemodynamic monitoring.[5]

The appearance of dementia or delirium should be considered a sign of inadequate oxygenation, ventilation, or impending shock rather than a baseline condition.

A study by Pellicane et al. demonstrated that the physiologic Trauma Score was unreliable in predicting mortality in the elderly.[6] Fifty-two percent of deaths in their study of 374 elderly trauma victims occurred in patients with normal trauma scores. Most of these patients died after developing sepsis or multiple organ failure from unrecognized shock. In addition, preventable complications occurred in 32% of all deaths and in 62% of all patients with multiple organ failure.[6]

Scalea et al. confirmed this observation of older patients who appear stable but are in occult shock.[5] They aggressively monitored the cardiac output of elderly patients with high-risk trauma injuries and found that almost one half of the patients with normal vital signs and no clinical

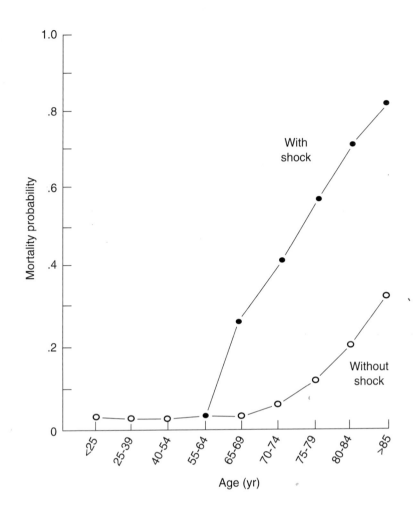

FIGURE 10–2 Mortality with and without shock. Modified from Osler T, et al. Trauma in the elderly. *Am J Surg.* 156: 537;1988. Reprinted with permission from *American Journal of Surgery.*

signs of shock had low cardiac output. When hemodynamics were aggressively monitored and treated, mortality of these high-risk patients fell from 85% to 47%. Thus, traditional trauma scoring systems and physiologic indicators may not be applicable in the elderly. Emergency physicians must have a high index of suspicion for occult shock and preventable complications of trauma. Thus early, aggressive monitoring must be considered for the elderly trauma victim.[5,6]

Hypothermia frequently complicates resuscitation of the elderly trauma patient.[2] Impaired thermoregulation combined with prolonged environmental exposure and resuscitation with room-temperature fluids or blood products contribute to hypothermia and can result in fatal arrhythmias and neurologic sequelae.[3]

Management of multiply injured patients is challenging and requires expeditious evaluation and definitive care by a team of specialists dedicated specifically to trauma care. Elderly trauma victims are particularly at risk of excess morbidity and mortality. Further data exist indicating that these patients are best served by early transfer to a major trauma center for definitive care and early rehabilitation.[7]

Data suggest more favorable outcomes result from Swan-Ganz catheter-guided hemodynamic optimization as soon as feasible.

FALLS

Falls are not a part of normal aging. A fall is a presenting clinical symptom that has its own etiology as well as its own consequences.

Falls are not a part of normal aging. A fall is a presenting clinical symptom that has its own etiology as well as its own consequences (Figure 10–3).

Falls are a special problem for the elderly and a significant cause of morbidity and mortality. Falls are common and occur in approximately one third of persons 65 years and older living independently at home each year. Falls occur even more frequently in nursing home residents, with a reported average annual incidence of 1.6-2.0 falls per patient year. Significant injury is common, with 10% resulting in fracture, dislocation, or lacerations requiring suturing. Both frequency of falls and severity of injury increase markedly with advancing decades. A fall may be more than an isolated incident and may represent accelerated general decline or progression of a pre-existing disease process. As many as 50% of elderly patients requiring hospitalization after a fall die within one year.[1–3,8–10]

The elderly victim of a fall may represent a considerable challenge for the emergency physician. Beyond the often arduous task of ruling out significant injury, the cause of the fall must be pursued to rule out a life-threatening underlying condition. In evaluating the independent patient, the important question of whether that person is now

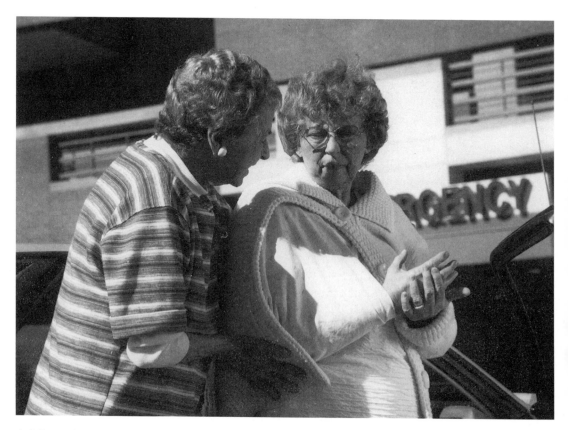

A fall may be more than an isolated incident and may represent accelerated decline or progression of a pre-existing disease process.

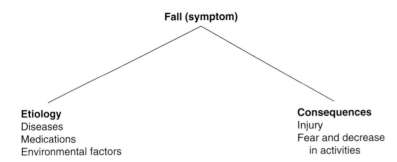

FIGURE 10–3   A fall is a clinical symptom rather than a natural part of aging.

able to care for himself or herself must be addressed along with an often difficult analysis of what resources may be available to provide additional care at home. The occasional need for the "social" admission of a patient who is just not doing well at home runs against the modern imperative to avoid hospitalization whenever possible. This imperative places great responsibility on the emergency physician to act as patient advocate at a time when advocacy often falls on deaf ears.

As many as 50% of those elderly who are hospitalized after a fall die within a year.

ETIOLOGY

Classification of falls by cause is a difficult undertaking and is perhaps more valuable as a tool for research and risk factor modification than as a clinical tool for the emergency physician. A commonly used categorization scheme lists causes as either *extrinsic* or *intrinsic*. Extrinsic causes include any part of the elderly person's environment that might contribute to the likelihood of a fall, such as poor lighting, absent handrails, loose rugs, or unstable furniture. Intrinsic causes are subdivided into those deficits that accompany normal physiologic aging (i.e., diminished visual acuity, hearing, balance, strength, reaction time) and those deficits resulting from disease conditions (i.e., cardiac, respiratory, neurologic, musculoskeletal, and iatrogenic).[8,11] However, it must be stressed that causation is usually multifactorial with considerable overlap between categories. For example, a dimly lit environment cluttered with numerous obstacles represents an *extrinsic* hazard. Whether an individual falls while negotiating that environment depends highly on a variety of *intrinsic* factors such as balance, gait, and vision.

The emergency physician must make the primary distinction between causes that may be immediately life threatening and all others. Often this is reduced to determining whether the patient has suffered an unexplained *syncopal* episode; that is, a sudden and brief loss of consciousness, and whether hospitalization is warranted. Syncope can be approached by considering four basic causes: (1) defective blood pressure control, (2) primary cardiac dysfunction, (3) diminished cerebral blood flow, and (4) metabolic and respiratory derangements.[12,13]

Defective blood pressure control includes orthostatic hypotension and vasovagal or vasomotor attacks. Orthostatic hypotension may be a natural consequence of aging but can be acutely worsened by hypovolemia, medication side effects, or vascular insufficiency. Vasovagal reactions result from carotid sinus hypersensitivity, visceral stimulation, or so-called "situational syncope." Situational syncope includes cough, micturition, postprandial, defecation, and emotional etiologies.

Primary cardiac dysfunction includes arrhythmias, heart failure, and outflow obstructions. Virtually all arrhythmias and conduction defects are more common in the elderly, who also are more likely to experience syncope as a result. Heart failure may accompany cardiomyopathy, ischemia, and infarct or may be a manifestation of hypertensive or valvular heart disease. Cardiac outflow obstruction is an uncommon cause of syncope but may result from aortic stenosis, septal hypertrophy, or atrial myxomas.

Disorders of cerebral blood flow causing syncope include vertebrobasilar insufficiency, subclavian steal syndrome, and rarely, basilar artery spasm in migraine headache presentations.

Metabolic and respiratory derangements causing syncope include hypoglycemic reactions, hyperventilation, and hypoxia secondary to respiratory failure.

In approximately 50% of cases of syncope in the elderly population no definitive diagnosis is made. Of those cases in which a diagnosis can be made, 80% could be established in the ED on initial presentation. A careful history, physical examination, and basic diagnostic testing should be sufficient to identify those patients in whom syncope carries the greatest risk.[12–14]

INITIAL ASSESSMENT AND STABILIZATION

The initial assessment of a patient who has fallen should include a primary survey to address the basic ABCs (airway, breathing, and circulation). It is important to remember that the fall may have resulted from a significant cardiovascular event and that the patient may be in imminent danger. If spine immobilization, including the use of stiff collars and backboards, is prolonged, it may position the patient in such a way as to compromise airway or breathing. Orthopedic injuries, especially hip fractures, may be accompanied by significant occult bleeding, and elderly patients tolerate hypovolemia and shock very poorly. Provisions should be made for resuscitation if needed, and the patient is not triaged from the main ED area without close monitoring. If the patient is in spine immobilization, priority is given to checking the spine for injury by physical examination and appropriate x-ray studies. Beyond the discomfort of spine immobilization, elderly patients are at increased risk of developing pressure sores after short intervals of immobilization. If prolonged immobilization is anticipated, the patient is logrolled and placed on an egg-crate foam mattress or equivalent.

It is important to remember that the fall may have resulted from a significant cardiovascular event and that the patient may be in imminent danger.

HISTORY

The history is of key importance in determining the cause of a fall and the range of potential injuries. Pre-hospital personnel, witnesses, and family members should be thoroughly interrogated. Knowing that the patient fell from a chair to a carpeted floor instead of being found at the bottom of a basement stairway will influence the extent of a search for occult injury. Determine what the patient was doing immediately before the fall. As a clue to orthostatic hypotension, determine whether the patient was seated, standing, or walking. Seek out prodromal symptoms. Did the patient feel dizzy, giddy, or light-headed before the fall, or were there palpitations to suggest an arrhythmia? Does the patient remember tripping? Was there a documented loss of consciousness, convulsions, post-ictal confusion, incontinence, or tongue biting?

A knowledge of the pre-fall functional status of the patient and of whether falls have occurred in the past is useful. If falls have occurred before, is there a change in pattern with regard to frequency and severity of injury? A history of increased frequency of falling may signal an important functional decline or progression of a disease process. The circumstances immediately following the fall are important in assessing etiology as well as injury. Did the patient need assistance getting up? Did the patient lie on the floor for a long time before assistance arrived?

Past medical history may suggest an etiology. Known or suspected cardiovascular disease evidenced by a history of diabetes, hypertension, angina, myocardial infarct, or stroke increases the possibility of syncope secondary to cardiac disease. A complete medication profile with an emphasis on finding the recent addition or deletion of drugs is important. Antihypertensive agents may affect vasomotor tone and the baroreflex, and diuretics can significantly deplete intravascular volume. These drugs often produce or aggravate orthostatic symptoms and thus promote falls. Hypokalemia and hyperkalemia predispose to cardiac arrhythmias and can occur when elderly persons are treated with diuretics and angiotensin converting enzyme (ACE) inhibitors. Hypokalemia is especially likely to precipitate arrhythmia in elderly persons taking digoxin. Commonly prescribed sedatives and hypnotics may produce cardiovascular symptoms or dysequilibrium or may dull reaction time needed to avoid falls and limit injury. Do not neglect to inquire about over-the-counter medications that may be omitted from a drug history offered by the patient and yet have significant toxic potential.[15]

When faced with an injured elderly patient, the emergency physician must look beyond the injuries themselves and consider the cause.

PHYSICAL EXAMINATION

The physical examination will focus on identifying injuries sustained in falling but must also seek clues to the cause of the fall. In addition to routine vital signs and a mental status screen (see Chapters 7 & 8), blood pressure and pulse should be obtained with the patient lying, sitting, and standing to detect signs of orthostatic hypotension. Dry mucous membranes, sunken eyes, decreased skin turgor, and decreased axillary sweat suggest dehydration. Maneuvers to provoke labyrinthine stimulation may reproduce symptoms of dizziness, suggesting an inner ear problem (see Figure 16–1). Although not specific, bruits in the neck may point toward cerebrovascular disease as an etiology. A loud bruit over the left subclavian artery can occur in subclavian steal syndrome, and exercising the left upper extremity may precipitate syncopal symptoms. Careful attention to the cardiac examination may reveal

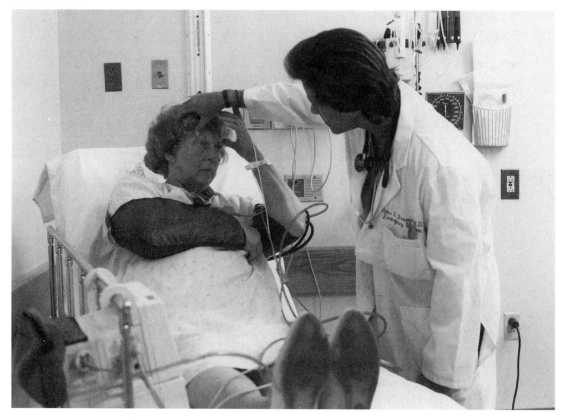

The circumstances immediately following the fall are important in assessing etiology as well as injury.

signs of congestive heart failure or arrhythmia. If orthostatic hypotension and anemia are present, a rectal examination may reveal a source of blood loss.

The neurologic examination focuses on detecting subtle indicators of stroke. Special attention should be paid to evaluation for gait and balance disturbances. Functional assessment should be matched with historic information to determine the presence of an acute decline.

DIAGNOSTIC TESTING

Diagnostic testing must be tailored to the individual's presentation. A witnessed trip-and-fall accident will require a less comprehensive evaluation than unexplained syncope. A complete blood count (CBC) may reveal significant anemia. Basic electrolytes, glucose, calcium, blood urea nitrogen (BUN), and creatinine are sufficient to screen for most important conditions. Toxicologic screening and blood alcohol levels may be informative. An electrocardiogram (ECG) to rule out arrhythmia, ischemia, or infarct is appropriate. If a neurologic examination reveals no marked global or focal deficits, a head computed tomography (CT) scan is unlikely to provide useful information.

TREATMENT AND DISPOSITION

Treatment of injuries sustained by a fall should be straightforward. The emergency physician should consider that wounds heal more slowly in the elderly and that sutures often must stay in place longer. The impact of joint or extremity immobilization must be considered in light of the patient's overall functional status. It is common for elderly patients to be unable to use crutches safely. An arm sling may contribute further to balance problems. It may be necessary to arrange for a cane, walker, or wheelchair. Keep in mind that devices to stabilize gait can be dangerous if used improperly, and referral for appropriate training should be made.

Arriving at a decision to hospitalize the elderly patient after a fall is often difficult. When injury or a significant functional decline has resulted, hospital admission is warranted to protect the patient from further injury and coordinate continuing care. If the patient had a fall related to a syncopal episode, and careful history, physical examination, and diagnostic studies available in the ED cannot rule out a serious and potentially unstable cardiovascular or neurologic condition, hospital admission for close monitoring is indicated.

Once a decision to discharge the patient is made, the emergency physician must be sure that timely and appropriate follow-up is possible. The morbidity of a fall often extends beyond injuries sustained. The elderly patient may be fearful of falling again and restrict activity, with a resulting loss of independence and social isolation. Any period of immobility will be accompanied by deconditioning that can contribute to a further decline in overall health and well-being. Coordination with community resources is important to guarantee timely and appropriate follow-up with primary care providers, visiting nurse specialists, and physical medicine and rehabilitation personnel. If special geriatric services exist within a community, the ED physician must have ready access for referral. The key point to remember is that interventions can be instituted to address the problem of falls in the elderly patient. Table 10–4 gives examples of possible interventions for falls as part of a comprehensive assessment in an office or clinic setting.

SPECIFIC INJURIES

HEAD TRAUMA

As a cause of trauma-related deaths in the elderly, head injury is second only to shock. Elderly patients presenting with head injury and a Glasgow Coma Scale score of 8 or less have a mortality in excess of 90%.[1,16]

Epidural hematomas are relatively rare in the elderly population. However, *subdural* hematomas are three times more frequent in the elderly. With aging, veins become more fragile and cerebral atrophy tends to stretch bridging vessels. Additionally, these individuals are more likely to have age-related clotting deficiencies or be therapeutically anticoagulated. These factors contribute to the higher incidence of subdural hematomas. Subdural hematoma in the elderly has been

Table 10–4 **Possible Interventions for Fall Risk Factors**

Risk Factors	Possible Interventions
Vision	
Medical	Refraction; cataract extraction
Rehabilitative	Balance and gait training; low-vision aids
Environmental	Good lighting; home safety assessment; architectural design that minimizes distortion and illusions
Hearing	
Medical	Cerumen removal; audiologic evaluation with hearing aid if appropriate
Rehabilitative	Training in hearing aid use
Environmental	Decrease of background noise
Vestibular dysfunction	
Medical	Avoidance of vestibulotoxic drugs; surgical ablation (rarely indicated)
Rehabilitative	Habituation exercises
Environmental	Good lighting (increased reliance on visual input); home safety assessment
Proprioceptive-cervical disorders; peripheral neuropathy	
Medical	Diagnosis and treatment of specific diseases such as spondylosis, vitamin B_{12} deficiency
Rehabilitative	Balance exercises; appropriate walking aid
Environmental	Good lighting (increased reliance on visual input); good footwear; home safety assessment
Central nervous system diseases	
Medical	Diagnosis and treatment of specific diseases such as Parkinson's disease, normal-pressure hydrocephalus
Rehabilitative	Physical therapy; balance and gait training; appropriate walking aid
Environmental	Home safety assessment; appropriate adaptations (e.g., high, firm chairs; raised toilet seats; grab bars in bathroom)
Dementia	
Medical	Avoidance of sedating or centrally acting drugs
Rehabilitative	Supervised exercise and ambulation
Environmental	Safe, structured, supervised environment
Musculoskeletal problems, including hip and knee weakness, ankle weakness, foot problems	
Medical	Diagnosis and treatment of specific diseases
Rehabilitative	Balance and gait training; muscle-strengthening exercises; back exercises; correct walking aid; correct footwear; good foot care (e.g., nails, calluses, bunions)
Environmental	Home safety assessment; appropriate adaptations
Postural hypotension	
Medical	Diagnosis and treatment of specific diseases; avoidance of offending drugs; careful medication review; rehydration; identification of precipitating situations (e.g., meals)
Rehabilitative	Tilt table (if severe); reconditioning exercises; graded-pressure stockings
Environmental	Elevation of head of bed
Depression	
Medical	Avoidance of antidepressants associated with greater anticholinergic effect
Medications, especially sedatives, phenothiazines, antidepressants	
Medical	Determination of lowest effective dose of essential medication; readjustment and discontinuation when possible; selection of shorter-acting medications
Acute illness; new or increased medications	
Medical	Diagnosis and treatment of specific diseases; starting of medications at low dose and increasing slowly
Environmental	Increased supervision during illnesses or with new medications

termed the *great imitator*. Cerebral atrophy leaves room for large hematomas, and symptoms may be insidious and nonspecific. Presentation may be as simple as mild headache, subtle mental status change, or a new gait disorder without other focal deficits. Often a prior history of trauma is lacking. A CT scan will show a hyperdense hematoma during the first 5-10 days. From 7-20 days the hematoma may become isodense and almost invisible radiographically. One must look for subtle clues of a mass effect such as ipsilateral ventricle compression and a flattening or a concavity at the white matter border.[5]

On occasion it is difficult to distinguish traumatic from spontaneous intracranial hemorrhage. As a rule, trauma tends to produce multiple hemorrhagic sites throughout the cortex. In contrast, spontaneous hemorrhages are often single, large, expansive, and more common in the basal ganglia, pons, or cerebellum.

A major consideration in the management of head injury is control of intracranial pressure (ICP). In the multiply injured patient, management of ICP is often complicated by significant blood loss and the need for fluid resuscitation. Cerebral blood flow depends on systemic arterial pressure and arterial P_{CO_2}. After normalization of blood pressure, intubation and hyperventilation to maintain a P_{CO_2} of 26-28 mmHg will further support cerebral blood flow. Administration of mannitol at a dose of 1 g/kg is further temporizing. Early consultation with a neurosurgeon to help coordinate management priorities is key. If the services of a neurosurgeon are not readily available, arrangements to transfer the patient to a designated trauma center should be made simultaneously with initial resuscitation.[1,2]

> *Elderly patients presenting with head injury and a Glasgow Coma Scale score of 8 or less carry a mortality rate in excess of 90%.*

CHEST INJURIES

With aging the chest wall becomes less elastic and more prone to fracture in major trauma. Rib fractures, pneumothorax, and hemothorax are more common. With multiple rib fractures adequate ventilation may be impaired by pain and changes in the mechanics of breathing. Resulting atelectasis and inefficient clearing of the airway put elderly patients at increased risk of pneumonia. As a rule, injury resulting in fracture of two or more ribs should be a criterion for hospitalization of the elderly patient. Epidural and intercostal anesthetic blocks provide pain relief and improve ventilatory function.

Pulmonary and cardiac contusions do not appear to occur with increased frequency with aging. Age-related stiffening of the aorta and large arteries of the chest does not appear to predispose the elderly to vascular injuries in trauma.[1,2]

> *Injury resulting in fracture of two or more ribs should be a criterion for hospitalization of the elderly patient.*

ABDOMINAL INJURIES

Significant intraabdominal injury occurs in up to 35% of multiply injured elderly patients. Mortality from such injuries may be four times higher than in young persons. Examination of the abdomen can be particularly unreliable because pain is often poorly localized and peritoneal signs may be subtle. The liberal application of diagnostic peritoneal lavage in the unstable, head-injured, or intoxicated patient is advocated. Abdominal CT scan is frequently useful in identifying occult injury and retroperitoneal hemorrhage. Occult injury to the mesentery and hollow viscera is not uncommon in the elderly trauma patient and may reflect increased visceral mobility and thinning of connective tissue elements of the viscera and vasculature.[1,2]

SPINE INJURIES

The elderly are more likely to have intravertebral disk and ligamentous injuries that are not readily apparent on plain radiographs.

Arthritis involving the spine is common in the elderly, and it is often difficult to determine whether poorly localized pain is related to acute injury or to an exacerbation of a chronic condition. In contrast to younger patients, older patients are more likely to have intravertebral disk and ligamentous injuries that are not readily apparent on plain radiographs. X-ray interpretation is further complicated by degenerative changes in the spine that occur with aging. Special attention should be paid to the integrity of the ring of C2 on lateral views and to open-mouth views of the odontoid and lateral masses of C1. Flexion and extension views of the cervical and lumbar spine may help identify ligamentous injury. It is often necessary to obtain a CT scan to definitively clear the spine of the older patient with pain and equivocal plain films.[1,2]

FRACTURES

Fractures occur in the elderly population with differing frequency, location, and pattern than in the younger population. For example, fractures typically are the result of low-energy impacts. Often the fracture involves bone weakening by osteoporosis or another pathologic condition such as Paget's disease, infection, malignancy, marrow dysplasias, osteomalacia, or metabolic derangements (e.g., hyperthyroidism and hyperparathyroidism). Osteoporosis is uncommon in African-Americans but occurs in 15% of Caucasian females over 65 years of age, and 30% will experience a related fracture by 75 years of age. Trabecular bone thins and weakens to a greater degree with aging then does cortical bone. Thus fractures involving the trabecular bone of the proximal humerus, wrist, tibia, pubic rami, vertebral bodies, and hip are more common in the elderly. Also, fracture is more common than joint dislocation. Fractures take longer to heal with aging as the remodeling process slows. Non-union and recurrent fractures are also more common.[17]

Fractures involving the trabecular bone of the proximal humerus, wrist, tibia, pubic rami, vertebral bodies, and hip are more common in the elderly.

Presentation of fractures may be atypical, such as pain with weight bearing and movement with otherwise non-diagnostic radiographs. Making a diagnosis of an incomplete fracture before a complete fracture occurs with the attendant increased morbidity is a priority. Complete fractures more commonly result in joint stiffness and decreased mobility than do incomplete fractures. Prolonged confinement to bed and immobility are accompanied by decreased functional status and deconditioning, which ultimately may predispose the patient to further injury or medical problems. Initial management of fractures in the elderly must be done with consideration of the impact of the injury *and* the treatment on the well-being of the individual. Long-term results should be balanced with a pragmatic consideration of short-term functional demands. For example, fracture reduction with prolonged limb immobilization may result in improved appearance without an appreciable impact on function and may subject the individual to unnecessary disability.

Age-related changes in bone structure often make non-displaced fractures difficult to diagnose on routine x-ray studies. Often the addition of oblique views is helpful when anteroposterior (AP) and lateral views are equivocal. Tomograms or CT scans may be a useful adjunct to routine studies, especially when evaluating potential spine, hip, and pelvis fractures. Depending on the index of suspicion for fracture, immobilization and follow-up bone scan are sometimes indicated.

Compartment syndrome is an important potential fracture complication that may occur as a result of the injury itself or from improper splinting or casting. Patients complaining of increasing pain and numbness distal to an injury should have compartment pressures measured and hospital admission considered for close monitoring.[1,2]

> *Age-related changes in bone structure often make non-displaced fractures difficult to diagnose on routine x-ray studies.*

Proximal Humerus

Fractures of the proximal humerus tend to result from falls with an outstretched hand and present with shoulder pain and immobility. Most fractures are minimally displaced and can be treated with a sling and swath. Displaced or comminuted fractures generally require consultation with an orthopedic surgeon for reduction. Rotator cuff injuries are common accompaniments. Inflammation after trauma produces adhesive capsulitis and long-term disability. Isolated cuff injuries are suggested when passive movement of the shoulder is benign, but active abduction and external rotation produce pain. Early introduction of range-of-motion exercises is very important, and referral for physical therapy should be part of discharge planning.[1,17]

Distal Radius

Fractures of the distal radius (Colles' fractures) also tend to result from forward falls with an outstretched hand and present with pain, tenderness, and swelling at the wrist. Bone impaction, angulation, and shortening are key features. When there is minimal displacement and functional demands are not a major consideration, these fractures can be treated definitively with a short arm cast. Closed reduction is often necessary and requires anesthesia either by a hematoma block or Beir block. The latter involves the use of pneumatic tourniquets and instillation of a significant volume of lidocaine into the venous circulation of the forearm. It requires specialized equipment and expertise to avoid the potential complication of releasing a lidocaine bolus into the central circulation, but it can be very effective. It is important to stress early mobilization of the shoulder, elbow, and fingers to avoid long-term loss of extremity function.[1,17]

Pelvic Ramus

Pain and inability to walk after a simple fall on level ground are typical of the history. Examination may reveal localized tenderness in the groin and pain with passive movement of the leg. X-ray studies usually demonstrate fracture of a single ramus, with the pubic ramus involved most commonly. The bony arches of the ilium provide the majority of structural weight bearing, and fracture of a single ramus is considered a stable fracture. Even with fracture of both rami restricted to one side, the weight-bearing arch of the pelvis remains essentially intact. Such fractures do not of themselves require urgent orthopedic consultation and hospitalization unless pain with ambulation affects the ability of the patient to care for himself or herself.[1,17]

The Hip

Fractures of the hip unfortunately are common in the elderly and carry significant morbidity and mortality. Femoral neck fractures are classified as occult, impacted, non-displaced, and displaced. Occult fractures may occur spontaneously or with minimal trauma, present as groin or medial knee pain with weight bearing, and have seemingly normal routine x-ray studies. Making the diagnosis of occult fracture is important to limit subsequent morbidity. CT scan or tomography is indicated when there is a high index of suspicion. Occult and impacted fractures carry the best prognosis because the circulation to the femoral head is usually not threatened. Bleeding from femoral neck fractures is usually contained within the joint capsule and is not a common source of significant blood loss. Intertrochanteric fractures typically result from falls on level ground. When displaced, the affected leg will be shortened and externally rotated. Significant hemorrhage will accompany such fractures and may cause shock.[1,17]

Tibial Plateau

Fractures of the tibial plateau are relatively common in pedestrian–motor vehicle accidents involving the elderly. The lateral bending force and angulation of the leg force the femoral condyle into the tibial articular surface with resulting fracture of underlying bone. The presentation includes knee pain and effusion with proximal tenderness to palpation of the tibia and inability to bear weight. Globules of fat in the aspirate of the knee effusion may be diagnostic. Neurovascular compromise can occur secondary to soft tissue swelling and, as a rule, such an injury warrants hospitalization for monitoring and pain control.[1,17]

Vertebral Body Compression

Osteoporosis is the major underlying cause of the vertebral body compression fractures that may occur spontaneously with lifting or bending forward or as a result of a simple misstep while walking. Acute back pain is worsened by movement, sitting, or standing and is generally well localized to percussion on examination. Neurologic deficits are rare, and many fractures occur gradually or are symptomatically silent, and are found incidentally on x-ray studies. Osteoporosis weakens the trabecular bone of the vertebral body, leaving the posterior supporting elements relatively intact, which accounts for the typical wedge-shaped deformity seen on x-ray evaluation. Hospitalization is often required for bed rest and pain control. Bracing of the back does not prevent subsequent deformity but can afford a degree of pain relief. Braces are most useful with lumbar and low thoracic fractures. The Jewett brace produces hyperextension by placing three-point stabilizers at the abdomen, chest, and fracture area. Lumbar fractures can be treated with a simple abdominal binder, which is generally better tolerated than the Jewett brace.[1,17]

SUMMARY POINTS

- Trauma is an important cause of morbidity and mortality in the elderly, and falls account for the majority of serious injuries.
- When faced with an injured elderly patient the emergency physician must look beyond the injuries and consider the cause. Was the injury related to a significant underlying condition or sudden disturbance in cardiovascular or neurologic function? Might there be toxins or drug side effects that contributed to the accident? Is this person living in an unsafe environment? And, perhaps most importantly, what impact does this injury have on the patient's functional status and ability to care for himself or herself? A priority is to prevent further injury whenever possible.
- Elderly persons experience prolonged disability and a high death rate from multiple trauma. The loss of major organ system functional reserve capacity and aging homeostatic mechanisms contribute to poor outcome. Basic principles of resuscitation apply, with the additional recommendation that all multiply injured elderly patients be transferred expeditiously to a level 1 trauma center for definitive care. Given the difficulty in assessing adequacy of resuscitation, elderly patients may benefit from early, invasive hemodynamic monitoring to optimize cardiac output and oxygen delivery.

CHAPTER AUTHOR

Rawden Evans, PhD, MD

REFERENCES

1. Levy DB, Hanlon DP, Townsend RN. Geriatric trauma. *Clin Geriatr Med.* 1993;9:601–620.
2. Martin RE, Teberian G. Multiple trauma and the elderly patient. *Emerg Med Clin North Am.* 1990;8:411–420.
3. Osler TM, Demarest GB. Geriatric trauma. In: Moore EE, Mattox KL, Feliciano DV, Eds. *Trauma.* 2nd ed. Norwalk, CT: Appleton & Lange; 1991: 703–714.
4. Jerrard DA, Cappadorro K. Burns in the elderly patient. *Emerg Med Clin North Am.* 1990;8:421–428.
5. Scalea TM et al. Geriatric blunt multiple trauma: improved survival with early invasive monitoring. *J Trauma.* 1990;30:129–136.
6. Pellicane JV, Byrne K, DeMaria EJ. Preventable complications and death from multiple organ failure among geriatric trauma victims. *J Trauma.* 1982;33:440–444.
7. Smith JS, Martin LF, Young WW, et al: Do trauma centers improve outcome over non-trauma centers: The evaluation of regional trauma care using discharge abstract data and patient management categories. *J. Trauma* 1990;30:1533–1588.

8. Kiel DP. The evaluation of falls in the emergency department. *Clin Geriatr Med.* 1993;9:591–599.

9. Nelson RC, Murlidhar AA. Falls in the elderly. *Emerg Med Clin North Am.* 1990;8:309–324.

10. Tinetti ME, Speechley M, Ginter SF. Risk factors for falls among elderly persons living in the community. *N Eng J Med.* 1988;319:1701–1707.

11. Lach HW, Reed AT, Arfken CL, et al. Falls in the elderly: reliability of a classification system. *J Am Geriatr Soc.* 1991;39:197–202.

12. Kapoor WN. Syncope in the elderly: a pragmatic approach. *Geriatrics.* 1983;38:46–52.

13. Olsky M, Murray J. Dizziness and fainting in the elderly. *Emerg Med Clin North Am.* 1990;8:295–307.

14. Day S, Cook E, Funkenstein H, et al. Evaluation and outcome of emergency room patients with transient loss of consciousness. *Am J Med.* 1982; 73:15–23.

15. Sloan RW. Principles of drug therapy in geriatric patients. *Am Fam Phys.* 1992;45:2709–2718.

16. Ellis GL. Subdural hematoma in the elderly. *Emerg Med Clin North Am.* 1990;8:281–294.

17. Miller MD. Orthopedic trauma in the elderly. *Emerg Med Clin North Am.* 1990;8:325–340.

SELECTED READINGS

Loberant N, Rose C. Imaging considerations in the geriatric emergency department patient. *Emerg Med Clin North Am.* 1990;8:361–398.

Robbins AS, Rubenstein LZ, Josephson KR, et al. Predictors of falls among elderly people: results of two population-based studies. *Arch Intern Med.* 1989;149:1628–1633.

11 *Abuse and Neglect*

LEARNING OBJECTIVES

1. Define elder abuse and neglect, and list types of abuse and neglect.
2. Identify the risk factors and etiologies for abuse and neglect.
3. Demonstrate the appropriate history and physical examination for an abused or neglected elderly patient.
4. Describe the options available for interventions for patients with suspected abuse or neglect.

"Elderly abuse is far from an isolated and localized problem involving a few frail elderly and their pathological offspring. The problem is a full-scale national problem which exists with a frequency that few have dared to imagine. In fact, abuse of the elderly by their loved ones and caretakers exists with a frequency and rate only slightly less than child abuse on the basis of data supplied by the states.[1]"

Abuse of the elderly has occurred throughout the ages, as determined by literary and historical sources. Until recently, however, research on domestic violence has focused primarily on child and spouse abuse. Among the first national forums to examine elder abuse and attempt to formulate effective legislation was the US House Select Committee on Aging. This committee conducted extensive hearings in 1978 and again in 1984 at which activists, experts, agency personnel, and victims of abuse defined the scope of the problem and proposed practical solutions. The committee eventually released two reports, *Elder Abuse: An Examination of a Hidden Problem* (1981) and *Elder Abuse:*

Although states spend an average of $22 per child for protective services, only $2.90 is spent for the abused elderly person.

A National Disgrace (1985), which together constitute an invaluable source of information on elder abuse and neglect.[1,2]

Through these congressional reports and the hearings that preceded them, the house committee has done much to educate and energize the professional community and the public. Although enactment of federal legislation concerning elder abuse has been slow, each of the 50 states now has abuse laws specific to elderly persons, the vast majority of which require physicians who have "reasonable cause to believe or suspect that elder abuse has occurred" to file a report.[3]

SCOPE OF THE PROBLEM

Each of the 50 states now has abuse laws specific to the elderly. The vast majority of these laws require physicians who have "reasonable cause to believe or suspect that elder abuse has occurred" to file a report.

Research suggests that elder abuse and neglect occurs in 2%-5% of the elderly population. One exploratory study of elderly residents of a Washington, DC, census tract found that nearly 4% were abused or neglected.[4] Another study in Illinois estimated that at least 5% of all older adults experience some type of mistreatment.[5] In the largest study to date, 3.2% of 2020 elderly Boston residents experienced abuse: 20 cases per 1000 were physically mistreated; 11 per 1000 were psychologically abused; and 4 per 1000 were neglected.[6] The investigators also demonstrated that spouse abuse was more prevalent (58%) than abuse by adult children (24%) and that economic status and age were not related to the risk of abuse. Among virtually all studies, women are reportably abused or neglected more often than men. However, in the Boston survey men reported more abuse but appeared to suffer less serious injuries and less emotional stress. This finding may account for the larger proportion of women than men among the victims reported to protective service agencies.

An informal survey of leaders of the American College of Emergency Physicians in May 1992 revealed abandonment to be a significant problem. The survey found a median of 24 elderly patients abandoned per ED each year.[7] Although the survey was not scientific, if extrapolated to the 5000 EDs across the United States, then approximately 100,000 elderly persons are being left at the ED door. Forty-six percent of the abandonment cases were people who lived alone and could no longer care for themselves. Another 41% were abandoned by a family member or caregiver, and 13% were abandoned by an institution.

It is unfortunate that incidence and prevalence rates of elder abuse have several methodologic limitations. A central problem in obtaining national incidence data is the absence of uniform legal statutes, reporting requirements, definitions, and methods of record keeping. Data collection has been limited by inconsistent operational definitions of elder abuse and varied sampling techniques that limit generalization.

There are close to 2 million cases annually of domestic elder abuse and neglect nationwide.

The National Aging Resource Center on Elder Abuse reported that in 1988 there were 140,000 reports of elder abuse received by 24 state protection agencies in the United States.[8] The center suggests that this number grossly underrepresents the actual incidence rate and speculates that for every report taken there are 14 unreported cases. If estimates of reportable cases are correct, there are close to 2 million cases annually of domestic elder abuse and neglect nationwide.

Table 11–1 **Problems in Recognizing and Reporting Abuse**

Ageism or unfavorable attitudes toward the elderly
Denial of abuse by the victim
Disagreement on definitions of abuse
Doctor-patient confidentiality issues
Health care professionals who avoid involvement
Inadequate societal resources to respond to identified cases
Lack of coordination of services
Only subtle signs of abuse (e.g., poor hygiene)
No established procedures for case detection
Professional and public lack of awareness
Relative isolation of victims
Risks of liability
Time-consuming nature of evaluation
Underfunded and overworked social workers
Weak or nonexistent surveillance or enforcement efforts

Underlying the growing concerns about elder abuse and neglect is the realization that this problem is just in its infancy. By the year 2000 the number of Americans ages 65-75 is expected to increase by 23% and the number of those 75 years of age and older by 40%.[9] This increased population will have longer life expectancies and will therefore require personal care for longer periods of time. In addition, the increasing geographic mobility and growing number of two-income families are trends that significantly reduce the number of caregivers available for elderly persons. Finally, one must realize that a number of barriers exist for health care workers in reporting elder abuse. Table 11–1 lists common problems in obtaining accurate information and reporting abuse.

DEFINITIONS

From the very beginning of scientific investigation into the nature and causes of elder abuse, definitions have been a major issue.[10] Lack of agreement on the precise meaning of elder abuse has made it impossible to compare research findings from early studies. Even greater variability is evident in state protective service laws. Without federal legislation for elder abuse, each state has established its own definitions, clinical criteria, and reporting systems. In the extreme, this can mean 50 variations on a single theme. Some states do not use the word *abuse,* and an act may be defined as abuse in one state but not in another. Neglect is defined even more broadly, with some state laws focusing on intent and others on consequences. Difficulties in compiling national incidence data and in transferring specific model programs between states are only some of the problems that stem from the lack of common definitions.[3]

In March, 1985, the Elder Abuse Prevention, Identification and Treatment Act (H.R. 1674) was introduced in Congress. This legislation served to clarify and standardize the definitions and language related to elder abuse (Table 11–2). The American Medical Association has described elder abuse and neglect as "actions or the omission of ac-

Personnel should suspect physical abuse when the patient presents with unexplained injuries or the history is inconsistent with the medical findings.

Table 11–2 **Definitions Relating to Elder Abuse**

Term	Definition
Abuse	Willful infliction of injury, unreasonable confinement, intimidation, or cruel punishment with resulting physical harm, pain, or mental anguish; or the willful deprivation by a caregiver of goods and services necessary to avoid physical harm, mental anguish, or mental illness
Physical harm	Bodily pain, injury, impairment, or disease
Exploitation	Illegal or improper acts of a caregiver using the resources of an elderly person for monetary or personal benefit, profit, or gain
Neglect	Failure of a caregiver to provide the goods or services necessary to avoid physical harm, mental anguish, or mental illness

From Jones J, Dougherty J, Schelble D. Emergency protocol for the diagnosis and evaluation of geriatric abuse. *Ann Emerg Med.* 1988;17:1006. Reprinted with permission.

tions that result in harm or threatened harm to the health or welfare of the elderly."[11] At least 33 different types of elder abuse (from endangerment to passive neglect) have been described in various studies, but all can be condensed into five primary categories: physical abuse, neglect, psychologic abuse, violation of personal rights, and financial abuse.[12]

PHYSICAL ABUSE

Physical abuse or battery involves acts of violence that may result in pain, injury, impairment, or disease.[13] This includes beatings, deliberate burns, sexual assault, force-feeding, and unreasonable physical restraint. In one study, 63% of the victims described being pushed, shoved, or grabbed; 45% had something thrown at them; 42% were slapped; and 10% were bitten or kicked.[14]

Emergency health care personnel should suspect physical abuse when the patient presents with unexplained injuries, or the history

Table 11–3 **Indicators of Possible Abuse**

Burns (cigarette, immersion, friction burns from restraints)
Conflicting or implausible accounts regarding how injuries occurred
Delay in seeking medical care for illness or injury
Evidence of improper administration of medication
Eye injuries or broken teeth
History of similar episodes or of other suspicious injuries in the past
Malnutrition or dehydration
Multiple injuries in various stages of healing
Patient brought to the ED by someone other than caregiver
Patient or caregiver's history of doctor shopping
Sexually transmitted disease
Unusual soft tissue injuries (bite marks, scalp hemorrhage)

provided by the patient or caregiver is inconsistent with the medical findings. Table 11–3 lists indicators of physical abuse.

NEGLECT

Neglect seems far more common than deliberate injury.[12,15] This occurs in situations (1) in which the well-intentioned caregiver is not capable of meeting the needs of the elderly individual or (2) that involve maliciousness. Examples include withholding personal care, medical therapy, or food. If an individual has been denied glasses, hearing aids, walkers, or other mechanical aids that will make life easier, the motive should be investigated. Non-ambulatory patients may be left unattended for long periods, resulting in vermin infestation and decubitus ulcers.

Victims of neglect tend to be in poorer health than victims of physical or psychologic abuse. As such, abuse by neglect is found more frequently in debilitated elderly patients and is more common than physical abuse in nursing home residents. Persons in good health are often able to do something about the deprivation, whereas bedridden persons cannot. A study by Kinsey and colleagues cites anecdotal evidence expanding these observations.[16] Physical abuse should be suspected in the presence of malnutrition, dehydration, poor personal hygiene, or lack of compliance with medical regimens.

Self-inflicted neglect presents ethical problems, because the elderly, unlike children, can choose their own lifestyle. Therefore self-neglect may stem from a person's decision not to accept funds, services, or medical care.[17] The right to self-determination is relinquished only if and when the individual is declared legally incapable or incompetent. Self-neglect will probably continue to be the type of abuse most often detected and the most challenging for emergency care providers to treat.

PSYCHOLOGIC ABUSE

Emotional or mental mistreatment occurs on a more subtle level but is not necessarily less damaging than physical abuse. Types of psychologic abuse include the following:

• Infantilization
• Derogation
• Social isolation
• Threats of institutionalization, abandonment, and homicide

Fear may be provoked when family members, who are aware of their power over the elderly person, use subtle or obvious pressures and threats to force the person to conform. Distinguishing this abusive behavior from hostile or resentful communication can be difficult.[18]

Psychologic abuse is difficult to detect, especially if the victim is suffering from mental impairment. Behavioral signs include the following:

• Passivity
• Withdrawal
• Depression
• Agitation

The victim may act confused, disoriented, and fearful or show signs of infantile behavior in the presence of the caregiver. At times, questions will be deferred to the caregiver, or when a stressful topic is broached, the victim may suddenly change the subject.

VIOLATION OF PERSONAL RIGHTS

Violation of personal rights occurs when caregivers or providers ignore the elderly person's inalienable or legal rights and capabilities to make decisions for himself or herself.[13] Typical examples of this behavior include the following:

- Refusal to grant privacy
- Denying self-determination or decision making regarding personal issues
- Forcible eviction and/or placement in a nursing home

FINANCIAL ABUSE

Financial abuse, or exploitation, typically occurs in one of two forms.[19] It may be the misuse of an elderly person's funds by another person, usually a caregiver or close relative, or a caregiver may withhold medical attention or refrain from making necessary expenditures for the elderly person's benefit. Money saved to provide for retirement needs may be used by the family for other purposes, sometimes with the result of depriving the victim of basic needs. Financial abuse should be suspected if any one of the following conditions is present:

1. The patient is suffering from substandard care in the home despite adequate financial resources.
2. Medical bills are not being paid.
3. The patient seems confused or unaware of his or her financial situation.

The elderly are particularly susceptible to this type of mistreatment, yet it may be the most difficult to identify.[13] The majority of victims suffer from more than one type of mistreatment. Not only does one incident lead to another, but the occurrence of one form of abuse or neglect appears to provoke other forms.[19]

ETIOLOGY AND RISK FACTORS

When I was a laddie
I lived with my granny
And many a hiding ma granny di'ed me
Now I am a man
And I live with my granny
And do to my granny
what she did to me.
　　Traditional rhyme

During the past 20 years, investigators have turned their attention toward identifying risk factors for the mistreatment of both the elderly and their caregivers. These risk factors are based on etiologic theories or explanations for the occurrence of elder abuse and neglect. It is unfortunate that these theories are generally based on small retrospective studies and nonrepresentative samples. However, awareness of such factors and the theories underlying them may help health care professionals understand, recognize, and prevent situations in which mistreatment may occur.

Perhaps the easiest theory of all to understand is that of the psychopathology of the abuser.[11] According to this theory, abusers have personality traits or character disorders that cause them to be abusive. A provider who is mentally retarded, has a psychiatric disorder, or is a substance abuser may not have the capacity to make appropriate judgments regarding the elderly person's needs. Interestingly, studies have shown that the most likely primary caregiver for an elderly relative is often the least socially integrated child in the family (e.g., unemployed).[20] A related explanation underlying elder mistreatment is that of transgenerational violence, which asserts that violence is a learned behavior in some families. In a Detroit study of 77 cases of elder abuse, 10.4% of the documented cases showed clear evidence of mutual abuse between family members.[21] In this vicious cycle, family members alternatively reinforce the abusive behavior of one another.

Transgenerational violence asserts that violence is a learned behavior in some families.

A third theory emphasizes stress as an important factor in elder mistreatment. Many duties and responsibilities that are associated with providing care for the elderly may place overwhelming demands on providers. They may have to give up previous lifestyles, social relationships, and possibly jobs to be home to care for the elderly person. These stressors may cause the abuser to lash out in anger or slowly transfer personal enmities to the elderly person as a scapegoat.[19] The abused person may have behavioral problems (e.g., nighttime shouting) that contribute to the stress at home.[12]

Theories of impairment and consequent dependency underlie much of the analysis of child abuse.[22] The inability of the victim to do some activities of daily living leads to dependency and consequent vulnerability to abuse and neglect by a caregiver. It has been suggested that as these needs increase, the burden and stress level of caregivers increase.[17] In one sample of 240 elderly clients referred for intensive home support because of significant unmet needs, 17% were reported to have been abused or severely neglected.[23] Evolving changes in the delivery of health care have increased pressure for shorter hospital stays and may result in early discharges of elderly patients. It is important to consider whether early discharge adds to home caregiver stress and contributes to elder abuse, since these patients may require extensive care at home and therefore be at high risk for abuse.[11]

Dependency makes the elderly vulnerable to abuse and neglect by a caregiver.

Other authorities point out that the caregiver may be dependent, especially economically, on the older adult.[13,24] This dependency may lead to resentment and, when combined with caregiver stress, may predispose to violence. Other potential causes for abuse and neglect include the following:

- A lack of knowledge (or misinformation) by caregivers
- Ageism
- Greed
- Social isolation of the victim
- Lack of community support

Table 11–4 **High-Risk Situations**

Alcohol or drug abuse or mental illness among family members

Caregiver demonstrates poor impulse control

Caregiver forced by circumstances to care for elderly person who is unwanted

Caregiver unemployed, without sufficient funds, or dependent on the elderly person for housing and money

Elderly person whose primary caregiver is under severe external stress (loss of job, personal illness, divorce)

Victim with problematic behavior: incontinence, shouting, paranoia

Victim socially isolated

Family with a history of domestic violence (spouse, child abuse)

Inadequate housing or unsafe conditions in the home

Increasing care needs because of progressive or unstable conditions, such as Alzheimer's disease, parkinsonism, or severe stroke, that exceed the caregiver's ability to cope.

Physical, functional, or cognitive problems in caregiver that may make providing proper care impossible

Most of the etiologic theories explaining elder mistreatment can also be applied to formal caregivers (e.g., nursing home personnel). Although abuse and neglect in institutional settings cannot be ignored, the vast majority of elder care is given by family members living in the same household. Seventy percent of the population older than 60 years of age reside with family members; 25% live on their own in the community; and only 5% reside in institutions.[20] With these statistics in mind, no should be surprised to learn that most abusers are relatives (i.e., a spouse, a child, a grandchild, or a sibling). Approximately 60% of the abusers (or neglecters) are spouses of victims, and about 24% are adult children.[6] In a review of the literature, Hudson and Johnson conclude that "pioneering studies have uncovered an important fact about elder abuse and neglect—they are primarily family affairs."[25]

Most abusers are relatives (i.e., a spouse, a child, a grandchild, or a sibling).

High-risk situations conducive to elder mistreatment are summarized in Table 11–4. Further study remains to be done to identify with precision the highest-risk groups and to identify marker conditions for mistreatment of the elderly.

PRE-HOSPITAL CONSIDERATIONS

Emergency medical services (EMS) personnel, as initial responders to calls for medical assistance, are in an ideal position to identify abuse or neglect. The elderly are more than four times more likely than non-elderly patients to use ambulance services for transportation to the ED; about 30% of elderly patients seeking emergency care arrive by EMS.[26] Paramedics can identify patients whose health, social, psychologic, and environmental circumstances place them at risk. The lack of necessary appliances such as walkers, canes, and bedside commodes, and the lack of necessities such as heat, food, and water, as well as unsafe conditions in the home may indicate mistreatment.

As discussed in Chapter 6 Gerson et al.[27] developed a program that used paramedics to identify at-risk elderly persons who may need help and refer them to the area agency on aging for assessment and, if necessary, for services. Paramedics are trained to observe the home situation and record problems that they believe warrant further investigation (see Figure 6–3). During the 9-month study period, the Akron Fire Department attended 6000 patients 60 years of age or older and identified 197 (3%) as needing assessment. Area agency on aging investigators confirmed problems in 98% of these cases on follow-up and were able to link many to appropriate community resources (e.g., homemaker services). Fifteen percent of patients were referred to adult protective services.

CLINICAL ASSESSMENT

The physician should ensure that a comprehensive medical examination is conducted, and that the results of the examination are documented, including the patient's statements, behavior, and appearance.[13]

If an immediate danger is not present, the comprehensive assessment need not be done in the ED environment but can be scheduled for a clinic or an office visit. Figure 11–1, endorsed by the American Medical Association (AMA), gives guidelines for such an approach.

CASE DETECTION

To intervene effectively and prevent cases of elder mistreatment, two major barriers must be overcome. First, emergency care providers must be aware that the problem exists and that, in the face of present economic and demographic conditions, its prevalence may be increasing. Second, the detection of elder abuse and neglect requires a high index of

At least 30 state statutes contain penalties for the failure to report abuse and range from fines of up to $1,000 to a maximum of 6 months' imprisonment.

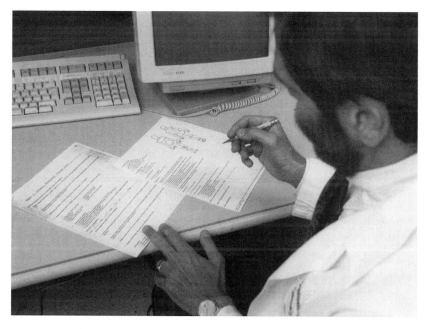

Physical injury is the most obvious type of abuse, and any ED protocol should call for the documentation of any bruises or burns.

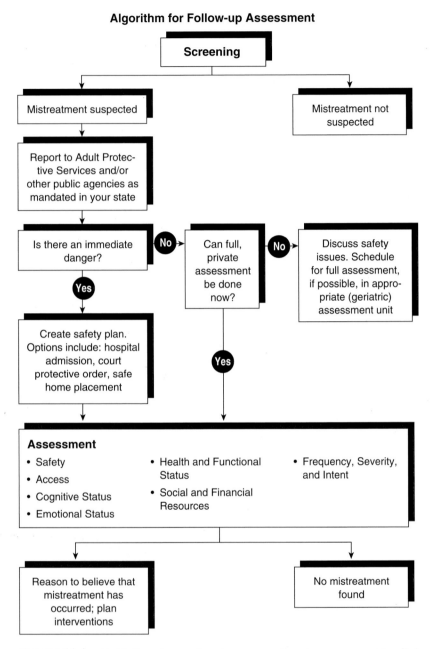

FIGURE 11-1   Guidelines for performing comprehensive assessment in clinic or office setting. (From Aravanis SC, Adelman RD, Breckman R, et al. Diagnostic and treatment guidelines on elder abuse and neglect. Chicago, IL: American Medical Association; 1992:13.)

suspicion. In some cases the victim reports the battering and requests some form of assistance. More often, the presentation is covert, requiring health care providers to take an active role in identifying the problem.

Every clinical setting should have guidelines to determine what information is necessary to assess and report cases of elder abuse and neglect. Providers are more likely to inquire about an elderly patient's bruises if they have training in detecting mistreatment and feel comfortable with a protocol for identifying and reporting suspected victims. Although several excellent protocols are available,[13,28,29] few have been subjected to reliability and validity tests. An interdisciplinary team has been successful in some settings.[15,22,30] In the ED, such a coordinated effort may include EMS personnel, nurses, physicians, local law enforcement officers, social workers, or mental health staff when available. These specialists may have important referral information for patients or family members—support groups and other services in the community that focus on aging parents, home care, family violence, substance abuse, and legal planning.

Figure 11–2 provides a framework to aid the health care provider in the crucial first steps of identification, assessment, and documentation of abusive and high-risk families.[12] The protocol consists of sections for the following information:

1. Obtaining the pertinent history/Psychosocial evaluation
2. Interviewing the potential abuser
3. Recording the physical examination
4. Diagnostics

Informed consent should be obtained with regard to several aspects of the evaluation, including taking photographs and the release of medical records to authorities.

OBTAINING THE HISTORY

How do physicians decide which patients may be victims of mistreatment? The AMA recommends that physicians now routinely ask every patient questions related to elder abuse and neglect.[13] Even if the patient has a cognitive impairment, it is reasonable to ask about mistreatment. Dementia does not necessarily prevent the older patient from describing recent events at home. A Mini-Mental State Examination should be conducted early during the interview to evaluate the patient's cognitive function. If patients score poorly, it may indicate that they are incapable of caring for themselves or of giving consent for intervention.

As with battered women, it is essential that part of the history be obtained while the patient is alone. Excusing the caregiver during the examination will provide privacy. Confidentiality of the interview should be stressed. Developing a level of trust to allow the patient to disclose abuse or neglect may be helpful. Questions that may be seen as threatening should be deferred until later in the interview.

Medically ill patients constitute the largest portion of abused elderly patients presenting to the ED.[12,31] Therefore, besides querying patients about the circumstances surrounding their injuries and asking psychiatric patients about their domestic situation, medical complaints should be explored as a screening device for domestic violence. While giving attention to the presenting complaint, the model protocol includes specific questions about the nature of the abusive situation. Many abuse victims can be identified simply by asking patients direct questions such as the following:

"Has anyone at home ever hurt you?"
"Are you afraid of anyone in your family?"
"Has anyone ever scolded or threatened you?"

Geriatric Abuse Protocol

MEDICAL AND PSYCHOLOGIC HISTORY (quote where possible)

1. **History of present illness or injury.** If patient, caregiver, or other informants (EMS, police) give different histories, document what is said by each.

2. **Past medical history.** Other current problems, severe cognitive and/or physical impairment requiring extended care, history of abuse or neglect, repetitive admissions because of injuries or poor health.

3. **Dependence on caregiver.** Financial, physical, or emotional support; social isolation.

4. **Recent household crises or conflicts.** Inadequate housing, financial difficulties, dysfunctional relationships.

5. **Can the patient relate instances of:**
   - ☐ Rough handling
   - ☐ Sexual abuse
   - ☐ Alcohol or drug abuse by family
   - ☐ Verbal or emotional abuse
   - ☐ Isolation or confinement
   - ☐ Misuse of property or theft
   - ☐ Threats
   - ☐ Gross neglect (fluids, food, hygiene)

6. **Interview with caregiver:**
   - ☐ Recent household conflicts
   - ☐ Knowledge of patient's medical condition; gives care and medicine required
   - ☐ Mental health of caregiver (abuse as a child, poor self-image, history of violent behavior)
   - ☐ Willingness and ability to meet elderly person's needs
   - ☐ Commission of any threatening or abusive acts
   - ☐ Demonstration of poor self-control (blaming the patient for being old or ill, denial, exaggerated defensiveness)

PHYSICAL ASSESSMENT

Temp _____   Pulse _____   Resp _____   BP _____   Weight _____

1. **General appearance (include condition of clothing).**

2. **Current mental or emotional status.** Mental status examination; behavior during examination (extremely fearful or agitated, overly quiet and passive, depressed).

3. **Physical neglect.** Dehydration or malnutrition, inappropriate or soiled clothing, poor hygiene, injury that has not received proper care, evidence of inappropriate care (i.e., neglected gross decubitus ulcers).

4. **Evidence of sexual abuse.** Torn, stained, or bloody underclothing; bruises or bleeding of genitalia, anal areas; signs of sexually transmitted diseases.

5. **Physical abuse findings (also mark on illustrations on the other side):**

   Head injuries
   - ☐ Absence of hair
   - ☐ Hemorrhaging below scalp
   - ☐ Broken teeth or eye injuries

Continued on following page.

FIGURE 11-2   Geriatric abuse protocol. (Adapted from Jones J, Dougherty J, Schelble D. Emergency department protocol for the diagnosis and evaluation of geriatric abuse. *Ann Emerg Med.* 1988;17:1007.)

5. **Physical abuse findings** *(Continued)*

Unexplained bruises
- ☐ Face, lips, mouth
- ☐ Torso, back, buttocks
- ☐ Bilaterally on upper arms
- ☐ Clustered, forming patterns
- ☐ Morphologically similar to striking object
- ☐ In various stages of healing

Unexplained burns
- ☐ Cigar or cigarette burns
- ☐ Immersion burns
- ☐ Friction from ropes or chains
- ☐ Pattern like electric iron, burner

Sprains or dislocations
- ☐

Lacerations or abrasions
- ☐ Mouth, lips, gums, bite marks

DIAGNOSTICS

1. **Color photos:** Label with name of patient, date, photographer, and witness. Include picture with ruler in plane of lesions and picture of patient's face.

2. **Laboratory confirmation (depending on type of injury or neglect present):**
   - ☐ Complete blood count
   - ☐ Partial thromboplastin time, prothrombin time, platelet count (easy bleeding)
   - ☐ Urinalysis, electrolyte panel (dehydration)
   - ☐ GC and chlamydia cultures, wet mount, VDRL (sexual abuse)
   - ☐ Radiologic screening for fractures
   - ☐ Metabolic screening for nutritional or endocrine abnormalities
   - ☐ Serum drug levels or toxicologic screens (overmedication or undermedication)

3. **Computerized axial tomography (CT) scan:** major changes in neurologic status or head trauma that could result in subdural hematoma.

ASSESSMENT
- ☐ No forms of abuse evident
- ☐ Psychologic abuse (verbal assault, threats, isolation)
- ☐ Material abuse or theft
- ☐ Physical abuse (deliberate inappropriate care, direct beating, sexual abuse)
  - ☐ physical neglect (determine causes)
  - ☐ age or frailty of caregiver
  - ☐ caregiver's lack of knowledge of patient's condition; failure to give care or medicine needed
  - ☐ physical or mental illness of caregiver
  - ☐ lack of support systems for the caregiver
  - ☐ financial difficulties

MEDICAL FINDINGS ARE CONSISTENT WITH:

AGENCY/AUTHORITIES CONTACTED:

FINAL DISPOSITION:

FIGURE 11–2 *CONTINUED*

"Are you receiving enough care at home?"

The provider should narrow the focus of the interview to the specific incident or incidents mentioned and obtain more detail, such as the precipitating factors for the abuse or neglect and how often these incidents are repeated. Determine how serious the danger is and what the older adult thinks can be done to prevent the mistreatment from recurring. Use quotations to record the patient's statements verbatim.

Questioning the patient about recent daily routines and activities may reveal a history consistent with abuse, confinement, isolation, environmental exposure, lack of needed appliances (e.g., walker, dentures) or supervision, or other types of neglect. A brief social history may reveal alcohol or drug abuse in the home or other instances of increased caregiver stress. Medical records might indicate previous suspicious injuries or evidence of neglect. Further, examining medication bottles and reviewing the medication history may reveal non-compliance or inappropriate medication, suggesting neglect or medication abuse.

INTERVIEWING THE CAREGIVER

In assessing the primary caregiver (when available), the provider should ask about lifestyle, family structure, and caretaking skills. Whether or not the family understands the patient's medical condition and the necessity of care and medication may be crucial in determining whether inadvertent or willful neglect is involved. Other factors in the caregiver's history include excessive use of alcohol or drugs, mental illness in the residence, alienation, social isolation, poor self-image, and behavior that reveals unmet dependency needs or senility.

The caregiver may resist an interview with the health care provider; however, if a protocol is introduced as a standard part of the examination and read by the interviewer, the caregiver may be less defensive or less likely to feel unjustly accused of wrongdoing. Harborview Medical Center in Seattle has developed a written script for interviews with potential elder abuse or neglect perpetrators.[29] The interview is designed to provide a picture of the family situation, available resources, and current emotional environment of the household (Figure 11–3).

PHYSICAL INDICATORS

Physical indicators have been described as "observable conditions that range from signs of physical neglect to obvious physical injury."[32] Because an adequate history of mistreatment is frequently not obtainable from the patient, one of the most important aspects of case detection is understanding physical indicators. Emergency care providers need to be aware of these signs because of the potential urgency of treating a patient's injury and the necessity of gathering hard evidence to legitimize and facilitate further interventional steps. The classic symptoms of child abuse do not always pertain to elder abuse cases. For example, improper skin hygiene or bruises in infants indicate abuse; in the elderly, diagnosis must be more circumspect. Because of decreased skin elasticity, minor trauma may result in significant ecchymosis, falsely implying abuse.

Interview with Possible Elder Abuse Perpetrator

"Thank you for waiting while I interviewed your mother. Now it's your turn. I need your help. I am doing a psychosocial assessment of your mother's current functioning and situation in order to determine what services are appropriate at this time. I would like to spend some time with you and have you tell me your perception of how things are."

- Tell me what you want me to know about your mother.
- What is her medical condition? What medicine does she take?
- What kind of care does she require?
- How involved are you with your mother's everyday activities and care?
- What do you expect her to do for herself?
- What does she expect you to do for her?
  — And do you do them?
  — Are you able to do them?
  — Have you had any difficulties? What?
- Please describe a typical day for yourself.
- How do you cope with having to care for your mother all the time?
- Do you have support or respite care?
  — Who and what?
  — Are there other siblings who help?
- What responsibilities do you have outside the home?
- Do you work?
- What are the hours?
- What do you do?
- Would you mind telling me your income? (if questions seem touchy to caregiver, say, "I just wondered if the pills she needs to take are affordable to your family." At the same time you are assessing the caregiver's degree of dependence on the elderly patient's income/pension/assets.)
- Is your mother's Social Security check deposited directly in the bank?
- Who owns your home? Do you pay rent? Whose name is on the deed?
- If you help your mother pay her bills, how do you do it? Is your name on her account? Do you have power of attorney? Does it have a durable clause? When did you get it?

Delicate questions to save for last:

- You know those bruises on your mother's arms (head, nose, etc.)? How do you suppose she got them? (Document response verbatim.) If possible, follow up with request that caregiver demonstrate how injury may have happened.
- Your mother is suffering from malnourishment and/or dehydration — or — your mother seems rather undernourished and thin; how do you think she got this way?
- Is there a reason for waiting this long to seek medical care for your mother?
- Caring for someone as impaired as your mother is a difficult task. Have you ever felt so frustrated with her that you pushed her a little harder than you expected? How about hitting or slapping her? What were the circumstances? (Record responses verbatim)
- Have you ever had to tie your mother to a bed or chair or lock her in a room when you go out?
- Have there been times when you've yelled at her or threatened her verbally?

FIGURE 11-3 Sample interview with possible elder abuse perpetrator. (From Tomita SK. Elder Abuse Diagnostic and Intervention Protocol. Harborview Medical Center. Seattle, WA. 1983.)

Physical injury is the most obvious type of abuse, and any ED protocol should call for the documentation of any bruises or burns. Completely undress the patient and look for unusual patterns that might reflect the use of an instrument (e.g., electrical cord, belt buckle), human bite marks, or confinement with ropes or chains. Injuries that appear in different stages of resolution must have multi-

ple explanations to account for them. Contusions of soft tissue can
be staged according to age:

Color of Lesion	Approximate Age
Swollen, tender	0–2 days
Red-blue	0–5 days
Green-yellow	5–7 days
Yellow-brown	10 days
Normal skin tone	3 weeks

Thermal injuries, both burns and cold injuries, can also be suspicious because of their shape and location. The injury may take the shape of common hot objects, such as curling irons, cigarette tips, and heating grills. Scald burns often fit one of three patterns:

1. Evidence of immersion without splash marks (the burn is often uniform in depth with a vivid demarcation between burned and unburned tissue)
2. A burn that spares flexed surfaces (the elbow is immersed into the water, and the antecubital fossa is spared)
3. A burn of the buttocks and genitalia from sitting in scalding water[18]

The presence of a neurologic deficit or abnormal mental status may be due to an unreported head injury. Head injuries, lacerations, abrasions to the face, and trauma to the eyes are frequently encountered in elder abuse and should be treated with a high index of suspicion.[32] Hair loss and ecchymoses at the roots suggest hair being pulled. Eye evaluation may disclose cataracts, or visual field deficits. Posttraumatic dentition, mandibular or maxillary fractures, oral burns, and poor dental hygiene should be subjected to a more detailed investigation. The neck may also reveal evidence of choking, particularly when linear marks are noted, and trachea patency must be confirmed.

Ambulation must be observed when possible; painful or unusual gait may reflect signs of sexual assault or occult injuries. As with children, multiple fractures should be suspected as abuse. Osteoporosis, falls, metastatic disease, and renal osteodystrophy should be differentiated in these patients from traumatic bone fractures.[17] Bilateral injuries to the upper extremities may indicate shaking or an attempt to ward off the abuser. Blunt abdominal trauma may present with Grey Turner's or Cullen's sign—the former sign is blue-green ecchymosis in the flank present 2-3 days after trauma, and the latter sign is blue periumbilical discoloration. Both indicate extravasation of intraabdominal hemolyzed blood.

Physical neglect should be suspected if the physical examination shows the aged patient is malnourished, dehydrated, or shows wasting of subcutaneous tissue. However, these problems are common among frail and immobile elderly persons and therefore are difficult to associate with abuse by the caregiver. Nail care may be a sensitive barometer of hygiene negligence. Except in debilitated patients, decubitus ulcers are usually preventable and their presence suggests neglect. Improper care of medical problems, untreated injuries, poor hygiene, and inappropriate dress for the weather require care to discriminate, if possible, the effects of poverty from those of neglect.[12] Either case necessitates involvement of social services.

The mental status examination may reveal the presence of oversedation, confusion, or agitation. Likewise, abused and neglected elderly persons may be withdrawn or display infantile behavior. Observe the interaction between the patient and caregiver. The patient may become fearful or demonstrate a sudden change in behavior when the caregiver is present, and may be reluctant to speak for himself or herself, especially while the abuser is present. Overt antagonism may be evident.[32] The caregiver may appear domineering, contrite or overly concerned or instead may show a lack of appropriate concern. Either the victim or abuser may have overt clinical signs (irritability, crying, silence) indicative of depression or social withdrawal.[17]

DIAGNOSTICS

Laboratory data are needed in the evaluation of the chief complaint, as well as for the assessment of cases of suspected elder mistreatment. The workup may include metabolic screening for nutritional, electrolyte, or endocrine abnormalities; hematologic and coagulation studies to assess abnormal bruising or bleeding tendencies; a urinalysis to rule out urinary system trauma; and a toxicologic or drug-level screen to determine overmedication or undermedication. The laboratory evaluation of the older patient suspected of having been sexually abused may include serology and cultures for sexually transmitted disease.

Radiologic studies appropriate for the short-term management of the patient must be obtained. Radiographs can be invaluable in identifying previously undetected fractures and may indicate the "age" of the trauma. All patients with suspected abuse plus any patient with documented radiologic injuries should have survey films taken. Special signs to look for include periosteal thickening and transverse or

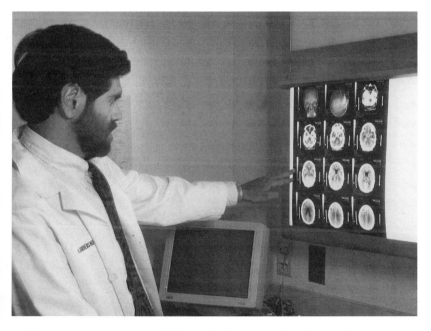

A CT scan may be necessary if there has been a major change in neurologic status.

oblique fractures of the midshafts of long bones and fingers. A computed tomography (CT) scan may be necessary if there has been a major change in neurologic status or head trauma.

CRISIS INTERVENTION

The first priority of the physician when mistreatment is detected or suspected is to assure the safety of the victim. The second is to report the case to the appropriate state agency.[13]

If an emergency health care provider suspects elder mistreatment, proper intervention will depend on the type of mistreatment, the severity, the victim's desire to remain at home, and the caregiver's interest in improving the home environment (Figure 11–4). Immediate action is needed for cases in which the magnitude of abuse and neglect

Decision Flow Chart for Abuse or Neglect of Elderly Patients

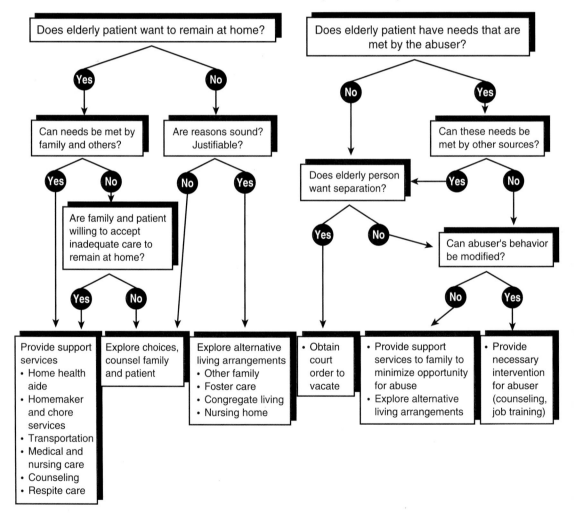

FIGURE 11–4   From O'Malley TA, Everitt DE, O'Malley HC, et al. Identifying and preventing family-mediated abuse and neglect of elderly persons. *Ann Intern Med.* 1983;98:998–1005.

may lead to permanent physical or mental damage. Hospitalization is warranted in high-risk situations and is more likely to be accepted as treatment for a specific problem (e.g., dehydration, decubitus ulcers) than as protection from further harm.[12] Hospitalization then provides adequate time and opportunity to define the actual care needs of the patient and arrange for necessary services. In a retrospective study of abused patients served by a chronic illness center, Lau and Kosberg[33] found that patients were subsequently institutionalized in 46% of cases. Support services were provided in 28% of cases, but intervention was refused in 26% of situations.

Hospitalization is more likely to be accepted as treatment for a specific problem, such as dehydration or decubiti, than as protection from further harm.

The elderly patient has the right to refuse protective services and may elect to return home with his or her family.[11,12] Unless a court issues a finding of incompetence and appoints a temporary guardian, the patient is assumed to be able to judge his or her own needs. This differs from child abuse, in which the government assumes the right to intervene, if necessary, without regard to the parents. When the elderly patient is discharged from the ED, the health care provider should attempt to modify the home situation by involving other family members to unburden the stressed caregiver, contact the appropriate reporting agency, and ensure involvement of social service authorities to guarantee a timely follow-up home visit (e.g., visiting nurse, social worker).[18] The key to getting help for non-consenting elderly patients is to gain the patient's trust or work with the family and significant others. In some cases, providers may be able to reach elderly persons by asking someone close to them to explain and advocate for needed services.

Once it has been determined whether the patient is capable of and willing to take action, a range of intervention alternatives may be considered. The community social services that should be available include the following:

1. Case management
2. Home health services
3. Alternative housing
4. Legal intervention
5. Police protection and cooperation
6. Counseling (for the abused individual and the abuser)

Although the family is often the source of the abuse, it is still potentially the most nurturing source of long-term care for the elderly person.[22] Efforts should be directed toward assisting the stressed caregiver to cope with the role and to prevent the occurrence of situations that might lead to abuse. Drug and alcohol programs may help those caregivers dependent on such substances. If additional skilled help is required for the care of the victim, this can be arranged with the local visiting nurses association or home health service of the hospital. Emergency care providers must take the responsibility of educating themselves about various local community social and health services available (Table 11–5). In some cases the steps that need to be taken to halt the abuse or prevent further abuse may be clear. In other cases it may be necessary to convene a team comprising various disciplines to brainstorm possible solutions and facili-

Table 11–5 **Common Social Problems of the Elderly and Referral Resources**

Problem	Resources	Problem	Resources

Isolation	Senior citizens' centers
	Senior grandparent
	    program
	Friendly visitor program
	Telephone reassurance
	    services
	Medical alert systems
		Emotional problems	Psychiatric emergency
			    services
			In-home counseling
			    programs
			Support groups
			Religious counseling
			    services

Transportation	Senior citizen paratransit
	    services
	Volunteer agencies
	County assistance office
	Medical transportation
	    services
		Caretaking issues	Community mental health
			    services
			Area agency on aging
			Homemaker/companion
			    services
			Chore services

Medication
    assistance
	Senior citizens' discounts
	Pharmaceutical company
	    samples
			Area home health
			    agencies
			Visiting nurses' services

Access to medical
    care
	Neighborhood health
	    centers
	Health maintenance
	    organizations
	Senior wellness programs
	Listing of physicians
	    accepting Medicare
		Caregiver relief
		
		Terminal illness
		
		Alcohol/drug
		    dependence
			Adult day-care centers
			Respite programs
			Hospice programs
			Bereavement support
			    services
			Geriatric treatment
			    programs

Nutrition	Meals on Wheels program
	Senior citizen lunch
	    programs
	County assistance (food
	    stamps)
		Inactivity/boredom	Alcoholics Anonymous
			Senior employment
			    programs
			Foster grandparent
			    program

Housing	Senior citizens' housing Retirement communities Emergency shelters		Retired senior volunteer program Voluntary agencies

Residential Care	Nursing home directory
	Boarding home listings
		Abuse, neglect,
		    exploitation
			Adult protective services
			Department of human
			    services

Financial assistance	Tax rebate programs Social Security Energy assistance relief Volunteer agencies		Victim assistance program

From McDonald AJ, Abrahams ST. Social emergencies in the elderly. *Emerg Med Clin North Am.* 1990;8:447.

tate decision making.[13] The patient's primary care physician can participate in ongoing management or at least provide follow-up after a referral has been made and serve as a monitor who can reactivate assistance if the situation deteriorates.

LEGAL IMPLICATIONS

All emergency care providers should become familiar with applicable elder mistreatment laws and the procedure for referring a suspected case. In most states there is a designated agency—generally the local adult protective services unit of the state department of social services—but in some areas it may be a private agency. Providers may be unaware of the mandatory reporting laws that have been enacted in 46 states and the District of Columbia, most within the past decade.[3] Only four states (Colorado, New York, Wisconsin, and Illinois) have voluntary reporting laws; that is, they state abuse "may be reported" instead of mandating that it "shall be reported." In every law the physician is either named specifically as a reporter or included with others as "any person with knowledge of, or who reasonably suspects abuse." At least 30 state statutes contain penalties for failing to report abuse, which range from fines of up to $1000 to a maximum of 6 months' imprisonment.

The issue of mandatory reporting of elder abuse and neglect is still being debated by practitioners in the field. Although mandatory reporting has proven to be a valuable tool in child abuse, some authorities maintain that it deters elderly people from seeking needed medical care and other assistance. Although these laws vary from state to state, they typically provide no funds that would allow for meaningful intervention in abuse or neglect situations.[3] Whereas the states spend an average of $22 per child for pro-

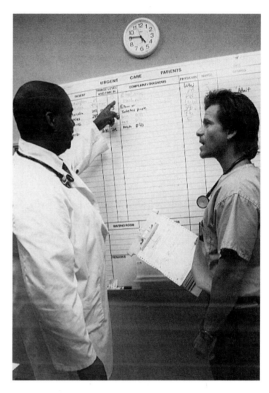

The detection of elder abuse and neglect requires a high index of suspicion

tective services, only $2.90 is spent for each elderly person.[11] Laws that mandate reporting but do not provide adequate resources or protective services may actually inflict harm by creating false expectations.

For physicians and other health care providers who are protected by privileged communication statutes, mandatory reporting of abuse and neglect presents another dilemma. It may be necessary to violate the law or to break the trust of a patient and possibly jeopardize a therapeutic relationship.[19] The AMA suggests that the provider explain to the patient that he or she is obligated to report suspected mistreatment and should strive to maintain a positive provider-patient relationship, keeping in mind the medical need for intervention.[13] The goal is not to punish the individual or family but to stop the abuse or neglect and to access help in the form of outside resources.

All states protect the health care provider from civil or criminal liability for the content of the report.[19] Most of these laws have added that the provider must have acted "in good faith" or performed his or her duties with "reasonable competence." On the other side of the issue is the question of whether a provider may be liable for not reporting suspected elder abuse or neglect. No tort as yet addresses this liability issue. However, based on the provider's responsibility concerning child abuse, the provider can be held responsible for subsequent abuse if the elderly person's ability to escape the situation has been questioned.[3,19]

The goal is not to punish the individual or family but to stop the abuse or neglect and to access help in the form of outside resources.

INSTITUTIONAL ABUSE AND NEGLECT

Institutional elder abuse and neglect refers to mistreatment that occurs in nursing homes, foster care, group homes, and other board and care facilities. In a recent study, 81% of nursing home staff members witnessed psychologic abuse within the previous year and 36% witnessed physical abuse during the same period.[34] Neglect was reported even more often than abuse. Examples include unauthorized use of physical or chemical restraints or the use of medication or isolation as punishment.[13] Abused burned adults are found more frequently in institutions and are more often male. In one study of 26 burn patients identified as victims of abuse or neglect, only two incidents occurred in private homes.[35] To cut costs, some institutions may provide food in lesser quantity and of poor nutritional value, thus further diminishing the resident's quality of life. Additionally, medications designated for older patients may be misappropriated by employees for personal use or street sale.[11] Dehydration and other types of neglect may be seen, and all of the various injuries reported in elder abuse may be found in the institutional setting.

Some authorities have attributed elder mistreatment in institutional settings primarily to poor working conditions, staff shortages, high turnover, and inadequate supervision and training. However, residents of nursing facilities are typically dependent, frail or chronically ill and are extremely vulnerable to abuse or neglect. Many are socially isolated and do not have regular visitors who can monitor their care. Cognitive, vision, and hearing impairments are common; the AMA reports that at least one half of all nursing home residents suffer from dementia.[13] Many communities do not have local long-term care ombudsman programs to help residents resolve problems and complaints.[36] Finally, elder mistreatment may be exacerbated by society's acceptance of abuse and neglectful behavior as inevitable in institutional facilities.

Residents of nursing facilities are typically dependent, frail or chronically ill and are extremely vulnerable to abuse or neglect.

Most states have legislation that addresses institutional abuse and neglect; such statutes are usually contained in domestic violence or adult protective service legislation. Currently, six states (Delaware, Georgia, Maryland, Massachusetts, Missouri, and Oregon) have laws specific to the institutional setting.[36] Twenty-four–hour abuse hotlines have facilitated reporting mistreatment in many communities. As established by the Older Americans Act in 1978, every state has an ombudsman program that provides visitation of nursing facilities to monitor long-term quality of institutional care.[13] Other agencies that have been designated to receive and investigate reports of institutional abuse include adult protective services or aging agencies, state Medicaid Fraud Control Units, state agencies for nursing home certification and licensure, and state health departments.[36] In addition, every nursing care facility must have a process for investigating reports of abuse, neglect, and misappropriation of resident property.

THE RESEARCH GAP

Honor thy father and mother [which is the first commandment with promise]; that it may be well with thee, and thou mayest live long on the earth. (Ephesians 6:2, King James Bible)

Few scientific studies have investigated elder abuse, especially if comparisons are made with the number of studies on child abuse carried out in the same period. Most of the existing knowledge about elder abuse is based on small studies, non-representative samples, informal surveys, and personal observations. Emergency care providers can play a valuable role in (1) encouraging and participating in research on risk factors, (2) procedures for case detection, (3) identifying and meeting the needs of elderly persons, (4) treatment modalities, and (5) prevention strategies. To understand the nature and scope of a complex social problem such as elder abuse, both national prevalence data and incidence data are needed. In addition, research studies focusing on causes of different types of abuse, as well as those linking research findings and public policy, are critical.[3]

Research grants on elder abuse are available from several sources. The National Aging Resource Center on Elder Abuse (NARCEA) in Washington, DC, awards four to five small grants each fiscal year to academic institutions, hospitals, professional associations, or individual researchers. Research funding is also available through the John A. Hartford Foundation (New York), Emergency Medicine Foundation (Dallas), and the American Association of Retired Persons (Washington, DC).

RESOURCES FOR PROVIDERS

The following list of resources has been adapted from the AMA's *Diagnostic and Treatment Guidelines on Elder Abuse and Neglect*[13] to assist emergency care providers in their evaluation and crisis interventions.

- **Area agencies on aging (AAA).** Provide supportive services, make referrals, and serve as advocates for the elderly (e.g., participation in committees and task forces). In some states, AAAs have an investigative role in elder mistreatment.
- **Adult protective services (APS):** Primary service agency with the legal responsibility to investigate reports of mistreatment in the home, community, or institution and to provide services that will increase the elderly victim's safety and well-being.
- **Community services and referral agencies:** Every clinical setting should maintain a directory of community resources to utilize for patient referral. Include the social services provided, hours of operation, eligibility requirements, costs of services, and criteria for admission to programs. Directory information may be obtained from local experts in social work, geriatrics, home nursing, law enforcement, mental health, and volunteer agencies.
- **Elder mistreatment protocols:** Additional protocols for the detection and assessment of elder mistreatment are available from the American Medical Association,[13] Mount Sinai Medical Center in New York,[28] or the Harborview Medical Center in Seattle.[29]
- **Law enforcement:** Where state law defines elder mistreatment as a crime (e.g., sexual assault or battery), health care providers may be required to report suspected abuse to the local police or sheriff. These officers are given more authority to intervene in cases of domestic violence.

- **Medicaid Fraud Control Units (MFCUs):** Located in the state attorney general's office, each MFCU is required by federal law to investigate and prosecute Medicaid provider fraud and patient abuse or neglect in health care facilities that participate in Medicaid.
- **National Aging Resource Center on Elder Abuse (NARCEA):** Established by a grant awarded to the American Public Welfare Association in September 1988. The purpose of NARCEA is to provide information, data, and expertise to professionals and the public on the problems of elder abuse and neglect. NARCEA (810 First Street NE, Suite 500, Washington, DC 20002) conducts training, provides technical assistance, publishes newsletters, operates an information clearinghouse, engages in research, and disseminates technical reports.
- **Ombudsman program:** Every state has a long-term ombudsman program to provide regular visitation and monitoring of nursing facilities. Information about the ombudsman program is provided through local area agencies on aging.
- **State elder abuse hotline:** Most states have instituted a 24-hour toll-free number for receiving reports of elder mistreatment. A list of state telephone numbers is available through the AMA.[13]
- **State legislation on elder abuse or neglect:** All emergency care providers should become familiar with their state laws that deal with elder abuse and neglect. Relevant legislation for individual states can be obtained from state legislators or from the American Association of Retired Persons, Criminal Justice Services Department, 601 E Street NW, Washington, DC 20049.
- **State licensure and survey agency:** This state agency, responsible for certification of nursing facilities, also has the authority to receive and investigate reports of abuse, neglect, and misappropriation of resident property by staff members.

SUMMARY POINTS

- Although a great deal is still unknown about why family members mistreat elder relatives and what can be done to prevent it, there have been a number of achievements. Definitional issues, if not completely resolved, have been clarified. The largest prevalence study to date estimated a 3.2% rate of abuse and neglect among the elderly population living in private homes.[6] Among the many risk factors that have been proposed, psychopathology of the abuser, dependency relationships between victim and abuser, and social isolation appear to be the most important.[37]
- Physicians are advised to incorporate routine questions related to elder mistreatment into their daily practice. The US government recommendation for the year 2000 that 90% of all hospital EDs have a protocol for identifying, treating, and properly referring elder abuse cases has already stimulated activity among emergency physicians on elder abuse issues.[38]
- A variety of programs have been developed to meet the needs of elderly victims and abusers, some of them representing new multidisciplinary models for service delivery. The inclusion of EMS personnel as part of the organizational network serving elderly victims represents a first step toward the prevention of elder abuse and neglect.

Physicians and other hospital-based providers can participate in the primary prevention of mistreatment by making referrals to appropriate community and social service centers. These achievements have also emphasized areas of research and practice to be addressed in the future.

CHAPTER AUTHOR

Jeffrey S. Jones, MD

REFERENCES

1. US House of Representatives Select Committee on Aging. *Elder abuse: an examination of a hidden problem.* Washington, DC: 97th Congress (Comm. Pub. No. 97-277), US Government Printing Office; 1981.
2. US House of Representatives Select Committee on Aging. *Elder abuse: a national disgrace.* Washington, DC: 99th Congress (Comm. Pub. No. 99-502), US Government Printing Office; 1985.
3. Brewer RA, Jones JS. Reporting elder abuse: limitations of statutes. *Ann Emerg Med.* 1989;18:1217–1221.
4. Block MR, Sinnott JD. *The battered elder syndrome: an exploratory study.* College Park, MD: Center on Aging, University of Maryland; 1979.
5. Poetner J. Estimating the incidence of abused older persons. *J Gerontol Social Work.* 1986;9:3–9.
6. Pillemer K, Finkelhor D. The prevalence of elder abuse: a random sample survey. *Gerontol.* 1988;28:51–57.
7. ACEP Survey. Elderly abandonment survey: the abandonment of the elderly in the emergency department. *Frontlines.* Fall 1992.
8. Tatara T. *Summaries of national elder abuse data: an exploratory study of state statistics.* Washington, DC: National Aging Resource Center on Elder Abuse; 1990.
9. Sanders AB. Care of the elderly in emergency departments: where do we stand? *Ann Emerg Med.* 1992;21:792–795.
10. Wolf RS. Elder abuse: ten years later. *J Am Geriatr Soc.* 1988;36:758–762.
11. Council on Scientific Affairs. Elder abuse and neglect. *JAMA.* 1987;257:966–971.
12. Jones J, Dougherty J, Schelble D. Emergency department protocol for the diagnosis and evaluation of geriatric abuse. *Ann Emerg Med.* 1988;17:1006–1015.
13. Aravanis SC, Adelman RD, Breckman R, et al. *Diagnostic and treatment guidelines on elder abuse and neglect.* Chicago, IL: American Medical Association; 1992.
14. Kosberg JI. Preventing elder abuse: identification of high-risk factors prior to placement decisions. *Gerontologist.* 1988;28:43–50.
15. Fulmer T, McMahon DJ, Baer-Hines M, et al. Abuse, neglect, abandonment, violence and exploitation: an analysis of all elderly patients seen in one emergency department during a six month period. *JEN.* 1992;18:505–510.
16. Kinsey LR, AR, Bragg DF. Abuse of the elderly—the hidden agenda, I: The caretakers and the categories of abuse. *J Am Geriatr Soc.* 1981;29:465–472.
17. Benton D, Marshall C. Elder abuse. *Clin Geriatr Med.* 1991;7:831–845.
18. Stewart C, Stewart C, Jones J, et al. Confronting the grim realities of elder abuse and neglect. *Emerg Med Reports.* 1991;12:179–186.
19. Palincsar J, Cobb DC. The physician's role in detecting and reporting elder abuse. *J Legal Med.* 1982;3:413–441.

20. Movsas TZ, Movsas B. Abuse versus neglect: a model to understand the causes of the treatment strategies for mistreatment of older persons. *Issues Law Med.* 1990;6:163–173.

21. Sengstock M, Liang J. *Identifying and characterizing elder abuse, final report submitted to the NRTA-AARP Andrus Foundation.* Detroit, MI: Institute of Gerontology, Wayne State University; 1982.

22. O'Malley TA, Everitt DE, O'Malley HC, et al. Identifying and preventing family-mediated abuse and neglect of elderly persons. *Ann Intern Med.* 1983;98:998–1005.

23. Shaughnessy PW, Kramer AM. The increased needs of patients in nursing homes and patients receiving home health care. *N Engl J Med.* 1990;322: 21–27.

24. Pillemer K. The dangers of dependency: new findings on domestic violence against the elderly. *Soc Probl.* 1985;33:146–151.

25. Hudson MF, Johnson TF. Elder neglect and abuse: a review of the literature. *Ann Rev Gerontol Geriatr.* 1986;6:81–134.

26. Strange GR, Chen EH, Sanders AB. Use of emergency departments by elderly patients: projections from a multicenter data base. *Ann Emerg Med.* 1992;21:819–824.

27. Gerson LW, Schelble DT, Wilson JE. Using paramedics to identify at-risk elderly. *Ann Emerg Med.* 1992;21:688–691.

28. *Elder mistreatment guidelines for health care professionals: detection, assessment, and intervention.* New York, NY: Mount Sinai/Victim Services Agency Elder Abuse Project; 1988.

29. *Elder abuse diagnostic and intervention protocol.* Seattle, WA: Harborview Medical Center; 1990.

30. Clark CB. Geriatric abuse intervention team in a family practice setting. *J Tenn Med Assoc.* 1984;77:535–536.

31. Goldberg WG, Tomlanovich MC. Domestic violence victims in the emergency department: new findings. *JAMA.* 1984;251:3259–3264.

32. Rathbone-McCuan E, Voyles B. Case detection of abused elderly parents. *Am J Psychiatry.* 1982;139:189–192.

33. Lau EE, Kosberg JI. Abuse of the elderly by informal care providers. *Aging.* 1979;300:10–15.

34. Pillemer K, Moore DW. Abuse of patients in nursing homes: findings from a survey of staff. *Gerontologist.* 1989;29:314–320.

35. Bowden ML, Grant ST, Vogel B, et al. The elderly, disabled, and handicapped adult burned through abuse and neglect. *Burns.* 1988;14:447–450.

36. Tatara T. *Elder abuse in the United States: an issue paper.* Washington, DC: National Aging Resource Center on Elder Abuse; 1990.

37. Wolf RS. Victimization of the elderly: elder abuse and neglect. *Rev Clin Gerontol.* 1992;2:269–276.

38. US Department of Health and Human Services. *National health promotion and disease prevention* (Pub. No. DHHS-PHS 91-50212). Washington, DC: US Government Printing Office; 1991.

12 Acute Myocardial Infarction

LEARNING OBJECTIVES

1. Identify types of presentation that may be seen in the elderly patient with an acute myocardial infarction (AMI).
2. Identify features of atypical chest pain or discomfort that may be associated with AMI in the elderly patient.
3. Distinguish symptoms of aortic dissection from symptoms of AMI.
4. Identify electrocardiogram (ECG) changes typically associated with AMI and changes that may be age related.
5. Describe parameters of a risk-benefit analysis in determining appropriate clinical management of the elderly patient with AMI.
6. Discuss age as a prognostic indicator for resuscitation from cardiac arrest.

*T*he greatest clinical challenges are not necessarily presented by rare disease, but by those common illnesses which present in an atypical manner.[1]

This quotation from an early review of coronary artery disease in the elderly population epitomizes the challenges that face the emergency physician in evaluating and treating the elderly patient with an AMI. Not only is AMI common in the elderly, but it is one of the significant examples in medicine of how a deadly disease may present subtly or atypically in that age group. The challenge for the emergency medicine physician is to quickly and accurately make this often difficult diagnosis and intervene when medically indicated with powerful therapeutic agents. These agents may be lifesaving but carry risks of significant side effects or complications.

INCIDENCE

More than half of AMIs occur in elderly persons, although they represent less than 13% of the general population. AMIs not only occur with increasing frequency, but also are associated with significantly increased complications, morbidity, and mortality as people age.[2-4]

PROGNOSIS

80% of the deaths from AMI occur in the elderly.

In contrast to patients younger than 55 years of age, who have an excellent likelihood of surviving an initial AMI, elderly individuals have a significantly worse prognosis. Goldberg and colleagues[4] noted that inhouse mortality for patients 65–74 years of age was double the mortality of those younger than 65 (16% to 8%) but half the mortality (32%) of patients older than 75 admitted for acute myocardial infarction. Although just over 50% of all initial AMIs occur in the elderly population, 80% of the deaths from AMI occur in this age group. AMI is by far the leading cause of mortality in the elderly (older than 65 years), accounting for two of three deaths from all causes in this age group.

The prognosis for elderly patients presenting with their first AMI has historically been quite grim, but it is improving. The risk of in-hospital death from AMI has decreased nearly 50% in the past 20 years. Pashos et al.[5] recently reviewed outcomes of all Medicare patients who presented with their initial AMI over the 4-year period 1987-1990. The 1987 cohort of over 218,000 patients had a 26% mortality at 30 days and 40% at 1 year. The 1990 cohort of 214,000 patients had a 23% and a 36% mortality, respectively, slightly better than a 10% improvement in both 30-day and 1-year figures over the 4-year period. Thus the prognosis of AMI in the elderly, although worse than the prognosis for AMI in younger adults, is improving.

PRE-HOSPITAL CONSIDERATIONS

The average delay between onset of symptoms of AMI and seeking medical help is 2-4 hours, but it is considerably longer among elderly persons.[6-8] It is during this delay that a significant portion of sudden deaths from coronary disease occur.[7] Thus the role of emergency medical services (EMS) dispatch and response becomes pivotal in the early recognition and treatment of AMI in this population. The EMS provider must be cognizant of the wide spectrum of symptoms, particularly in this age group, in addition to classic chest discomfort that potentially represent AMI and treat the patient accordingly.

A succinct history and directed physical examination may provide information that the patient has symptomatic ischemic heart disease

(IHD). EMS personnel often can obtain critical information about the patient that otherwise may not be available, including the patient's functional status, medications, and advance directives. Suspicion of AMI is based to a large extent on history and symptoms; in the elderly patient the presentation is often atypical or subclinical, or AMI may not be noted because of aphasia, delirium, or dementia. All patients with a pre-hospital history consistent with or suspicious for symptomatic IHD should be assumed to be having an AMI.

Age itself is an independent risk factor for coronary artery disease.

Since the incidence of serious arrhythmia during the first hours of symptoms is significant, the EMS provider should, immediately on suspicion of the diagnosis, begin cardiac monitoring as well as obtain intravenous (IV) access at one or preferably two compressible sites such as the antecubital fossa. Oxygen is administered by mask or nasal cannula at a flow rate of 4-6 L/min. Lower flow rates may be considered in patients with chronic obstructive pulmonary disease (COPD) because of CO_2 retention but should not be used at the expense of adequate oxygenation.[7] Pulse oximetry may be a useful adjunct in measuring oxygen supply. Vital signs are monitored serially and frequently.

Patients with persistent chest pain consistent with symptomatic IHD are given fast-acting sublingual nitroglycerin (if blood pressure is adequate). Morphine sulfate may also be useful at IV doses of 1-3 mg administered over 1-5 minutes until symptoms are relieved or it must be limited secondary to hypotension. These therapeutic agents routinely lower blood pressure and often precipitate clinically significant hypotension, thus mandating frequent (every 2-4 minutes) vital sign monitoring.

Pre-hospital prophylactic use of lidocaine for ventricular ectopy varies by protocols established in EMS jurisdictions. Routine prophylactic lidocaine is no longer recommended; its use should be reserved for symptomatic ventricular arrhythmias, ventricular tachycardia, or ventricular fibrillation.[7] (See Emergency Department Management.)

Certain EMS jurisdictions have current protocols that call for use of thrombolytic therapy in the field, typically after confirmation of AMI by transmission of a 12-lead ECG to the receiving hospital.[8]

Prompt and rapid transport to the nearest appropriate ED is indicated. Communication with the receiving ED is helpful to prioritize patient care to prepare for this life-threatening condition.

INITIAL ED ASSESSMENT AND STABILIZATION

The individual presenting with signs and symptoms of symptomatic IHD should receive imme-

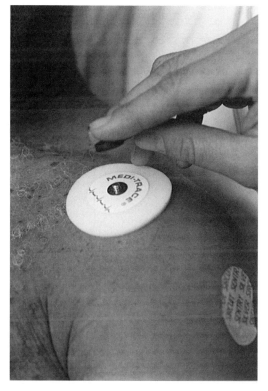

The patient presenting with signs and symptoms of symptomatic IHD should receive immediate triage to a high-acuity monitored area.

diate triage to a high-acuity monitored area, immediate vital signs, and 12-lead ECG interpreted by the ED physician. If oxygen has not been administered, give the patient 4-6 L/min by nasal cannula. Obtain IV access in at least two sites. Consider the second IV site to be a peripheral dual-lumen IV catheter, which would provide a total of three ports.

The physician should perform a brief, targeted history and directed rapid physical examination. The elderly presenting with AMI or unstable angina are more likely than their younger cohorts to have clinically significant bradydysrhythmia, ventricular dysrhythmia, hypoperfusion, congestive heart failure, or acute pulmonary edema. Protocols following the current advanced cardiac life support (ACLS) guidelines[7] should be in place and adjusted for age.

HISTORY

The history is the single most important aspect available to the emergency care provider for the initial identification of patients with symptomatic myocardial ischemia. The history may contain the only information that discriminates this disease from a multitude of other diseases (Table 12–1). Clinically, the history is sufficient by itself to initiate admission to an intensive care unit.

AMI may manifest in the elderly person in four ways: (1) classic anginal chest pain, (2) chest discomfort or pain atypical of the classic presentation, (3) signs or symptoms that may not be classically associated with myocardial ischemia, and (4) asymptomatic presentation.

Table 12–1 **Suggestions for History Taking in Elderly Patients**

1. Obtain history from paramedics about the environment in which the patient was found, including the initial clinical presentation.
2. Interview the patient directly and alone, but confirm information with paramedics and family members when they are available.
3. Initiate the interview with general questions, and follow with specific questions that clarify. Pursue the information you need for medical decision making. Although the patient may offer peripheral and tangential information, your task is to determine the information that will allow you to discriminate IHD from other diagnoses. This requires tenacity, patience, and good judgment to guide patients without forcing their responses.
4. Do not anticipate only the classic symptoms and signs of IHD in the elderly population. Approximately 40% of patients in their 70s and the majority (60%) of patients in their 80s do not have classic symptoms.
5. Determining the presence of risk factors for IHD is only helpful when the patient does *not* carry the diagnosis of symptomatic angina or previous myocardial infarction, because that patient's risk for IHD is already 100%. Even if the elderly patient does not have a previous diagnosis of IHD, the absence of risk factors does not rule out the potential for IHD.
6. Some patients, particularly frail or aphasic elderly individuals or persons with dementia or delirium, may not be able to give a history that will discriminate IHD from other diagnoses. Often determining changes in the patient's activities of daily living will give important clues to the underlying etiology.

Reprinted from Rosen P, et al. Emergency Medicine: Concepts and Clinical Practice. St. Louis: Mosby-Year Book, Inc.; 1992:1318–1319.

CLASSIC CHEST PAIN

The classic chest pain syndrome associated with IHD, described in 1912 by Herrick,[9] consists of crushing, substernal, dull pain, with or without radiation to arm(s), neck, or jaw. It is unfortunate that the likelihood of the elderly person presenting with classic symptoms decreases with age[10,11] (Table 12–2 and Figure 12-1).

The likelihood of the elderly patient presenting classically decreases with age.

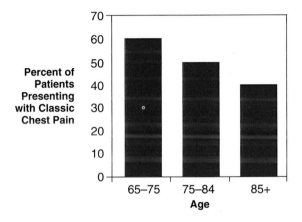

FIGURE 12–1   Liklihood of classic chest pain during initial myocardial infarction. Adapted from: Applegate WB et al. Acute myocardial infarction in elderly patients. *South Med J.* 1984;77:1127-1129. Bayer AJ et al. Changing presentation of myocardial infarction with increasing old age. *J Am Geriatr Soc.* 1986;34:263-266.

Table 12–2 **Signs and Symptoms Other than Chest Pain During Initial Presentation of Myocardial Infarction**

	Age (yr)					
	<70 (n = 125)	70-74 (n = 243)	75-79 (n = 181)	80-84 (n = 140)	85+ (n = 88)	Total (n = 777)
Symptom	No. (%)	No. (%)	No. (%)	No. (%)	No. (%)	No. (%)
Short of breath	47 (37.6)	104 (42.8)	74 (40.9)	66 (47.1)	38 (43.2)	329 (42.4)
Syncope	11 (8.8)	20 (8.2)	27 (14.9)	30 (21.4)	16 (18.0)	104 (13.4)
Stroke	2 (1.6)	5 (2.1)	9 (5.0)	12 (8.6)	6 (6.8)	34 (4.4)
Delirium	4 (3.2)	6 (2.5)	15 (8.3)	11 (7.9)	17 (19.3)	53 (6.8)
Weakness	9 (7.2)	17 (7.0)	14 (7.7)	8 (5.7)	9 (10.2)	57 (7.3)
Giddiness	7 (5.6)	16 (6.6)	7 (3.9)	7 (5.0)	4 (4.5)	41 (5.3)
Palpitations	5 (4.0)	4 (1.6)	3 (1.7)	2 (1.4)	1 (1.1)	15 (1.9)
Vomiting	23 (18.4)	51 (21.0)	33 (18.2)	24 (17.1)	14 (15.9)	145 (18.7)
Diaphoresis	45 (36.0)	79 (32.5)	49 (27.1)	24 (17.1)	12 (13.6)	209 (26.9)
Arterial embolus	1 (0.8)	2 (0.8)	0	0	0	3 (0.4)

Adapted from Bayer AJ et al. Changing presentation of myocardial infarction with increasing old age. *J Am Geriatr Soc.* 1986;34:263–266. Reprinted with permission.

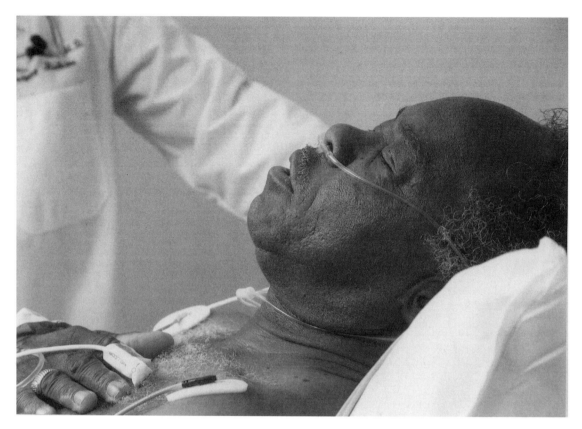

Clinically, the history is sufficient by itself to initiate admission to an intensive care unit.

ATYPICAL CHEST PAIN OR DISCOMFORT

Atypical pain presentations may include prominent abdominal, back, shoulder and upper extremity, throat and neck, pleuritic, or chest wall pain. The patient may actually deny pain, rather preferring to describe the symptoms as a discomfort, pressure, tightness, or indigestion. The quality or character of the pain, such as sharp vs. dull, is less likely to discriminate symptomatic IHD from other diseases, because elderly persons may interpret sharp pain as severe pain. Quantification of pain may be helpful by asking the individual to rate the pain on an intensity scale of 1-10. The reproducibility of the chest pain by physical examination techniques is helpful but does not exclude cardiac ischemia as the etiology. The duration of chest pain may be discriminatory because chest pain that lasts but seconds is rarely due to symptomatic IHD. Likewise, chest pain syndromes that last for days usually are not associated with cardiac ischemia. However, the elderly person may not recall periods when the pain was significantly diminished or absent, thus giving the clinician compromised information.

PRESENTATIONS WITHOUT PAIN

A truly asymptomatic patient who is having an AMI is very unusual, even in the elderly population. Typically there is some manifestation of

Table 12–3 **Signs and Symptoms Associated with Atypical Presentations of Symptomatic Heart Disease in Elderly Persons**

Dyspnea	Palpitations
Pre-syncope	Numbness
Syncope	Paresthesias
Diaphoresis	Acute neurologic deficit
Nausea	Flulike syndrome
Vomiting	General malaise
Hypotension	Acute confusion or delirium
Bradycardia	Falls
Indigestion or heartburn	Sudden inability to ambulate
Exhaustion	Acute functional decline
Inability to take deep breath	

40% of patients over 65 years of age with infarcts, documented by ECG and enzymes, did not complain of pain.

symptoms that precipitate a visit to the primary physician or the ED. Most of the time, atypical presentations without pain often have other symptoms or signs that the vigilant emergency physician will detect (Table 12–3). They may be the emergency medical provider's only initial clue of AMI.

Muller reported recently that 40% of infarcts in a series of patients over 65 years of age were not considered painful by patients who were admitted with ECG and enzymatic evidence of AMI.[12]

Acute confusion or delirium as the sole presenting issue represents a significant number (13-22%) of AMI presentations in the oldest age group or in those patients with chronic mental impairment caused by organic brain syndromes or dementia.[11,13]

"SILENT" MYOCARDIAL INFARCTION

The silent AMI may not give the patient any identifiable presenting complaint or concern of significant magnitude to warrant accessing health care. Logically, if the patient were truly asymptomatic, he or she would have no reason to seek emergency medical care and thus would not ever be seen in an ED during the peri-infarct period. However, well-designed studies have found ECG evidence of myocardial infarction (MI) on routine evaluations of patients observed prospectively. Kannel et al.[14] observed 5000 men and women, aged initially between 30 and 62 years, over a 30-year period. During that time, 700 infarcts occurred. Thirty-one percent of patients 65-74 years of age and 39% of patients 75 years of age or older had infarcts as measured by new Q waves or loss of R waves that were found on routine, every-other-year ECGs (Table 12–4). Retrospective history revealed nearly 50% of these were without symptoms that could be recalled.

Atypical presentations of AMI do not portend a benign course. Lee et al.[15] noted that 25% of all patients (50% of the elderly patients) discharged from the ED with an atypical presentation who subsequently were diagnosed with an AMI died within 3 days of initial presentation or were found to have experienced a sudden death episode in the field.

Table 12–4 **Percentage of Unrecognized Myocardial Infarctions by Age and Sex**

	Men		Women	
Age (yr)*	Total Infarcts	Percent Unrecognized	Total Infarcts	Percent Unrecognized
30–44	14	28.6	1	0.0
45–54	67	17.9	17	41.2
55–64	189	25.4	59	30.5
65–74	134	29.1	95	34.7
75–84	62	41.9	56	35.7
85–94	3	33.3	11	45.5
Total	469	27.7	239	34.7

Reprinted with permission The New England Journal of Medicine. Kannel WB, Abbott RD. Incidence and prognosis of unrecognized myocardial infarction: an update on the Framingham Study. *N Engl J Med*. 1984;311:1144–1147. Copyright 1984. Massachusetts Medical Society.
*Age at infarction.

PHYSICAL EXAMINATION

Before the era of diagnostic tests such as echocardiography or coronary artery angiography, the clinician had to place greater importance on the physical examination, including auscultation of the heart, to confirm or exclude symptomatic IHD. Subsequently, reliance on technology portended a lesser role for physical examination in the setting of IHD. Such technology is not readily available in an ED setting; thus the emergency clinician must rely on a directed but limited physical examination. The general appearance of the patient may give important clues to the patient's underlying condition and acuity. The patient may appear anxious, agitated, or confused; the posture may be bolt upright or the patient may be writhing in pain and the skin may be pale or diaphoretic. A few seconds of observation from a short distance may be very helpful.

Initial vital signs should be confirmed by the clinician, including blood pressure in both arms. Radial and femoral pulses are evaluated routinely. Internal jugular venous pressure may give an important clue to the etiology of the presentation and the hemodynamic status of the patient. The patient is examined for evidence of right- or left-sided heart failure, new or changing murmurs, and hypoperfusion. The pulmonary examination should include auscultation of the lung fields as well as inspection of the chest wall. An abdominal examination may reveal clues to an extracardiac etiology to the

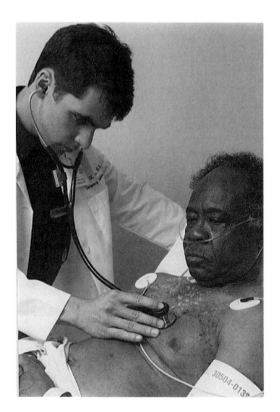

The patient is examined for evidence of right- or left-sided heart failure, new or changing murmurs, and hypoperfusion.

presentation, such as gallbladder disease, peptic ulcer disease, or aortic abdominal aneurysm.

Hypotension may indicate relative hypovolemia or cardiogenic shock. In the hypotensive elderly patient the clinical examination is less sensitive and specific than analysis of data obtained through Swan-Ganz catheterization in determining the cause of the hypotension.

DIFFERENTIAL DIAGNOSIS

An expansive differential diagnosis of chest pain is beyond the scope of this discussion. Because of the atypical presentation in the elderly population, AMI should be in the differential diagnosis of the presenting signs and symptoms of atypical chest pain, chest discomfort, dyspnea and shortness of breath, pre-syncope and syncope, acute or worsening confusion, indigestion or heartburn, acute neurologic deficit, flulike syndrome, general malaise, falls, and acute functional decline.

Aortic dissection should always be considered in the differential diagnosis of AMI in the elderly patient.

Aortic dissection should always be considered in the differential diagnosis of AMI in the elderly patient, particularly in those patients with hypertension or a condition such as Marfan's syndrome that has a predisposition for dissection. The pain is often described as immediately intense, long lasting, and shearing, tearing, or ripping in quality. It is often characterized as different in quality from angina in patients who have a history of angina. Radiation of the pain varies with the area of the dissection, but suspicion should be heightened in patients with pain radiating to the posterior area of the neck, interscapular area, back, or abdomen, particularly if the pain migrates. Syncope is a quite common (5%) presenting sign in aortic dissection. In 20% of patients an acute neurologic deficit is the predominant presenting complaint. ECG changes may occur that suggest regional myocardial ischemia or infarction in 10-40% of cases of aortic dissection.

DIAGNOSTIC TESTS

ELECTROCARDIOGRAM

The initial ECG is most useful when it clearly demonstrates pathology such as left bundle branch block, Q waves, or ST-T wave changes consistent with regional ischemia or infarct that are new when compared to a recent ECG. *The absence of changes consistent with infarct or ischemia does not exclude AMI.*[16] Indeed, 50% of patients older than 65 did not have an ECG diagnostic for ischemia or infarct at the time of presentation.[10]

The absence of ECG changes consistent with infarct or ischemia does not exclude symptomatic ischemic heart disease.

Age-related changes in the ECG are frequent and include reduction in QRS voltage, prolongation of the PR interval, and T-wave flattening. The elderly often have ECGs with evidence of prior MI, bundle branch block, ventricular hypertrophy, early repolarization with J-point elevation, paced ventricular beats, premature ventricular contractions, or atrial dysrhythmia. Comparison ECGs when available may be very helpful. A normal ECG, an ECG with nonspecific ST-T wave changes, or an abnormal ECG unchanged from prior ECGs does not rule out ischemia or infarct.

ENZYME CHANGES

The diagnosis of AMI traditionally can be confirmed when the total creatinine kinase (CK) elevates to a particular threshold (typically five times the upper limit of normal values) and then normalizes. Absolute elevation of the MB fraction above a particular threshold also is evidence of an AMI. These thresholds vary from institution to institution. However, in the elderly population, strict interpretation of these traditional thresholds is problematic for at least two reasons. First, the usual baseline serum concentrations of CK may be significantly less than standards for "normal," particularly if the patient is alcoholic, frail or thin. Thus the peak in total CK associated with AMI may fall within normal limits in this population. However, the absolute value of the CK-MB fraction should be diagnostic. The second concern relates to the rapid clearance of CK from the serum and the often significantly long delays in patients seeking medical care with often atypical symptoms of AMI. Here, the initial serum CK, when obtained, may be after the temporal peak. In this circumstance, serum lactate dehydrogenase (LDH) may be useful. LDH is found in many tissues. However, the LDH_1 isoenzyme is quite specific to myocardium. LDH is elevated within 24-48 hours, peaks at 3-6 days, and returns to baseline at 8-14 days in AMI. In patients who may have delayed presentation, the LDH_1/LDH_2 ratio may be the only serologic marker diagnostic of AMI (Table 12–5).

50% of elderly patients do not have an ECG diagnostic for ischemia or infarct at the time of presentation of their initial MI.

CHEST RADIOGRAPHS

The chest radiograph may be helpful in determining the source of non-ischemic chest pain that is within the differential diagnosis of IHD, including pulmonary embolism, pericardial disease, pneumonia, or aortic dissection. However, portable chest radiographs are notorious for neither discriminating the etiology of the patient's symptoms nor predicting hemodynamic compromise in the setting of IHD.

EMERGENCY DEPARTMENT MANAGEMENT

ED management of unstable angina and AMI in the elderly population may be guided by current ACLS standards[7] and the *Clinical Practice Guideline* edited by Braunwald et al.[17] As in any decision about the ap-

Table 12–5 **Enzymatic Changes in AMI**

CK-MB	Elevation within 4–6 hr
	Peak in 12–20 hr
	Return to baseline in 36–48 hr
LDH (LDH_1/LDH_2 ratio > 1 indicative of AMI)	Elevation within 24–48 hr
	Peak in 3–6 days
	Return to baseline within 8–14 days

From Cannon LA, Marshall JM. Cardiac disease in the elderly population. *Geriatr Emerg Care.* 1993;9(3):499–525.

propriateness of a given diagnostic test or therapeutic intervention, the emergency physician must weigh the risks of side effects and complications with the benefits.

> Whereas the therapeutic approach to young adult patients with acute MI has evolved to rapid interventional therapy, clinicians are somewhat reluctant to pursue a similar tact for their elderly patients. To an extent, this is counterintuitive since the prognosis for elderly cardiac patients is worse than for young adults. . . . Age is, therefore, best considered as an impetus to pursue prompt therapy rather than a reason to avoid it.[18]

Although certain therapies in the elderly have relative or absolute contraindications for a variety of reasons, the elderly patient should no longer be excluded *a priori* from consideration of a therapeutic intervention because of age.[19]

Patients with decision-making capacity may refuse any therapy, and their desires should be honored. The patient's decision of do not attempt to resuscitate (DNAR) does not prevent the emergency physician from utilizing aggressive interventional therapy when medically indicated.

ANTIPLATELET THERAPY

Aspirin has been shown to reduce mortality and morbidity of AMI in elderly patients, independent of other therapeutic interventions. Low-dose aspirin (75-150 mg) may be as efficacious as full strength (325 mg) with fewer side effects. Unless the elderly patient has a known hypersensitivity to aspirin, 160 mg should be administered in the ED.[20]

NITRATES

Nitrates may reduce preload and afterload, improve left ventricular function, relieve coronary artery spasm, reduce myocardial oxygen demand, limit infarct size, and lower the incidence of infarct-related complications and mortality. Pooled data from six studies (elderly and non-elderly individuals included) utilizing IV nitroglycerin noted an overall mortality reduction of 33%.[21]

Caution is advised with nitrate use, because nitrates may cause significant hypotension secondary to age-related anatomic and physiologic changes in the cardiovascular system.

MORPHINE SULFATE

Morphine is useful for treating symptomatic IHD and acute pulmonary edema. Caution must be exercised, because morphine is associated with respiratory depression and hypotension, particularly when the patient is elderly and volume depleted. Hypotension is very common in the setting of multiple pharmacologic interventions. Initial IV dosage is 1-3 mg over 3-5 minutes and titrated to relief of pain or onset of hypotension.

BETA-BLOCKERS

Early beta-blockade during AMI in the elderly population is associated with a 23% reduction in mortality.[22] Contraindications for use of beta-blockade include bradyarrhythmia, atrioventricular conduction abnor-

Aspirin has been shown to reduce mortality and morbidity of AMI in elderly patients, independent of other therapeutic interventions.

Early beta-blockade during AMI is associated with a 23% reduction in mortality.

malities, left-sided heart failure, and COPD. Significant side effects during the peri-infarct period include congestive heart failure, heart block, hypotension, and bronchospasm. Gurwitz et al.[23] found that in a significant number of elderly patients, beta-blockade is not utilized even when not contraindicated. IV beta-blockers that are more rapid in onset and have a shorter half-life may be of greater utility for elderly persons with an AMI than longer acting IV or oral beta-blockers.

HEPARIN

Optimal use of heparin for the elderly AMI patient is not established.[17,22] Revascularization is more likely with coadministration of heparin, but the risks of significant hemorrhage increase.

LIDOCAINE

Routine prophylactic use of lidocaine is not recommended by current ACLS standards.[7] Sustained or symptomatic ventricular ectopy is an indication to use lidocaine, but the bolus, maintenance dose, and total dosage are recommended to be cut in half for elderly patients. Side effects may include seizure, hypotension, and acute mental status changes.

THROMBOLYTICS

Thrombolytic therapy in the elderly patient with AMI is not contraindicated solely on the basis of chronologic age.[16,17,24,25] Thrombolytic therapy in elderly patients should follow the same criteria used for younger patients: namely, it is based on the patient's clinical presentation, appropriate ECG changes, and functional status, as well as on relative and absolute contraindications.

In several, but not all, European thrombolytic trials, mortality and morbidity were reduced in elderly patients given thrombolytic therapy (Table 12–6). Non–intracerebral hemorrhagic bleeding complications, although significant, are usually arguably less important, because they can be treated quite effectively without long-term morbidity. Intracerebral hemorrhage represents a small (0.2-2.1%) but definite increased risk in this population, approximately twice the rate for patients younger than age 65.[26]

As recently as 1987, 90% of all patients[27] and more than 95% of the elderly (99% of those older than age 75) patients[28] with AMI did not receive thrombolytic therapy for various reasons. Dorey et al.[19] identified five reasons that patients are not treated with thrombolytic therapy: liability exposure for iatrogenic complications, advanced age, nondiagnostic ECG, specific contraindications, and excessive delay in initiation of therapy. All of these reasons are directly or closely associated with advanced age. Pashos et al.[5] estimated an increase in utilization of thrombolytic therapy in Medicare patients from 4% to 11% over a 4-year period ending in 1990.

REVASCULARIZATION WITH PERCUTANEOUS TRANSLUMINAL CORONARY ANGIOPLASTY AND CORONARY ARTERY BYPASS GRAFTING

The decision to perform percutaneous transluminal coronary angioplasty (PTCA) and coronary artery bypass grafting (CABG) is made in

Table 12–6 **Thrombolytic Therapy in Elderly Persons: Results of Selected Trials***

	No.	Mortality (%)			
		Active	Control	Difference	% Change
Streptokinase					
GISSI-1	11,709				
≤ 65 yr	7608	5.7	7.7	–2.0	–26.0
66–75 yr	2886	16.6	18.1	–1.5	–8.3
> 75 yr	1215	28.9	33.1	–4.2	–12.7
ISAM	1741				
< 70 yr	1454	5.1	6.6	–1.5	–22.7
70–75 yr	287	13.0	9.6	+3.4	+35.4
ISIS-2	17,187				
< 60 yr	7720	4.2	5.8	–1.6	–27.6
60–69 yr	6056	10.6	14.4	–3.8	–26.4
≥ 70 yr	3411	18.2	21.6	–3.4	–15.7
≥ 80 yr	401	20.1	34.2	–14.1	–41.2
rt-PA					
ASSET	5031				
≤ 65 yr	3352	5.4	6.3	–0.9	–14.3
66–75 yr	1679	10.9	16.4	–5.5	–33.5
APSAC					
AIMS	1257				
< 60 yr	751	4.0	6.1	–2.1	–34.4
60–70 yr	506	9.9	21.3	–11.4	–53.5
Pooled totals	36,925				
Younger	26,941	6.2	8.4	+2.2	–25.7
Older	9984	17.2	20.7	–3.5	–16.9

From Forman DE, Gutierrez Bernal JL, Wei JY. Management of acute myocardial infarction in the very elderly. *Am J Med.* 1992;93:315–326. Reprinted with permission of American Journal of Medicine.
**GISSI-1*, Gruppo Italiano per lo Studio della Streptochinasi nell'Infarto Miocardico; *NS*, not significant; *ISAM*, Intravenous streptokinase in acute myocardial infarction; *ISIS-2*, Second International Study of Infarct Survival; *rt-PA*, recombinant tissue plasminogen activator; *ASSET*, Anglo-Scandinavian Study of Early Thrombosis; *APSAC*, anisoylated plasminogen streptokinase activator complex; *AIMS*, APSAC Intervention Mortality Study.

settings other than the ED. These therapies may benefit select elderly patients, since approximately 90% of elderly patients in studies such as TIMI are ineligible for thrombolytics.

Like thrombolytic therapy, the utilization of PTCA and CABG, based on the most current information, should not be proscribed on age alone. Many studies have found that in stable elderly patients, including the oldest individuals, these procedures are tolerated quite well. However, in unstable patients, significant complications and in-hospital mortality are increased. These interventions are best tolerated in those patients with a more youthful physiologic age. In select elderly populations, successful revascularization rates are similar to those in much younger populations.[29–31]

The elderly who have the highest mortality and morbidity following an MI benefit the most from early thrombolytics.

DISPOSITION PLAN

The actual diagnosis of AMI in elderly persons is often determined after the patient is admitted for symptomatic IHD. The history alone is sufficient to initiate admission to a monitored hospital bed. Neither serologic markers, radiographic data, nor ECGs are sufficiently sensitive in the elderly to discharge patients based on non-diagnostic findings.

ELECTROCARDIOGRAM CHANGES

Patients with ECG changes diagnostic for AMI should be given aspirin, heparin, and thrombolytic therapy, and they should be considered for revascularization early in their ED course if pain is not relieved by nitrates or morphine sulfate and their ECG changes are not resolved. (See Emergency Department Management.) Admission to an intensive care unit is indicated.

COMPLICATIONS CONSISTENT WITH AMI BUT WITHOUT ECG CHANGES DIAGNOSTIC FOR AMI

In the setting of continued significant symptoms, congestive heart failure, dysrhythmia, hypotension, or severe hypertension, the patient should be admitted to an intensive care unit.

HISTORY CONSISTENT WITH SYMPTOMATIC IHD

Consideration is given to treating patients with a history consistent with symptomatic IHD the same as patients with unstable angina. Those patients who are currently asymptomatic, without ECG changes, and medically stable and have a significant history consistent with unstable symptomatic IHD should be admitted to a monitored bed.

There remains a significant portion of elderly patients who do not fit in either of these categories who are evaluated in the ED. These are often the older and frailer of the elderly population, who may have significant functional or cognitive impairment or aphasia and thus are unable to communicate adequately. The emergency clinician should closely look for changes in the patient's activities of daily living (ADLs) and appreciate that such changes may be the only key to an underlying, life-threatening problem such as AMI, infection, or an acute condition of the abdomen. Admission for observation may be indicated in these circumstances.

CARDIAC ARREST

There was no overall difference in resuscitation success or survival to hospital discharge when elderly patients were compared to non-elderly patients.

The outcome of cardiac arrest in elderly persons has been the subject of some debate and conflicting data in the medical literature. Whereas some studies have concluded that the elderly have poor outcomes following cardiac arrest, other studies show no difference in outcome compared to non-elderly patients. Many of the studies showing poorer outcome for elderly persons do not differentiate the effects of age from other factors such as comorbid diseases, dependent lifestyle, and medications.

In the largest study assessing survival from cardiac arrest in older patients, the Belgium Cerebral Resuscitation Study Group analyzed 2776 out-of-hospital cardiac arrests. They found that age had no effect on hospital admission, survival to discharge, or neurologic outcome.[32] Similar results were obtained by Longstreth et al.[33] in a study of 1405 patients age 70 years and older in cardiac arrest. They found no overall difference in resuscitation success or survival to hospital discharge when elderly patients were compared to non-elderly patients. In fact, 24% of patients 70 years or older with ventricular fibrillation survived to hospital discharge.

In a study of in-hospital cardiopulmonary resuscitation, Bedell et al.[34] determined factors prognostic of hospital discharge and 6-month survival. Although a number of medical conditions such as pneumonia, renal failure, and cancer were associated with poor survival, age did not influence survival after cardiopulmonary resuscitation.[34]

In a series of studies Tresch et al.[35,36] helped to characterize the type of arrest and hospital course following successful resuscitation. Figure 12–2 demonstrates the changing pattern of presenting rhythms for patients with out-of-hospital cardiac arrest as a function of age. Only 44% of patients 70 years and older presented in ventricular fibrillation, compared to 58% of younger patients. Pulseless electrical activity (or electromechanical dissociation) was progressively more common in older age groups. In another study, Tresch found that long-term survival from cardiac arrest was similar for both younger and older patients following hospital discharge (Figure 12–3). Although more older patients were likely to die during hospitalization, the length of hospital stay, length of intensive care unit stays, residual neurologic deficits, and neurologic deaths were no different when younger and older patients were compared (Table 12–7).

The delay in presentation was the number one cause of patient exclusion from thrombolytic therapy protocols.

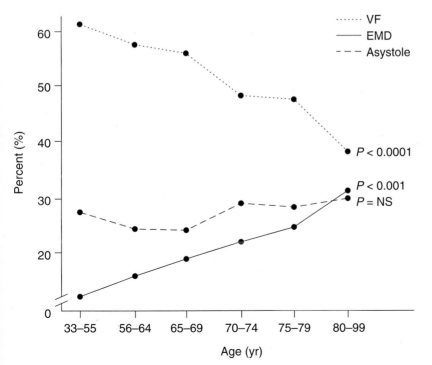

FIGURE 12–2

Difference in prevalence of initial documented out-of-hospital rhythm among age-groups. *EMD,* Electromechanical dissociation; *VF,* ventricular fibrillation; *NS,* not significant. (From Tresch DD, Thakur R, Hoffmann RG, Brooks HL. Comparison of outcome of resuscitation of out-of-hospital cardiac arrest in persons younger and older than 70 years of age. *Am J Cardiol.* 1988; 61:1120–1122. Reprinted with permission of American Journal of Cardiology.)

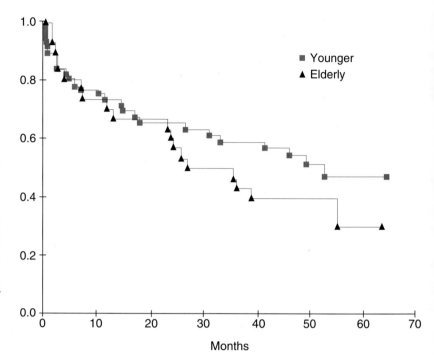

FIGURE 12–3

Comparison of actuarial survival curves of the two age-groups. (From Tresch DD, Thakur RK, Hoffman RG, et al. Should the elderly be resuscitated following out-of-hospital cardiac arrest? *Am J Med.* 1989;86:145–150. Reprinted with permission of American Journal of Medicine.

Table 12–7 **Hospital Course**

	Elderly (n = 112)	Younger (n = 102)	P Value
Total patients (no.)	112	102	NS*
Mean hospital stay (days)	13.5 ± 16.5	17.1 ± 18.1	NS
Mean intensive care stay (days)	4.7 ± 4.9	5.6 ± 6.6	NS
Patients discharged—survivors (no.)	32 (29%)	48 (47%)	<0.001
Mean hospital stay (days)	28.3 ± 18.9	25.6 ± 16.7	NS
Mean intensive care stay (days)	6.1 ± 5.9	7.2 ± 7.0	NS
Neurologic impairment (no.)	10 (32%)	11 (22%)	NS
Nursing home placement (no.)	5 (16%)	6 (13%)	NS
Comatose (no.)	2 (6%)	4 (8%)	NS
Deaths (no.)	80 (71%)	54 (53%)	<0.001
Within 2 days of hospitalization (no.)	37 (46%)	21 (39%)	NS
Neurologic deaths (no.)	40 (49%)	25 (46%)	NS

From Tresch DD, Thakur RK, Hoffman RG, et al. Should the elderly be resuscitated following out-of-hospital cardiac arrest? *Am J Med.* 1989;86:145–150. Reprinted with permission of American Journal of Medicine.
*NS, Not significant.

Thus age by itself is not a poor prognostic indicator for resuscitation from cardiac arrest or for long-term survival or neurologic outcome. All older patients in cardiac arrest should have full resuscitation protocols instituted using ACLS guidelines unless there is a clear advance directive specifying that the patient does not want cardiopulmonary resuscitation instituted.

RESEARCH AND TREATMENT PROTOCOLS

Significant and lifesaving advances have been made in treatment of patients with cardiovascular disease over the past 25 years. Examples include percutaneous transluminal coronary angioplasty (PTCA), coronary artery bypass grafts (CABG), and thrombolysis. Medications commonly used today to treat AMI, such as the calcium channel antagonists, the beta-adrenergic antagonists, and thrombolytics, were developed and approved by the US Food and Drug Administration (FDA) quite recently; for example, thrombolytic therapy was approved less than a decade ago. The elderly population, particularly the oldest of the population, were summarily excluded from these early research protocols. Age-based exclusions have been extremely common in research protocols in all areas of AMI management and have been the source of recent review,[19,37] editorial commentary,[38,39] and study.[18,22] Gurwitz and colleagues[18] in a recent review of the English language literature found 214 randomized, prospective studies from 1960 to 1991 on pharmacotherapy for AMI (Figures 12–4 and 12–5). They found that fully 60% of the studies excluded patients older than age 75 and concluded that such exclusions "limit the ability to generalize study findings to the patient population that experiences the most morbidity and mortality from acute myocardial infarction." Despite National Heart, Lung, and Blood Institute and American College of Cardiology conferences on improving enrollment of the elderly in AMI outcome research, physicians must continue to base most clinical care decisions for elderly patients predominantly or exclusively on data extrapolated from younger populations.

Significant comorbid conditions such as diabetes, congestive heart failure, hypertension, and chronic obstructive pulmonary disease are increasingly common among the elderly population and have historically excluded affected patients from most AMI research protocols. Ninety-

> *Age-based exclusions have been extremely common in research protocols in all areas of AMI management.*

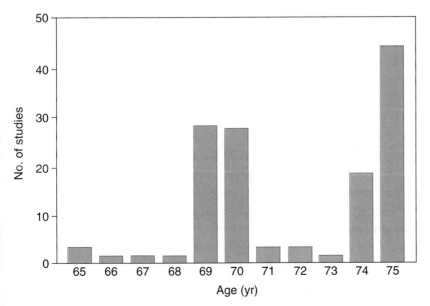

FIGURE 12–4
Distribution of maximum ages for subject inclusion among studies with age-based exclusions ($n = 130$). (From Gurwitz JH, Col NF, Avorn J. The exclusion of the elderly and women from clinical trials in acute myocardial infarction. *JAMA*. 1992; 268(11):1417–1422. Copyright 1992, American Medical Association.)

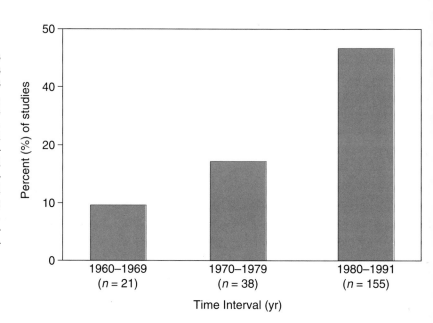

Figure 12–5
Percentage of studies
with age-based exclusions
for three time intervals
(1960 through 1969,
1970 through 1979, and
1980 through 1991).
(From Gurwitz JH, Col
NF, Avorn J. The exclu-
sion of the elderly and
women from clinical tri-
als in acute myocardial
infarction. *JAMA.* 1992;
268[11]:1417–1422.
Copyright 1992, Ameri-
can Medical Associa-
tion.)

four percent of elderly patients presenting to an ED for evaluation in one recent multicenter study had one or more significant comorbid conditions.[40]

The spectrum of a population with risk for AMI should be studied to determine who will benefit from an intervention. Unnecessarily restrictive exclusion criteria limit the generalizability of research results.

Chronologic age traditionally has been either an absolute or a relative contraindication for certain therapies that may have utility in patients with AMI. Increasingly, specialists from varied disciplines in geriatric emergency care are critical of that tradition. These authors are noting that functional status rather than absolute chronologic age is the better measure of the appropriateness or inappropriateness of a given therapy.[18,22]

Members of the SAEM Geriatric Task Force strongly concur, appreciating the heterogeneous nature of the elderly population. Further, the decision to utilize a given therapeutic intervention or diagnostic test should be based on a risk/benefit analysis founded on an increasing body of scientific evidence established on patients with similar age, comorbid conditions, and functional status.

SUMMARY POINTS

- AMI is the leading cause of death in the elderly population.
- Although elderly persons may present with classic chest pain associated with ischemia, it is common for them to present atypically. Those persons older than age 85, in fact, are unlikely to present with classic chest pain.
- AMI should be suspected in elderly patients presenting with atypical chest discomfort, congestive heart failure, dyspnea, acute mental status changes, or acute functional decline.
- Diagnostic tests performed in the ED are less likely to confirm myocardial ischemia or infarction in elderly persons.
- The elderly are more likely to present with shock, congestive heart failure, or acute pulmonary edema.

- Medical decision making in elderly patients presenting with AMI is not simple. Therapy should be based on physiologic age, functional status, known risks and benefits, and the patient's wishes, if known. Medical decision making should not be based on chronologic age. Decisions should be made quickly, because elderly patients often delay coming to the ED.
- Medications such as beta-blockers, aspirin, and narcotics are often withheld from elderly patients because of physician reticence, not because of specific absolute or relative contraindications.
- Thrombolytic therapy and anticoagulation can be well tolerated by the elderly patient with AMI, with a significant reduction in death and disability. The small but significant risk of hemorrhage and other complications should be discussed with the patient.
- Patients must have the decision-making capacity to understand the risks and benefits of these therapies before their administration.

CHAPTER AUTHOR

Norm Kalbfleisch, MD, FACEP

REFERENCES

1. MacDonald JB, Presentation of acute myocardial infarction in the elderly: a review. *Age Aging.* 1984;13:196–200.
2. Kapantais G. *Characteristics of persons dying of disease of the heart: preliminary data from the 1986 Mortality Followback Survey.* Advance data from vital and health statistics, No. 172. Hyattsville, MD: National Center for Health Statistics; 1989.
3. American Heart Association. *1993 heart and stroke facts.* Dallas, TX.
4. Goldberg RJ et al. The impact of age on the incidence and prognosis of initial acute myocardial infarction: the Worchester heart attack study. *Am Heart J.* 1989;117(3):543–549.
5. Pashos CL et al. Temporal changes in the care and outcomes of elderly patients with acute myocardial infarction, 1987 through 1990. *JAMA.* 1993;270:1832–1836.
6. Kowalenko T et al. Prehospital diagnosis and treatment of acute myocardial infarction: a critical review. *Am Heart J.* 1992;123:181–190.
7. Cummins O, Ed. *Textbook of advanced cardiac life support.* Dallas, TX: American Heart Association; 1994.
8. Weaver WD et al. Myocardial infarction triage and intervention project: phase I: patient characteristics and feasibility of prehospital initiation of thrombolytic therapy. *J Am Coll Cardiol.* 1990;15:925–931.
9. Herrick JB. Clinical features of sudden obstruction of the coronary arteries. *JAMA.* 1912;59:2015–2019.
10. Applegate WB et al. Acute myocardial infarction in elderly patients. *South Med J.* 1984;77:1127–1129.
11. Bayer AJ et al. Changing presentation of myocardial infarction with increasing old age. *J Am Geriatr Soc.* 1986;34:263–266.
12. Muller RT. Painless myocardial infarction in the elderly. *Am Heart J.* 1990;119:202–204.
13. Black DA. Mental state and presentation of myocardial infarction in the elderly. *Age Aging.* 1987;16:125–127.
14. Kannel WB et al. Incidence and prognosis of unrecognized myocardial infarction. *N Engl J Med.* 1984;311:1144–1147.
15. Lee TH et al. Clinical characteristics and natural history of patients with acute myocardial infarction sent home from the emergency room. *Am J Cardiol.* 1987;60:219–224.

16. Cannon LA, Marshall JM. Cardiac disease in the elderly population. *Geriatr Emerg Care.* 1993;9(3):499–525.

17. Braunwald E, Mark DB, Jones RH, et al. *Unstable angina: diagnosis and management.* Clinical practice guidelines No. 10. AHCPR Publication No. 94-0602. Rockville, MD: Agency for Health Care Policy and Research and the National Heart, Lung and Blood Institute. Public Health Service, US Department of Health and Human Services; March 1994.

18. Gurwitz JH et al. The exclusion of the elderly and women from clinical trials in acute myocardial infarction. *JAMA.* 1992;268:1417–1422.

19. Dorey AJ et al. Thrombolytic therapy of acute myocardial infarction: keeping the unfulfilled promises. *JAMA.* 1992;268:3108–3114.

20. Dalen JE, Goldberg RJ. Prophylactic aspirin and the elderly population. *Clin Geriatr Med.* 1992;8(1):119–126.

21. Yusef S. Effect of intravenous nitrates on mortality in acute myocardial infarction: an overview of the randomized trials. *Lancet.* 1988;1:1088–1092.

22. Forman DE. Management of acute myocardial infarction in the very elderly. *Am J Med.* 1992;93:315–326.

23. Gurwitz JH et al. Beta-blocker therapy in acute myocardial infarction: evidence for underutilization in the elderly. *Am J Med.* 1992; 82(12):1626–1630.

24. Williamson BD et al. Should older patients with acute myocardial infarction receive thrombolytic therapy? *Drugs Aging.* 1992;2(6):461–468.

25. Gurwitz JH. Coronary thrombolysis for the elderly? *JAMA.* 1991;265:1720–1723.

26. Gore JM et al. Intracerebral hemorrhage, cerebral infarction, and subdural hematoma after acute myocardial infarction and thrombolytic therapy in the Thrombolysis in Myocardial Infarction Study: thrombolysis in myocardial infarction, phase II, pilot and clinical trial. *Circulation.* 1991;2:448–459.

27. Grines CL et al. A comparison of immediate angioplasty with thrombolytic therapy for acute myocardial infarction. *N Engl J Med.* 1993;328:673–679.

28. Smith SC. Outlook after acute myocardial infarction in the very elderly compared with that in patients aged 65 to 75 years. *J Am Coll Cardiol.* 1990;16(4);784–792.

29. Forman DE. Coronary angiography and revascularization in very old patients early after myocardial infarction: early and long-term results. *J Am Coll Cardiol.* 1992;19:378A.

30. Lee TC. Emergency percutaneous transluminal coronary angioplasty for acute myocardial infarction in patients 70 years of age or older. *Am J Cardiol.* 1990;66:663–667.

31. Loop FD. Coronary artery bypass graft surgery in the elderly: indications and outcome. *Cleve Clin J Med.* 1988;55:23–34.

32. Van Hoeyweghen RJ, Bossaert LL, Mullie A, et al. Survival after out-of-hospital cardiac arrest in elderly patients. *Ann Emerg Med.* 1992;21:1179–1184.

33. Longstreth WT, Cobb LA, Fahrenbruch CE, Copass MK. Does age affect outcomes of out-of-hospital cardiopulmonary resuscitation? *JAMA.* 1990;264:2109–2110.

34. Bedell SE, Delbanco TL, Cook EF, Epstein FH. Survival after cardiopulmonary resuscitation in the hospital. *N Engl J Med.* 1983;309:569–576.

35. Tresch DD, Thakur R, Hoffman RG, Brooks HL. Comparison of outcome of resuscitation of out-of-hospital cardiac arrest in persons younger and older than 70 years of age. *Am J Cardiol.* 1988;61:1120–1122.

36. Tresch DD, Thakur RK, Hoffman RG, Olson D, Brooks HL. Should the elderly be resuscitated following out-of-hospital cardiac arrest? *Am J Med.* 1989;86:145–150.

37. O'Connor CM, Califf RM. Aggressive therapy of acute MI in the elderly. *Hosp Pract.* 1992:59–76.

38. Gurwitz JH et al. Diagnostic testing in acute myocardial infarction: does patient age influence utilization patterns? *Am J Epidemiol.* 1991;134: 948–957.
39. Wenger NK. Exclusion of the elderly and women from coronary trials: is their quality of care compromised? *JAMA.* 1992;268:1460–1461.
40. Singal BM et al. Geriatric patient emergency visits, I: comparison of visits by geriatric and patients. *Ann Emerg Med.* 1992;21:802–807.

SELECTED READING

Goldberg RJ et al. Patient delay and receipt of thrombolytic therapy among patients with acute myocardial infarction from a community-wide perspective. *Am J Cardiol.* 1992;70:421–425.

13 Acute Abdominal Pain

LEARNING OBJECTIVES

1. Identify factors contributing to delayed presentation among the elderly.
2. Identify factors that contribute to the difficulty of obtaining an accurate history from an elderly patient.
3. Demonstrate an adequate history and physical examination for the elderly patient presenting to the ED with abdominal pain.
4. Explain why abdominal guarding or muscular rigidity may be lacking with serious intraabdominal pathologic conditions with peritoneal irritation.
5. Identify chest disorders that may present as acute abdominal pain.
6. Describe the characteristics of life-threatening diseases that may present as abdominal pain in older patients.

Abdominal pain in the elderly patient is of great importance to emergency physicians. In a recent survey of practicing emergency physicians, 78% reported more difficulty in managing elderly patients with abdominal pain than younger adult patients.[1] Abdominal pain received the highest difficulty rating of the seven clinical presentations included in this study.[1] As the population ages, the overall number of elderly patients presenting to the ED with abdominal pain will steadily increase.

The emergency phase of care for the patient with abdominal pain is crucial to the final outcome. Inappropriate discharge of a surgical condition is an obvious concern, but the role of the emergency physician in admitted patients is also prominent. The mortality of elderly patients with abdominal pain admitted to the hospital through the ED doubles if the diagnosis is incorrect at the time of admission.[2,3] For a condition such as acute mesenteric ischemia, incorrect admission to a medical service is associated with a dismal outcome.[4] In a similar fashion the mortality for small bowel obstruction in the elderly patient is increased with incorrect placement of the patient on a medical service.[5] A delay in diagnosis increases the complication rate in both appendicitis and cholecystitis.[6,7]

Emergency physicians report that elderly patients with abdominal pain consume more of their time and require more ED resources compared to younger adults with abdominal pain.[1] This perception is supported by studies examining the spectrum of acute abdominal pain in elderly patients and the extent of care required for these patients. Admission rates of 51% and 63% have been reported for patients 65 years of age or older presenting to the ED with abdominal pain.[8,9] The corresponding rates of required surgery for the patients reported in these studies were 33% and 42%. The rate of subsequent operation for elderly patients with acute abdominal pain in the ED is double that of younger patients.[8] More sobering is the nine-fold higher mortality among elderly ED patients presenting with a complaint of abdominal pain.[8]

Certainly, acute abdominal pain in the elderly patient represents an issue of significance to persons practicing emergency medicine. This chapter reviews key aspects of the approach to the elderly patient with acute abdominal pain including history taking, the physical examination, the diagnostic evaluation, required emergency treatment measures, and the correct disposition of such a patient. Specific entities that will be reviewed because of their importance in the elderly include appendicitis, cholecystitis, peptic ulcer disease, intestinal obstruction, diverticulitis, mesenteric ischemia, and abdominal aortic aneurysms.

> *The rate of subsequent operation is double that of younger patients. More sobering is the 9-fold higher mortality rate among elderly emergency department patients.*

PRE-HOSPITAL CONSIDERATIONS

There is a paucity of literature on the pre-hospital aspects of acute abdominal pain in the elderly. Important points, however, can be drawn from other sources. The fact that over one half of elderly patients presenting to the ED with abdominal pain are eventually admitted to the hospital, with a significant percentage requiring surgery,[8,9] should encourage a conservative approach to such patients in the pre-hospital environment. Accurate triage of elderly patients with abdominal pain is difficult for physicians,[2] and pre-hospital providers should keep this in mind when dealing with such a presentation.

Familiarity with the presentation of a ruptured aortic aneurysm is essential, because this represents a potentially lethal process whose dramatic nature of onset will likely cause the patient or family to access the pre-hospital care system.[10] Early notification of the receiving facility should allow for timely mobilization of the resources and personnel required to properly care for these patients. In addition to standard management of patients in hypovolemic shock, the patient with a recognized ruptured abdominal aortic aneurysm may benefit from the application of the MAST (military anti shock trousers) suit.[11]

EMERGENCY DEPARTMENT INITIAL ASSESSMENT AND STABILIZATION

INITIAL APPROACH

Occasionally an elderly patient with acute abdominal pain, such as a patient with a ruptured abdominal aortic aneurysm, may be very unstable. In these situations the usual process of emergency stabilization with attention to airway, oxygen exchange, and the restoration of adequate circulation is pertinent.

Most patients will present in a less severe fashion, and a careful triage evaluation is essential to avoid a poor outcome (Table 3–1). Those persons performing the initial assessment should be aware of the high rate of serious disease even in the face of a seemingly benign presentation.[12]

Attention to vital signs is important, because they may be a clue to the true seriousness of the patient's condition. Continuous cardiac monitoring should be considered, especially in those patients presenting with upper abdominal pain, because myocardial ischemia may present as an abdominal complaint.[13] It is practical to routinely establish venous access and draw blood specimens for testing at the time of pre-

Table 13–1 **Approach to the Elderly Patient with Abdominal Pain**

Unstable patient
Consider: MI, aortic catastrophe
Assess: heart, lungs, abdominal aorta, peripheral pulses
Initial diagnostics: ECG, plain radiography of chest and abdomen

Stable patient (Evaluation)
Sudden onset: consider MI, vascular catastrophe, perforation, cecal volvulus
Severe pain with relatively normal examination: consider mesenteric ischemia
Abdominal pain or tenderness (location)
Upper: consider MI, biliary or peptic disease, pancreatitis, chest disease
Mid abdominal: consider bowel obstruction, infarction, early appendicitis
Lower: consider appendicitis, diverticulitis, urinary tract disease
Distention: consider volvulus, obstruction, colonic pseudo-obstruction
Repetitive vomiting: consider small bowel obstruction
Respiratory signs: consider MI, pulmonary embolus, other chest disease,
   metabolic acidosis

General diagnostic considerations
Laboratory studies: CBC with differential, urinalysis, amylase or lipase,
   electrolytes, renal function tests
ECG and plain radiographs of chest and abdomen

General therapeutic considerations
Intravenous rehydration
Nasogastric decompression
Pain relief, reassurance
Broad-spectrum antibiotics if peritonitis suspected

Table 13–2 **Confounding Factors in Obtaining a History**

Memory deficits	Stoicism
Change of mental status (acute or chronic)	Altered pain perception
	Communication problems: speech,
Reluctance to report symptoms	hearing

Data from Bender JS. Approach to the acute abdomen. *Med Clin North Am*. 1989;73: 1413–1422; Fenyo G. Diagnostic problems of acute abdominal diseases in the aged. *Acta Clin Scand*. 1974;140:396–405; and Vogt DP. The acute abdomen in the geriatric patient. *Cleve Clin J Med*. 1990;57:125–130.

sentation, because laboratory studies are almost invariably requested in elderly patients with acute abdominal pain.[14]

It is essential for the emergency physician to answer several questions regarding the abdominal pain. These include whether the cause of the pain is a surgical or non-surgical condition; whether the patient needs an operation; if required, how rapidly is surgery needed; and, finally, what is the proper disposition of the patient not requiring immediate surgery. The answers to these questions must be sought through a careful history and physical examination and an appropriate diagnostic evaluation.

HISTORY

The difficulties in assessment of the elderly patient with acute abdominal pain are exemplified by the factors confounding the recording of a proper history in these patients (Table 13–2). The history is frequently the cornerstone of the diagnosis in patients with abdominal pain, but, unfortunately, its attainment often is difficult in elderly patients.[3,12,14] Memory deficits may frustrate the physician and obscure the nature and time of onset of the abdominal pain.[12] Alterations in mental status or mental capacity of an acute or chronic nature may hamper investigative efforts.[3,14] Other factors contributing to difficulties in obtaining an accurate history include a reluctance to report symptoms, stoicism, altered perception of pain, and communication problems related to abnormal hearing and speech.[3,12,14]

Altered pain perception makes it difficult to diagnose an acute abdomen in an elderly patient.

Altered pain perception is considered to be a major contributing factor to the diagnostic difficulties.[3] This phenomenon is not well studied in abdominal conditions, but reports on the atypical nature of MI, including completely painless presentations,[15,16] support the presence of altered pain perception in elderly patients. In patients with endoscopically proven peptic ulcer disease, 35% of those older than 60 years reported no abdominal pain as opposed to only 8% of younger patients with this condition.[17]

When time allows, the history-taking process in any patient with abdominal pain is facilitated by an ordered approach (Table 13–3) and by allowing patients sufficient time to adequately describe what they are feeling.[18] The following areas should be covered:

Table 13–3 **Systematic History of Abdominal Pain**

Time of pain onset	Prior episodes
Mode of onset	Associated symptoms: nausea, vomit-
Progression since onset	ing, anorexia, diarrhea, constipation
Location of pain	Medications, including over-the-
Character of pain	counter
Pattern of radiation or referral	Past surgeries
Factors influencing pain	Other medical problems
Worsening: motion, cough, walking,	Social history, especially alcohol use
car ride?	Review of symptoms, especially
Improving: therapies attempted?	cardiopulmonary and genitourinary

Time of onset

A pain awakening someone from sleep is almost always of some significance.[19] The length of time the pain has been present is important to ascertain, because it has been suggested that abdominal pain
lasting 6 hours or more usually requires surgical intervention.[19]

In elderly patients, pain that had been present for less than 48
hours was more likely to require surgery than more chronic pain.[8]
However, many elderly patients with abdominal surgical conditions
will present in a delayed manner. This has been demonstrated for
appendicitis,[6,20] small bowel obstruction,[5] cecal volvulus,[21] sigmoid
volvulus,[22] and intussusception.[23] Unfortunately, as mentioned, memory deficits can obscure the timing of symptom onset.[12]

Mode of onset

A sudden onset of severe abdominal pain at any age, especially if accompanied by weakness or fainting, is likely to be a serious surgical
condition.[3] In the elderly patient the usual considerations with such
a history are a ruptured aortic aneurysm, an aortic dissection, perforation of a peptic ulcer, or volvulus.[24] Disturbingly, this classic pattern for some of these conditions does not always apply to the elderly. Fenyo[2] reported that only 47% of patients older than 70 years
with perforated ulcers presented with a history of sudden onset of
abdominal pain. Whereas cecal volvulus usually presents in an elderly patient with the acute onset of severe, colicky abdominal
pain,[21] the presentation of sigmoid volvulus is usually one of a gradual onset of pain.[22]

Despite these discrepancies, the acute onset of severe abdominal
pain should alert the physician to a potentially serious problem. If
this mode of onset is associated with relatively unimpressive findings
on physical examination of the abdomen, the primary consideration
must be an abdominal vascular accident.[24]

A less acute but still fairly abrupt onset is suspicious for surgical
diseases such as cholecystitis but includes non-surgical entities such
as renal colic. A more gradual onset of pain does not allow for easy
distinction between surgical and medical causes of abdominal pain.[18]

Progression since onset

A sustained improvement of an untreated abdominal pain is generally reassuring that the pain is of a non-surgical nature. The classic pattern of pain migration is very helpful in making the diagnosis of acute appendicitis.[25] However, in a retrospective study, this typical migration of pain was recorded in only 35% of patients older than 70 years with proven appendicitis.[2]

Location of the pain

The innervation patterns of the abdominal contents and the parietal peritoneum are not altered with aging. Therefore the location of perceived pain for specific disease entities should not differ among age groups. The diagnostic problems in elderly patients more commonly occur from the underreporting of pain or of its severity. For example, in acute cholecystitis the location and pattern of pain radiation are quite similar to younger patients with the disease.[12] However, the presentation of acute cholecystitis may be deceptively benign, leading to inadequate management.[7] Likewise, pain from acute appendicitis is usually present in the right lower quadrant, but its description may be atypical.[20]

Character of the pain

If the reported pain is severe the physician should be alerted to a serious cause of the pain.[24] Excruciating pain may herald the presence of mesenteric ischemia, a perforated ulcer, a dissecting or ruptured aortic aneurysm, or compromise of visceral circulation by gastric or colonic volvulus.[18] Fortunately, in all age groups, these conditions generally present with a degree of pain consistent with their severity.[4,21,26–29]

In many cases the underreporting of pain severity or atypical descriptions of the pain create significant difficulty for the physician evaluating the elderly patient with abdominal pain.[3,29,30] Any abdominal pain must therefore be carefully evaluated. In addition to the atypical nature of the presentation of acute cholecystitis[7] and appendicitis[20] mentioned above, special consideration must be taken to avoid the misdiagnosis of intestinal obstruction. A clear history of the abdominal pain is often difficult to obtain,[29] and the pain is often vaguely described and poorly localized.[31]

Abdominal guarding or muscular rigidity may be lacking in the face of serious intra-abdominal pathology with peritoneal irritation. This well-recognized phenomenon is partially attributed to the relatively thin abdominal musculature in elderly patients.

Pattern of radiation or referral

The referral pattern of biliary tract disease is often quite helpful in establishing the diagnosis, and this does not seem to be affected by aging.[12] Other patterns of referral have not been well studied in the elderly; however, radiation to the groin or testicle should raise the suspicion for pain of urinary tract origin.[19]

Factors influencing the pain

In any patient aggravation of abdominal pain by coughing, walking, or other types of movement suggests a pain of parietal origin (irritation of the parietal peritoneum) and usually indicates a surgical lesion.[24] Questioning the effects of the transport to the ED on the pain is useful, because the patient with peritoneal irritation may indicate increased pain with jarring of the vehicle caused by unevenness of the roadway. Whether symptoms consistent with peritoneal irritation are reliably reported by an elderly patient with peritonitis is not addressed in the literature. A review of any therapies attempted by the patient should also be conducted.

Previous episodes of the pain

Although recurrent episodes of a similar abdominal pain are considered more indicative of a medical condition,[32] serious pathologic conditions, including mesenteric ischemia,[33] can present as recurrent pain in the elderly patient. Significant numbers of patients with acute cholecystitis will give a prolonged history of remissions and exacerbations.[13] Generally, most serious acute abdominal disease in elderly patients will have a short clinical history.[13] If a medical evaluation occurred with a previous episode, every effort should be made to uncover the results of that investigation.

Associated symptoms

There is a great deal of overlap in gastrointestinal symptoms between surgical and non-surgical abdominal conditions. An important point to remember is that, in surgical causes, the abdominal pain nearly always precedes vomiting, whereas the converse is true in roughly 75% of patients with abdominal pain from gastroenteritis or of a non-specific origin.[8,24] One important exception to this guideline is Boerhaave's syndrome, in which severe pain after vomiting or retching results from esophageal rupture.[34]

Abdominal pain nearly always precedes vomiting in surgical cases. The opposite is true for gastroenteritis and for pain of non-specific origin.

The presence of vomiting will vary with the illness. In the elderly patient the incidence of vomiting in specific conditions is as follows:

- Generally present: small bowel obstruction
- Frequent (50-60%): appendicitis,[6,20] cholecystitis,[13,35] mesenteric ischemia,[33] and cecal volvulus[21]
- Less common (20-30%): large bowel obstruction[31] and sigmoid volvulus[22]
- Uncommon (<20%): perforated ulcers[36]

The character and quality of the vomitus may reveal important clues to the underlying condition. Vomiting that progresses from gastric contents to bilious to feculent is virtually diagnostic for the presence of small bowel obstruction.[19] Repetitive retching with little or no vomitus is characteristic of gastric volvulus.[29]

Anorexia is an important symptom in appendicitis, and the presence of hunger is considered reason to doubt the diagnosis.[19] The exact incidence of anorexia in elderly patients with appendicitis has not been defined; however, one retrospective study stated that it was present in only 34% of patients.[37]

Diarrhea and urinary tract symptoms can occasionally occur in the elderly patient with appendicitis.[20,37] Diarrhea has also been reported in about one half of the patients with mesenteric ischemia.[33] Disturbingly, one in five patients with large bowel obstruction of any cause will report diarrhea.[31]

Additional history

A review of systems, especially covering cardiopulmonary and genitourinary symptoms, is important to elucidate factors that may point to a non-surgical cause for the abdominal pain or complicate the management of the patient. A review of current medications, including over-the-counter preparations, and the previous surgical and medical history is essential. The social history, particularly in regard to alcohol abuse, must not be neglected.

PHYSICAL EXAMINATION

The physical examination proceeds in the same manner as for younger patients, but the physician must be alert for subtle signs of a serious nature. The abdominal examination may be complicated by the patient's stoicism or unwillingness or inability to report tenderness and the less pronounced muscular response to inflammation.[3,12,29] The focus of the physical examination will be the abdomen, but attention to the vital signs and adjacent organs is important. The following areas are essential to address:

General appearance and attitude of the patient

The ill-appearing elderly patient with abdominal pain is an immediate cause for concern. With a mortality of 8% to 14% in elderly patients presenting to the ED with abdominal pain,[2,8] such a patient must be evaluated on a priority basis. The appearance of the patient with abdominal pain can be deceiving, leaving the physician to make incorrect assumptions about the patient's condition.[12] The patient who lies still and is reluctant to move should be suspected of having peritoneal irritation.[19]

Vital signs

Obtaining a rectal temperature should be routine in the elderly patient with abdominal pain.[3] The lack of fever, however, is of little value in excluding serious abdominal processes, because even infectious causes of abdominal pain commonly present without an elevated temperature.[12,29] Hypotension is a critical concern and should raise the immediate suspicion of a ruptured abdominal aortic aneurysm[28] or another serious process. Tachypnea is a non-specific finding in the acutely ill patient but should alert the physician to a possible intrathoracic cause of the abdominal pain.[38]

Abdominal inspection and auscultation

Distention is very common but not universal in cases of large bowel obstruction, including cecal and sigmoid volvulus.[21,22,31] Auscultation for bowel sounds rarely adds to the data base, although high-pitched "rushes" may be heard in small bowel obstruction.[3]

Abdominal palpation

Warm hands, a gentle manner, and communication with the patient will enhance the abdominal examination. The examination should be conducted with the thighs flexed to ensure abdominal relaxation, and palpation should proceed from areas where the least tenderness is expected.[19] Gentle palpation is usually sufficient, and the use of one finger may aid in localization of the tenderness. Muscular guarding or rigidity is a key finding, but this may be voluntary. To eliminate the voluntary component of the abdominal musculature, the patient's abdomen can be palpated during deep inhalation.[19]

Palpation of the abdomen in the elderly patient will generally be a useful clue to the underlying diagnosis. Although appendicitis may present atypically, tenderness is nearly always found in the right lower quadrant.[2,26] Elderly patients with acute cholecystitis will most often have tenderness localized to the region of the gallbladder.[12] In a similar fashion, acute pancreatitis in older patients will generally present with epigastric tenderness.[12]

In the older patient, abdominal guarding or muscular rigidity may be lacking in the face of serious intraabdominal pathologic conditions with peritoneal irritation.[3] This well-recognized phenomenon is partially attributed to the thin abdominal musculature in the elderly.[12,29] As an illustration, in patients older than 70 years, only 21% of those with a perforated ulcer presented with epigastric rigidity.[2] The emergency physician must carefully assess the patient for even minor increases in abdominal wall muscle tone, because this may indicate a serious underlying problem.

Traditional testing of rebound tenderness involves sudden release of the palpating hand, and this is distressing to the patient. Peritoneal irritation is better tested by light percussion of the abdomen or by gentle rocking of the bed or pelvis.[18,19] The presence or absence of special signs such as the obturator or psoas sign is not documented for elderly persons, and their performance should be conducted in this light.

Further examination

All hernial orifices should be carefully examined with special attention to the femoral canal in the elderly female patient with abdominal pain.[12] Failure to detect an external hernia early in the care of the patient can be fatal.[5]

The rectal examination, an essential part of the physical examination in the elderly patient with abdominal pain, provides information regarding possible appendicitis, diverticulitis, and mesenteric ischemia. Also, intraabdominal cancer frequently may present as non-specific abdominal pain.[39]

Assessment of the femoral pulses may be revealing in cases of a dissecting aneurysm.[27] Attention to the heart, lung, and back examination is important to exclude the presence of a non-abdominal cause of the pain. Genital and pelvic examinations should be routinely conducted in a search for another cause of the presenting symptoms. An examination of the skin may uncover herpes zoster.

Table 13–4 **Causes of Abdominal Pain in Elderly Patients**

Cause	Percent
Biliary colic or cholecystitis	12–41
Nonspecific abdominal pain	9.6–23
Bowel obstruction	7.3–14
Perforated viscus	2.3–7
Incarcerated hernia	4–9.6
Appendicitis	3.5–6.7
Diverticulitis	3.4–7
Pancreatitis	2–5.1

Data from Fenyo G. Acute abdominal disease in the elderly: experience from two series in Stockholm. *Am J Surg.* 1982;143:751–754; Bugliosi TF, Meloy TD, Vukov LF. Acute abdominal pain in the elderly. *Ann Emerg Med.* 1990;19:1383–1386; and Fenyo G. Diagnostic problems of acute abdominal diseases in the aged. *Acta Chir Scand.* 1974;140:396–405.

SPECIFIC CONDITIONS

In addition to reviewing the general approach to acute abdominal pain in the elderly patient it is useful for the emergency physician to be aware of certain aspects of specific disease conditions in the elderly (Table 13–4). Elderly patients presenting to the ED with abdominal pain are twice as likely to have a lesion requiring surgery as compared to younger patients.[8] Knowledge of the specific presenting patterns of acute abdominal disease in elderly patients is essential for persons practicing emergency medicine. Table 13–5 identifies diagnostic traps of some of the conditions discussed here.

Table 13–5 **Diagnostic Traps in the Elderly Patient**

Appendicitis

Delayed presentation is common (20% > 3 days)
Migration of pain may be lacking
Anorexia may be absent
Nausea or vomiting in one half or less
Normal temperatures common
WBC count less than 10,000 in 20%
Elevated bilirubin common
Plain radiographs misinterpreted as small bowel obstruction

Perforated peptic ulcer

One half do not report sudden onset of pain
Pain may be generalized or also in lower quadrants
Epigastric rigidity may be absent
Lack of free air on plain films

Large bowel obstruction

Diarrhea frequently reported
Severe obstipation may be lacking
Vomiting often absent
Gradual onset of pain in volvulus, especially sigmoid
Colonic pseudo-obstruction

Acute mesenteric ischemia

Most report gradual onset of pain
Prior episodes can be reported
Hard evidence lacking early on
Guaiac-negative stool early on
Laboratory abnormalities are late findings

Abdominal aortic aneurysm

Back pain present in only one half
Syncope as primary complaint
Hypotension ascribed to other causes
Aorta not palpable
Hematuria may be present

APPENDICITIS

If an elderly patient presents to the ED with abdominal pain and the appendix has not been surgically removed, consideration of appendicitis is prudent. Diagnostic problems are frequently encountered in the elderly patient with appendicitis. Horattas et al.[6] reviewed 96 patients age 60 years or older with surgically proven appendicitis and found that only 51% carried that diagnosis at the time of admission. Even at the time of surgery, appendicitis was a consideration in only 70% of these patients. The physician can be misled in the other direction, since nearly one third of laparotomies for appendicitis in elderly patients will reveal another condition or no disease.[12]

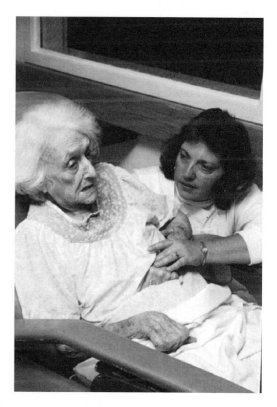

A major issue in the elderly patient with appendicitis is a consistent delay in seeking medical care. This factor is thought to contribute to the higher perforation rate and associated complications in elderly patients with appendicitis.[6,12,20,37] A large percentage of elderly patients with appendicitis will present more than 48 hours after the onset of symptoms.[6,20,37] Up to 20% will present after 3 days of symptoms, with 8% delaying medical evaluation for over 7 days.[37]

Abdominal pain is a consistent feature of appendicitis in the elderly patient, generally occurring in the right lower quadrant. However, its description may be vague, or the pain may be poorly localized.[6,20] A significant, potentially misleading, historical item is the lack of the classic migratory pattern for the abdominal pain. Separate studies indicate that only 35%[12] to 48%[37] of elderly patients will report this progression of their pain.

Nausea and vomiting are expected in only 40% to 50% of elderly patients with appendicitis.[6,12,20,37] Information on the incidence of anorexia is, unfortunately, limited, with a retrospective report indicating that this was noted in only 34% of patients over 60 years of age.[37] As with younger patients, the presence of diarrhea and urinary tract symptoms does not exclude the presence of acute appendicitis.[37]

If an elderly person presents with abdominal pain and the appendix has not been surgically removed, consideration of appendicitis is prudent.

The physical examination in elderly patients with acute appendicitis is notable for the potential lack of fever, with anywhere from 20% to 50% of patients presenting with a temperature less than 37.5° C. Tenderness in the right lower quadrant is a frequent finding and is present in 80% to 90% of these patients. Muscular rigidity and rebound tenderness have been reported to range from only 20% to over 80%.[12,37] The rectal examination has been reported to reveal pain from a low of three percent to a high of 53% in elderly patients with appendicitis.[20,37]

Laboratory testing is potentially misleading, because a white blood cell (WBC) count below 10,000 has been consistently reported in 20%

of elderly patients with acute appendicitis.[6,20,37] The addition of a differential count may be of some value, because Horattas et al. found that a band count higher than 10% in those with a WBC count below 10,000 increased the number of patients identified from 80% to 92%.[6] Other laboratory studies may also be misleading, because an elevated bilirubin level may be found in 17% of elderly patients with appendicitis, raising the possibility of biliary tract disease.[6] Abdominal radiographs rarely contribute to the diagnosis and, in fact, have been implicated in therapeutic delays, because these studies often show an ileus or a small bowel obstruction.[6,12]

In addition to appreciating the potential for any one of the presenting features of appendicitis to be missing or obscured, it is important for the emergency physician to realize that the elderly patient will generally not fit the classic diagnostic picture of acute appendicitis. Horattas et al. found that only 20% of their patients had all the symptoms of nausea or vomiting, fever, right lower quadrant tenderness, and an abnormal complete blood count.[6]

The emergency management of suspected appendicitis, as opposed to the diagnosis, is not complex and generally involves intravenous fluid therapy and broad-spectrum antibiotics when there is evidence of perforation.

ACUTE CHOLECYSTITIS

Mortality of 10% to 14% is typical of acute cholecystitis in the elderly.

In case series of elderly patients presenting to the hospital with abdominal pain, acute cholecystitis is consistently the most frequent diagnosis of a surgical nature, occurring in 12% to 41% of these patients.[2,9,12,13] The physician must not underestimate the seriousness of this disease in elderly patients, since mortality of 10% to 14% is typical of acute cholecystitis.[7,35,40]

The presenting features of acute cholecystitis in older patients are typical of the disease in younger patients and include epigastric or right upper quadrant pain with radiation to the back or shoulder area.[12,13] Nausea or vomiting is reported by roughly one half of all elderly patients with acute cholecystitis.[13,35] Chills or fever also are noted frequently by these patients.[13,35]

On physical examination, local tenderness over the gallbladder is usually present, whereas a palpable mass and muscular guarding are less frequent findings. Jaundice may be present in 23% to 30% of elderly patients requiring emergency surgery for acute cholecystitis.[7,13,35] Fever is variable, and the temperature may be normal in 30% to 40% of patients.[7,12,35]

Laboratory testing is even less useful than in appendicitis, because 30% to 35% of patients with acute cholecystitis will have a WBC count less than 10,000.[7,13] Plain radiographs of the abdomen are of little use, and the usual testing includes ultrasound or a nuclear medicine study.[7,13] Ultrasonography offers the advantage of a rapid turnaround, whereas nuclear medicine studies yield more information as to the presence of acute infection.

The emergency physician will generally have an easier time with cholecystitis in the elderly patient as opposed to other abdominal conditions. The diagnostic accuracy for cholecystitis is the highest of all acute abdominal conditions in elderly patients presenting to the ED.[2] Several important issues do exist, however, that are important for emergency physicians to realize. A clinical presentation of fever, jaundice, and mental disorientation without significant abdominal findings has been described in elderly patients.[7] Additionally, the elderly patient with acute biliary tract disease can be deceptively well appearing but should be aggressively treated to avoid excess morbidity. Adequate resuscitation and prompt operation are advocated for the management of acute cholecystitis, since the elderly patient is unlikely to improve with conservative management and operative delay increases the complication rate.[7,40] This problem is highlighted by the frequent and costly delay in diagnosing and appropriately operating on patients with perforation of the gallbladder.[17]

The emergency management will primarily consist of parenteral fluid therapy and antibiotics along with nasogastric decompression.

Prompt surgical intervention is advocated for acute cholecystitis, because the elderly patient is unlikely to improve with conservative management.

PERFORATED PEPTIC ULCER DISEASE

The most frequent serious manifestation of peptic ulcer disease encountered in elderly patients is gastrointestinal hemorrhage.[41] This section will cover the most serious, painful manifestation of peptic ulcer disease in elderly patients, namely, perforation. The emergency physician must be aware of several diagnostic traps in evaluating patients who may have this condition.

The most significant issue in the history is the frequent lack of an acute onset of upper abdominal pain. Fenyo reported that only 47% of patients older than 70 years with a perforated ulcer will give a history of a sudden onset of abdominal pain.[2] Patients with a perforated ulcer will generally present to the hospital within a few hours of the perforation, although the presentation can occasionally be delayed 1 to 2 days.[42] The pain will generally be severe, constant, and present to some degree in the epigastrium.[13] Generalized abdominal pain may occur in cases of free perforation, although atypical locations for pain, including the lower quadrants, are possible.[12,13] Vomiting is generally not a significant feature of perforated ulcer.[36]

On physical examination, tenderness is expected in the epigastrium but also may be generalized or maximal in the lower quadrants.[13] Fever is likely to be absent, and muscular guarding is not a consistent finding.[12,13] Fenyo reported that only 21% of elderly patients with perforated ulcer had epigastric rigidity.[2]

An extremely important issue in the diagnostic workup is to realize that plain radiography will not reveal free intraperitoneal air in roughly 40% of patients with a perforated ulcer.[12,42] Patients who do not have free air identified are less likely to receive an early operation and therefore have a higher mortality.[42] In one series of elderly patients with acute abdominal pain, missed perforation of a viscus was the most frequent fatal misdiagnosis.[3] In each of these missed cases no free air was evident on the admission radiographs.

If the clinical picture is suspicious the instillation of 400-500 ml of air via a nasogastric tube and repeating of the upright chest radiograph and abdominal series may reveal free air.[42] The left lateral decubitus film is considered by some to be more accurate for detecting free air

The absence of free air on plain radiographs results in a missed diagnosis and delayed operation in as many as 40% of perforated ulcers.

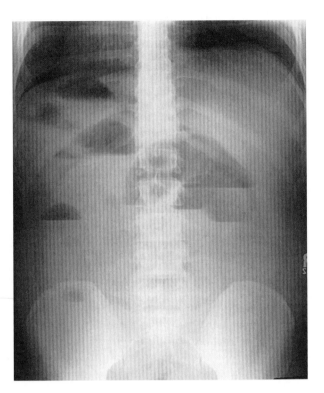

Upright radiograph revealing air fluid level

and is especially useful in the unstable patient who cannot tolerate the upright position.[43] Although not specifically studied for perforated ulcer, computed tomography (CT) can demonstrate small amounts of intraperitoneal air and should be considered if the plain films are normal and a question exists about the diagnosis or management of the elderly patient with epigastric pain.

Once the patient with a perforated ulcer is identified, he or she should receive fluid resuscitation, nasogastric decompression, and broad-spectrum parenteral antibiotics.

SMALL BOWEL OBSTRUCTION

The diagnosis of small bowel obstruction is usually not difficult in the elderly patient, because the cause and presenting features are fairly typical of the disease in other age groups.[5,13] The diagnosis can be obscured, however, by unclear descriptions of the pain.[29,31] Other than a higher frequency of prior surgery, elderly patients do not appear to be at any greater risk of small bowel obstruction from adhesions or hernias than younger patients.[44] Small bowel obstruction is a frequent cause of abdominal pain in elderly patients and is quite serious, since it carries a mortality of 14% to 35%.[3,5,45]

The principal manifestations of small bowel obstruction in this population include pain, usually colicky in nature, nausea, vomiting, and abdominal distention.[5,13] When an incarcerated hernia is the cause of the obstruction the diagnosis is usually easy.[12] The most common reason for misdiagnosis of this condition is the failure to properly interpret the abdominal radiographs.[3,5] Such a delay in diagnosis is fre-

Small bowel obstruction in the elderly patient has a mortality rate of 14% to 35%.

quently fatal. Small bowel obstruction is second only to appendicitis in abdominal conditions of a surgical nature for which patients are improperly discharged home from the ED.[8]

Management of small bowel obstruction in the ED will generally include nasogastric decompression and intravenous fluid therapy.

LARGE BOWEL OBSTRUCTION

The principal causes of large bowel obstruction in the elderly are carcinoma, volvulus, and diverticulitis, diseases that all have a higher incidence in this age group.[31,45] The large majority of cases are caused by carcinoma, and sigmoid volvulus is generally two to three times more frequent than cecal volvulus.[31,45–47] Mortality for large bowel obstruction is high, averaging around 40%.[31,45] Of diagnostic significance is the fact that up to 19% of patients with large bowel obstruction of any cause will report diarrhea, and only about one half will complain of severe constipation or obstipation.[31]

The presenting symptoms of large bowel obstruction secondary to carcinoma are commonly present for several days before presentation, and the abdominal pain may be poorly described.[31] Vomiting is present in less than one half of the patients, and the patient should be questioned regarding rectal bleeding, changes in bowel habits, weakness, fatigability, and weight loss.[31,48]

The presentations of sigmoid volvulus and cecal volvulus differ somewhat. Volvulus of the cecum typically presents with an acute onset of severe, colicky pain.[21] A history of previous abdominal surgery is noted in about two thirds of these patients, and roughly one quarter will report a previous similar episode.[46] Constipation, nausea, and vomiting are reported in about one half the patients, and diarrhea occurs in 14%.[46] The majority of patients will have a distended and tympanitic abdomen.[21] The presence of fever and evidence of peritonitis or leukocytosis should suggest gangrenous bowel or perforation.[21,46]

Sigmoid volvulus will commonly present in a delayed fashion with a more gradual onset of pain and distention.[22] Nausea and vomiting are present in only about one third of the patients, whereas constipation is present in one half to three quarters.[22,46] As with cecal volvulus, diarrhea may be present, occurring in 8% to 16% of these patients.[22,46] A previous episode of a similar pain is reported by 44%, whereas about one half have had previous abdominal surgery.[46] Abdominal distention is also the primary physical examination finding in sigmoid volvulus, and fever, peritoneal signs, and leukocytosis indicate the possibility of gangrenous bowel.[22,46]

A large series reported that around 10% of patients with volvulus of either type were institutionalized,[46] whereas a smaller series only found this in sigmoid volvulus.[47]

Plain radiographs of the abdomen will be diagnostic for cecal volvulus in just over one third of the cases.[21,46] The plain radiographs in cecal volvulus will most likely be interpreted as small bowel obstruction, and supplementary study with a barium enema may aid in securing the diagnosis.[21] The plain abdominal radiographs in sigmoid volvulus have been considered diagnostic 37%[46] to 71%[22] of the time.

A significant complication of large bowel obstruction is perforation and the attendant risk of generalized peritonitis and fatal sepsis. This

Large bowel obstruction, with a mortality rate of 40%, is accompanied by a report of diarrhea in only 19% of cases and constipation in only about 50% of cases.

was noted in eight percent of a series of 300 patients with large bowel obstruction of various causes.[31] A cecal diameter of 10 cm in this series was not useful as a predictor of potential perforation. In fact, cecal diameters of up to 20 cm were identified that responded to routine decompressive measures.[31]

The general emergency management of large bowel obstruction includes fluid resuscitation and nasogastric decompression. Further management is generally in the hands of a surgeon and may include colonic decompression through a sigmoidoscope or rectal tube.[29,31]

The emergency physician should be aware of colonic pseudo-obstruction, also known as Ogilvie's syndrome.[49] This entity presents as massive gaseous distention of the colon in an elderly patient with systemic illness and poor mobility.[50-52] The patient may present with abdominal pain, vomiting, and either diarrhea or constipation. Importantly, there is often no mechanical obstruction or it consists only of feces[49-52] that can be easily bypassed with the colonoscope.[53] The physical examination is remarkable for a distended, tympanitic abdomen that is usually not tender. The rectal examination is a clue to the diagnosis, since it may reveal constipation or a markedly dilated, cavernous rectum.[49,52] The major reason emergency physicians should be alerted to this condition is to avoid unnecessary surgery in an ill elderly patient.[52]

DIVERTICULAR DISEASE

Diverticulosis is a common condition in this population, with up to 50% at risk for developing this disease.[54] Diverticulitis, which is acute inflammation and infection of the diverticula, is a common cause of abdominal pain in the elderly ED patient. Diagnostic accuracy for diverticulitis is only about 50%, quite low in comparison to other abdominal conditions in this age group.[2]

Diverticulitis is often a clinical diagnosis with left lower quadrant pain, distention, and constipation or diarrhea the common presenting symptoms. The physical examination will reveal tenderness in the left lower quadrant, mild fever, and occasionally a mass.[12,13,44,54] The WBC count may be normal in one half of the patients.[13] Diverticulitis can be misdiagnosed in women as a pelvic mass of gynecologic origin.[55] Plain radiography may reveal a complication of diverticulitis, such as obstruction or perforation.[12,13] Barium enema examination or colonoscopy is contraindicated in acute diverticulitis, but a CT scan may be helpful if the diagnosis is unclear.[44,54]

The management of diverticulitis is often conservative, and in milder cases outpatient antibiotics are often prescribed despite little evidence of their efficacy.[54] In more severe cases, hospitalization, nasogastric tube drainage, intravenous fluids, and antibiotics to cover gram-negative organisms are indicated.[30,54] Surgery is indicated for suspected perforation, abscess formation, fistula, or obstruction.[54]

ACUTE MESENTERIC INFARCTION

Mesenteric infarction is generally a disease of older patients and represents a significant challenge for emergency physicians. The management of this condition is frequently suboptimal, with diagnostic delays leading to increased mortality.[4,26,33,44] Mesenteric ischemia has a very high mortality and along with ruptured abdominal aortic aneurysm represents one of the most lethal diagnostic possibilities in the elderly patient with acute abdominal pain.[14,45] An aggressive approach to these patients is required, because early diagnosis is associated with improved outcomes.[56]

The spectrum of mesenteric ischemia includes several distinct entities with about one half of the cases caused by occlusion of the superior mesenteric artery from a thrombus or embolus, roughly one quarter caused by non-occlusive infarction, and the remainder divided among inferior mesenteric artery occlusion, mesenteric venous thrombosis, aortic dissection, and mesenteric arteritis.[26] The diagnosis of mesenteric infarction requires a recognition of the patient at risk for the disease and an understanding of the clinical presentation.

In general, the patients who are at greatest risk include those with underlying cardiovascular disease or hypotension or hypovolemia from any cause.[44] Specifically, mesenteric arterial embolization most commonly occurs in patients with atrial fibrillation or a recent MI.[57,58] Mesenteric arterial thrombosis classically occurs in patients with significant atherosclerosis but is equally likely to occur in situations in which cardiac output is low and atherosclerosis is not prominent.[33]

Non-occlusive mesenteric infarction is common, and the underlying precipitant is generally a low cardiac output state from cardiovascular disease, especially congestive heart failure. Other causes of non-occlusive infarction include hypotension from sepsis or dehydration.[33,56] Digitalis therapy, probably through a vasoconstrictive effect on the mesenteric vessels, appears to play an independent role in non-occlusive mesenteric infarction.[33] Mesenteric venous thrombosis occurs most frequently in the setting of a hypercoagulable state, and the patient may have experienced a previous episode of deep venous thrombosis. Mesenteric venous thrombosis also occurs in the setting of liver disease, probably because of disturbances in portal blood flow.[33,59]

The principal manifestation of mesenteric ischemia is severe abdominal pain that is initially of a visceral nature and poorly localized. The pain may be refractory to narcotic analgesia.[26,57] The pain, particularly if an embolus is the cause, may be quite sudden in onset.[56] However, a gradual onset of pain is more common in the overall spectrum of mesenteric infarction.[33] The pain is usually present in the mid-abdomen, but atypical locations including the epigastrium and hypogastrium are possible and may relate to the vessels involved.[30] Prior episodes of abdominal pain, possibly related to eating (intestinal angina), may be reported by the patient, especially if mesenteric arterial thrombosis is the cause.[29,30]

Associated gastrointestinal symptoms are common in patients with mesenteric infarction, with nausea and anorexia occurring in 80%, vomiting in 60%, and diarrhea in about 50% of patients.[33] Some form of acute gastrointestinal emptying is considered part of a triad in patients with superior mesenteric artery embolism.[30] The other components of this triad include pain and the presence of significant cardiac disease.

The physical examination in mesenteric ischemia will reveal an essentially normal abdomen early in the course of the disease.[58] The presence of severe abdominal pain in an elderly patient in the face of a rel-

Mesenteric ischemia and ruptured AAA are among the most lethal diagnostic possibilities with abdominal pain presentations.

atively normal abdominal examination should prompt the physician to consider mesenteric infarction as a diagnostic possibility. Distention, severe tenderness, and evidence of peritonitis are inevitable as the disease progresses and intestinal necrosis and perforation ensue.[33,56–58] The ischemic process can be manifested in guaiac-positive stools in roughly 60% of cases.[58] Theoretically, the stool should be free of blood early in the illness before significant intestinal mucosal compromise.

The laboratory evaluation in mesenteric infarction is generally not helpful in making an early diagnosis. The onset of major laboratory abnormalities indicates significant disease progression.[30,33] Plain radiographs of the abdomen are usually normal early in the disease.[30] The principal purpose of laboratory and radiologic evaluation is to rule out other causes of acute abdominal pain.[26,30]

The critical issue regarding mesenteric infarction for the emergency physician is to aggressively pursue the diagnosis based on a suggestive history in an at-risk patient before the development of obvious physical examination, laboratory, or radiologic abnormalities. If one waits for "hard evidence" to develop it is invariable that intestinal necrosis has occurred and the patient's chance of survival will have been reduced dramatically.[30] Although the overall mortality of mesenteric infarction is generally around 70%, Boley et al.[56] reported a 90% survival rate in patients with this disease who had angiography before the development of peritonitis.

The emergency management of the patient with suspected mesenteric infarction will be dominated by an effort to secure an early angiographic study. Correction of hypovolemia by fluid resuscitation, nasogastric decompression, and parenteral antibiotics may all be helpful while awaiting angiography.[30]

The seriousness of mesenteric infarction has prompted the recommendation that this diagnosis be considered in any elderly patient with unexplained gastrointestinal symptoms.[33] The high mortality justifies this approach, because patients whose diagnosis is initially missed will probably die.[4]

The seriousness of mesenteric infarction has prompted the recommendation that this diagnosis be considered in any elderly patient with unexplained gastrointestinal symptoms.

ABDOMINAL AORTIC ANEURYSM

Rupture of an abdominal aortic aneurysm, along with acute mesenteric infarction, tops the list of fatalities per case in elderly patients with acute abdominal pain.[45] The mortality is 70% in the best of situations where a rapid diagnosis is followed by immediate transfer to the operating room.[10] The diagnosis can be difficult, further complicating the care of these patients. In one retrospective series the initial misdiagnosis rate was 30%.[28]

The incidence of abdominal aortic aneurysm is steadily rising, mainly because of the increasing median age of the population. The incidence in men increases rapidly after 55 years of age, with a peak of 5.9% at 80 years, whereas in women the incidence rises sharply after 70 years, peaking at 4.5% at 90 years.[60] An increased number of elderly patients presenting with rupture can be expected, and emergency physicians must therefore be aware of the presentation and management of this condition.

Ideally, an abdominal aortic aneurysm will be detected on a routine examination and the patient referred for elective repair, since the mortality in this situation usually is low, about four percent.[60] It is generally recommended that patients with unruptured aneurysms greater than 5 cm undergo elective repair,[60] with some authors recommending that patients with unruptured aneurysms larger than 6 cm be hospitalized for early repair.[30] The emergency physician who routinely encounters a large number of elderly patients on a daily basis should consider an assessment of the abdominal aorta in all of these patients. Suspicious cases can be evaluated by further study, such as an ultrasound, and referred to a vascular surgeon as necessary.

When the abdominal aorta ruptures, the classic symptom expected by physicians is back pain.[60] In actual series of patients, abdominal pain alone or in combination with back pain is a more common complaint.[28] Abdominal pain will be present in 70% to 80% of these patients, whereas back pain will be noted by just over 50%.[28] The diagnosis of ruptured abdominal aortic aneurysm must be considered in any elderly patient, especially men, with back or abdominal pain. The pain of a ruptured abdominal aortic aneurysm can be atypical or radiate to the flanks, hips, groin, or external genitalia.[29] Syncope may also be part of the presenting picture, and elderly patients with syncope should be questioned for the presence of abdominal or back pain.

Hypotension in combination with abdominal or back pain is an important clue to the presence of a ruptured aortic aneurysm. This has been reported in 70% to 96% of patients with hypotension and abdominal or back pain.[10,28] Exsanguination is uncommon, however, since there is usually an initial tamponade effect of the retroperitoneum in patients arriving at the hospital alive.[60] The emergency physician will often encounter patients who have developed an initial "warning leak" who will then go on to free rupture and fatal exsanguination if not diagnosed quickly and surgery is not performed.

The key finding on physical examination beyond the presence of hypotension is a pulsatile abdominal mass. The aorta that ruptures is generally greater than 5 cm in diameter, and many will be even larger at the time of rupture.[60] The ruptured aorta is usually tender.[29] Unfortunately, in many cases, often because of the size of the patient's abdomen, the aorta may not be palpable. This is problematic, since it may hamper the diagnosis of this condition. In patients initially misdiagnosed the aorta was palpable in only 26% as compared to 72% of those correctly diagnosed on presentation.[28]

The emergency management of patients with a ruptured aortic aneurysm focuses on rapid diagnosis and disposition to the operating room. Any delay places the patient at an increased risk of dying. When the physical examination or history is suggestive and the patient is unstable, immediate operation without confirmatory testing is mandatory.[60] The role of plain radiography is controversial, but one study did indicate that some evidence of a ruptured aortic aneurysm was present on 90% of supine abdominal films.[61] The principal signs were a calcified aneurysm, loss of a psoas shadow, or loss of a renal outline. If the diagnosis is unclear and the patient is stable, abdominal ultrasonography may delineate the size of the aorta, whereas CT imaging is more useful to detect rupture.[60] If such testing is to occur, the emergency physician should alert the vascular surgeon and operating theater of the patient's potential diagnosis.

Hypotension in combination with abdominal or back pain is an important clue to the presence of a ruptured aortic aneurysm.

Regarding misdiagnosis, erroneously suspected conditions in order of decreasing frequency are renal colic, diverticulitis, gastrointestinal hemorrhage, acute MI, back pain, and sepsis.[28] Renal colic frequently presents with severe flank or back pain, but an obvious clue in over one half of the aneurysms misdiagnosed as renal colic was an episode of hypotension that was wrongly ascribed to a vagal episode or developing sepsis.[28] The emergency physician must consider this possibility whenever an elderly patient is suspected of having renal colic.

Emergency management includes obtaining large-bore venous access in multiple sites. The availability of at least six units of packed red cells for transfusion should be established. However, fluid resuscitation should be undertaken cautiously in the conscious and adequately perfusing patient, because elevation of the blood pressure may lead to loss of the retroperitoneal tamponade and profound hemorrhage and death.[60] One report of interest demonstrated a drop in mortality for patients with a ruptured abdominal aneurysm when the MAST suit was applied during transport to the hospital or in the ED.[11] All included patients had a blood pressure below 80 mm Hg, and the mortality dropped to 25% with application of the MAST suit from 100% in historical controls treated with fluids and immediate operation.

OTHER ABDOMINAL CONDITIONS

The preceding discussion covers the major diagnostic categories of elderly patients with abdominal pain but is obviously not comprehensive. Further entities of importance in this population include aortic dissection, gastric volvulus, pancreatitis, intussusception, and ischemic colitis.

Aortic dissection, although it generally has its origins in the thoracic region, may cause abdominal pain directly or through mesenteric infarction. This disease occurs primarily in males and patients with hypertension at a median age of 59 years.[27] Acute gastric volvulus presents with the sudden onset of upper abdominal pain and repetitive nonproductive retching. The inability to pass a nasogastric tube is a clue to the diagnosis of this condition.[29]

Elderly patients with pancreatitis will present in a manner similar to younger patients, with severe upper abdominal pain, nausea, vomiting, and epigastric tenderness of varying degrees.[12,13,62] Given the retroperitoneal location of the pancreas, the abdominal tenderness may not be impressive, but some degree is usually present.[12,13] Diagnostic difficulty in the elderly patient with pancreatitis does not occur from the clinical picture but from dependence on laboratory testing that may not be confirmatory.[12]

Intussusception, although primarily a disease of childhood, does occur in the elderly. In this group, intussusception generally presents as bowel obstruction, and the symptoms can be quite prolonged.[23] The majority of these cases occur in the small intestine with a tumor as the precipitant. Ischemic colitis is an uncommon disorder of the elderly, but it should be considered when a patient presents with an initial episode of colitis.[62] Clinically, ischemic colitis is difficult to distinguish from other forms of colitis and it generally occurs in patients with severe peripheral vascular disease.

NON-ABDOMINAL CAUSES OF ABDOMINAL PAIN

The list of medical conditions that can present as acute abdominal pain is extensive, and a detailed systematic evaluation is important in the elderly patient with abdominal pain.

Probably the most serious mistake is to attribute the symptoms of myocardial infarction to an abdominal condition. An electrocardiogram and pertinent history should be considered in all elderly patients with acute abdominal pain, particularly upper abdominal pain.[13] Other chest diseases that may present as an abdominal condition include pneumonia, pulmonary emboli, empyema, tuberculosis, bacterial endocarditis, and congestive heart failure with hepatic congestion.[29,38]

Genitourinary disease, particularly renal colic and pyelonephritis, is a common cause of abdominal pain and may lead to an unnecessary laparotomy.[12,13] In elderly men a thorough genitourinary examination is important, not only to look for hernias but also to examine the patient for testicular torsion and epididymitis.

Other conditions that can present with acute abdominal pain in the elderly include herpes zoster, diabetic ketoacidosis, hypercalcemia, addisonian crisis, hyperthyroidism, hemochromatosis, tabes dorsalis, and retroperitoneal or rectus sheath hematomas associated with anticoagulant therapy.[29,32]

> *The most __serious__ mistake is to attribute symptoms of MI to an abdominal condition.*

DIAGNOSTIC TESTING

Most elderly patients with acute abdominal pain presenting to the ED will undergo laboratory testing.[14] This will routinely include a complete blood count, urinalysis, electrolytes, renal function tests, liver functions and a serum amylase or lipase level. The specific diagnostic tests required for different conditions vary but a few general points are worth emphasizing.

The WBC count, although helpful, should never be used to exclude the presence of significant abdominal disease. Remarkably, of patients older than 65 years with abdominal pain from a condition requiring surgery, only 39% had a WBC count greater than 10,000.[8] In the elderly patient, a differential cell count, if not done routinely, should sometimes be requested specifically, because this may increase the yield of patients with abnormal laboratory results.[6] A low hemoglobin level or low microcytic indices may be useful clues to underlying malignancy, a common factor in abdominal pain in the elderly patient.[48]

Serum amylase determinations are frequently normal in patients of all age groups with pancreatitis, and a serum lipase level will be of added benefit in this situation.[63] The urinalysis is important given the frequency of genitourinary problems presenting with abdominal pain.

The utility of plain abdominal radiographs is controversial, with some authors feeling they are overused[64] and others advocating their routine use.[65] They are almost universally helpful in small bowel obstruction.[5,65] The failure of these films to detect free air in up to 40% of

> *In one series of eldelry patients with acute abdominal pain, missed perforation of a viscus was the most frequent fatal misdiagnosis. In each of these missed cases, there was no free air evident on the admission radiographs.*

cases of ulcer perforation[12,42] has been mentioned, and it is wise to remember that these studies may confound the diagnosis of appendicitis.[6,12] More complex studies such as ultrasound, CT scanning, and barium enema all have a place in the evaluation of acute abdominal pain in the elderly patient. Their use is mentioned in the discussion of the preceding disease entities.

DISPOSITION

The proper disposition of an elderly patient with abdominal pain requires an accurate assessment as to the nature of the patient's condition and will depend on the suspected diagnosis. For those patients in whom the diagnosis is uncertain, serial evaluations in an observed setting are an extremely valuable strategy.[19]

It can be quite difficult to diagnose accurately conditions such as appendicitis in the early phases of the disease if an elderly patient presents at this stage. The two most common causes of abdominal pain of a surgical nature for which patients are discharged inappropriately from the ED are appendicitis and small bowel obstruction.[8] Instructing the patient to return if the pain or vomiting does not resolve in a brief period of time, such as 6-8 hours, or if vomiting that was not previously present occurs, can help to identify these conditions before serious morbidity.[18]

Emergency physicians should be aware that in patients older than 50 years who are evaluated in the ED and found to have "non-specific" pain, more than 10% will be diagnosed with cancer within 1 year.[39] Obviously, referral for continued care and further evaluation is appropriate in such patients.

SUMMARY POINTS

The elderly patient with acute abdominal pain is a great challenge to the emergency physician, and each such patient must be carefully evaluated. The following key points are essential to remember:

- The rate of required admission and subsequent surgery is very high in the elderly patient presenting to the ED with acute abdominal pain.
- Pain perception and the physical examination may be altered in older patients, creating diagnostic difficulties for the emergency physician.
- In the elderly patient with appendicitis, anorexia, leukocytosis, or the classic migration pattern of pain may be lacking, however, right lower quadrant tenderness is generally present.
- Elderly patients with cholecystitis can appear deceptively well but should undergo surgery on an urgent basis.
- The sudden onset of pain, epigastric rigidity, and evidence of free air on plain radiography are lacking in large percentages of elderly patients with a perforated ulcer.
- Large bowel obstruction of any cause may be present despite the patient's report of diarrhea.
- Colonic pseudo-obstruction should be suspected in patients appearing to have large bowel obstruction who have a non-tender

abdomen or a cavernous rectal vault.

- Acute mesenteric infarction must be suspected in any elderly patient with abdominal pain, particularly if underlying cardiovascular disease or hypotension of any cause is present.
- The patient with suspected mesenteric infarction must undergo angiography before the development of "hard evidence."
- A ruptured aortic aneurysm must be considered in any elderly patient with acute abdominal or back pain. A pulsatile mass will often not be detectable on physical examination.
- When renal colic is suspected, care should be taken to exclude the possibility of a ruptured abdominal aortic aneurysm.

CHAPTER AUTHOR

Robert M. McNamara, MD

REFERENCES

1. McNamara RM, Rousseau E, Sanders AB. Geriatric emergency medicine: a survey of practicing emergency physicians. *Ann Emerg Med.* 1992;21: 796–801.
2. Fenyo G. Acute abdominal disease in the elderly: experience from two series in Stockholm. *Am J Surg.* 1982;143:751–754.
3. Bender JS. Approach to the acute abdomen. *Med Clin North Am.* 1989;73:1413–1422.
4. Cooke M, Sande M. Diagnosis and outcome of bowel infarction on an acute medical service. *Am J Med* 1983;75:984–992.
5. Bender JS, Busuito MJ, Graham C, Allaben RD. Small bowel obstruction in the elderly. *Am Surg.* 1989;55:385–388.
6. Horattas MC, Guyton DP, Wu D. A reappraisal of appendicitis in the elderly. *Am J Surg.* 1990;160:291–293.
7. Morrow DJ, Thompson J, Wilson SE. Acute cholecystitis in the elderly. *Arch Surg.* 1978;113:1149–1152.
8. Brewer RJ, Golden GT, Hitch DC, et al. Abdominal pain: an analysis of 1,000 consecutive cases in a university hospital emergency room. *Am J Surg.* 1976;131:219–224.
9. Bugliosi TF, Meloy TD, Vukov LF. Acute abdominal pain in the elderly. *Ann Emerg Med.* 1990;19:1383–1386.
10. Johansen K, Kohler TR, Nicholls SC, et al. Ruptured abdominal aortic aneurysm: the Harborview experience. *J Vasc Surg.* 1991;13:240–247.
11. Gustafson RA, McDowell DE, Savrin RA. The use of the MAST suit in ruptured abdominal aortic aneurysms. *Am Surg.* 1983;49:454–459.
12. Fenyo G. Diagnostic problems of acute abdominal diseases in the aged. *Acta Chir Scand.* 1974;140:396–405.
13. Ponka JL, Welborn JK, Brush BE. Acute abdominal pain in aged patients: an analysis of 200 cases. *J Am Geriatr Soc.* 1963;11:993–1007.
14. Vogt DP. The acute abdomen in the geriatric patient. *Cleve Clin J Med.* 1990;57:125–130.
15. Bayer AJ, Chadha JS, Farag RR, et al. Changing presentation of myocardial infarction with increasing old age. *J Am Geriatr Soc.* 1986;34:263–266.
16. Cocchi A, Franceschini G, Incalzi RA, et al. Clinico-pathological correlations in the diagnosis of acute myocardial infarction in the elderly. *Age Ageing.* 1988;17:87–93.
17. Clinch D, Banerjee AK, Ostick G. Absence of abdominal pain in elderly patients with peptic ulcer. *Age Ageing.* 1984;13:120–123.

18. Davidson SJ, McNamara RM. Surgical causes of abdominal pain. In: Harwood-Nuss AL, Ed, *The clinical practice of emergency medicine.* Philadelphia, PA: JB Lippincott Co.; 1991:113–117.

19. Silen W, Ed. *Cope's early diagnosis of the acute abdomen.* 17th ed. New York, NY: Oxford University Press; 1987.

20. Owens, BJ III, Hamit HF. Appendicitis in the elderly. *Ann Surg.* 1978;187:392–396.

21. Andersson A, Bergdahl L, Van Der Linden W. Volvulus of the cecum. *Ann Surg.* 1976;181:876–880.

22. Anderson JR, Lee D. The management of acute sigmoid volvulus. *Br J Surg.* 1981;68:117–120.

23. Stubenbord WT, Thorbjarnarson B. Intussusception in adults. *Ann Surg.* 1970;172:306–310.

24. Way LW. Abdominal pain. *In:* Sleisinger WH, Ed. *Gastrointestinal disease.* 3rd ed. Philadelphia, PA: WB Saunders; 1983.

25. Menaker GJ. The physiology and mechanism of acute abdominal pain. *Surg Clin North Am.* 1962;42:241–248.

26. Ottinger LW. Mesenteric ischemia. *N Engl J Med.* 1982;307:535–537.

27. Crawford ES. The diagnosis and management of aortic dissection. *JAMA.* 1990;264:2537–2541.

28. Marston WA, Ahlquist R, Johnson G Jr, et al. Misdiagnosis of ruptured abdominal aortic aneurysms. *J Vasc Surg.* 1992;16:17–22.

29. Phillips SL, Burns GP. Acute abdominal disease in the aged. *Med Clin North Am.* 1988;72:1213–1224.

30. Balsano N, Cayten CG. Surgical emergencies of the abdomen. *Emerg Med Clin North Am.* 1990;8:399–410.

31. Greenlee HB, Pienkos EJ, Vanderbilt PC, et al. Acute large bowel obstruction. *Arch Surg.* 1974;108:470–476.

32. Steinheber FU. Medical conditions mimicking the acute surgical abdomen. *Med Clin North Am.* 1973;57:1559–1567.

33. Pierce GE, Brockenbrough EC. The spectrum of mesenteric infarction. *Am J Surg.* 1970;119:233–239.

34. Callaghan J. The Boerhaave syndrome. *Br J Surg.* 1972;52:41–44.

35. Huber DF, Martin EW, Cooperman M. Cholecystectomy in elderly patients. *Ann Surg.* 1983;146:719–722.

36. Diethelm AG. The acute abdomen. *In:* Sabiston DC, Ed. *Sabiston's textbook of surgery.* 12th ed. Philadelphia, PA: WB Saunders; 1986.

37. Freund HR, Rubinstein E. Appendicitis in the aged: is it really different? *Am Surg.* 1984;50:573–576.

38. Cope JR, Abrams PH. Chest disease presenting as an acute abdomen. *Am Surg.* 1979;45:364–365.

39. DeDombal FT, Matharu SS, Staniland JR, et al. Presentation of cancer to hospital as "acute abdominal pain." *Br J Surg.* 1980;67:413–416.

40. Glenn F. Surgical management of acute cholecystitis in patients 65 years of age and older. *Ann Surg.* 1981;193:56–59.

41. Levrat M, Pasquier J, Lambert R, et al. Peptic ulcer in patients over 60. *Am J Dig Dis.* 1966;11:279–285.

42. Maull KI, Reath DB. Pneumogastrography in the diagnosis of perforated peptic ulcer. *Am J Surg.* 1984;148:340–345.

43. Roh JJ, Thompson JS, Harned RK, Hodgson PE. Value of pneumoperitoneum in the diagnosis of visceral perforation. *Am J Surg.* 1983; 146:830–833.

44. Kauvar DR. The geriatric acute abdomen. *Clin Geriatr Med.* 1993;9: 547–558.

45. Blake R, Lynn J. Emergency abdominal surgery in the aged. *Br J Surg.* 1976;63:956–960.

46. Ballantyne GH, Brandner MD, Beart RW, et al. Volvulus of the colon: incidence and mortality. *Ann Surg.* 1985;202:83–92.

47. Wertkin MG, Aufses AH. Management of volvulus of the colon. *Dis Colon Rectum.* 1978;21:40–45.

48. Calabrese CT, Adam YG, Volk H. Geriatric colon cancer. *Am J Surg.* 1973;125:181–184.

49. Ogilvie H. Large intestinal colic due to sympathetic denervation: a new clinical syndrome. *Br Med J.* 1948;1:671–673.

50. Geelhoed GW. Colonic pseudo-obstruction in surgical patients. *Am J Surg.* 1985;149:258–265.

51. Gilchrist AM, Mils JO, Russel CF. Acute large bowel pseudo-obstruction. *Clin Radiol.* 1985;36:401–404.

52. Hyatt R. Colonic pseudo-obstruction: an important complication in hospitalized elderly patients. *Age Ageing.* 1987;16:145–152.

53. Nakhgevany KP. Colonoscopic decompression of the colon in patients with Ogilvie's syndrome. *Am J Surg.* 1984;148:317–320.

54. Almy TP, Howell DA. Diverticular disease of the colon. *N Engl J Med.* 1980;302:324–331.

55. Walker JD, Gray LA Sr, Polk HC Jr. Diverticulitis in women: an unappreciated clinical presentation. *Ann Surg.* 1977;185:402–405.

56. Boley SJ, Sprayregan S, Siegelman SS, et al. Initial results from an aggressive roentgenological and surgical approach to acute mesenteric ischemia. *Surgery.* 1977;82:848–855.

57. Ottinger LW, Austen WG. A study of 136 patients with mesenteric infarction. *Surg Gynecol Obstet.* 1967;124:251–261.

58. Sachs SM, Morton JH, Schwartz SI. Acute mesenteric ischemia. *Surgery.* 1982;92:646–653.

59. Harward TR, Green D, Bergan JJ, et al. Mesenteric venous thrombosis. *J Vasc Surg.* 1989;9:328–333.

60. Ernst CB. Abdominal aortic aneurysm. *N Engl J Med.* 1993;328:1167–1171.

61. Loughran CF. A review of the plain abdominal radiograph in acute rupture of abdominal aortic aneurysms. *Clin Radiol.* 1986;37:383–387.

62. Altman DF. Gastrointestinal diseases in the elderly. *Med Clin North Am.* 1983;67:433–445.

63. Clavien PA, Robert J, Meyer P, et al. Acute pancreatitis and normoamylasemia. *Ann Surg.* 1989;210:614–620.

64. Greene CS. Indications for plain abdominal radiography in the emergency department. *Ann Emerg Med.* 1986;15:257–260.

65. Lee PW. The plain x-ray in the acute abdomen: a surgeon's evaluation. *Br J Surg.* 1976;63:764–766.

14 *Infections*

LEARNING OBJECTIVES

1. Explain the significance of functional decline in the diagnosis of an infectious process.
2. State examples of how typical infectious processes among community-dwelling elderly people differ from those of nursing home residents.
3. Summarize physiologic changes that place the elderly at greater risk of infection.
4. Identify pathogens implicated in community-acquired pneumonia and in pneumonia acquired by persons recently hospitalized or living in a nursing home.
5. Identify factors that complicate both diagnosis and management of urinary tract infection (UTI) in the elderly.

Fever and concern about infection are common reasons for ED visits by the elderly, and it should be noted that they are more prone to infection and secondary complications. An aging immune system, when accompanied by chronic conditions such as diabetes, dementia, malnutrition, cardiovascular disease, chronic lung disease, cancer, and alcohol abuse, places the older individual at greater risk of serious infection (Table 14–1). When threatened by infection elderly persons face a higher morbidity and mortality than younger adults. Infection involving multiple organisms is not uncommon and may be further complicated by antibiotic resistance. Evaluation of the elderly patient with fever in the ED is often time consuming, is more demanding of resources, and very frequently results in hospitalization.[1–5]

Table 14–1 **Age-Related Risk Factors That Increase Susceptibility to Infection**

Decreased pulmonary function and cough reflex
Decreased gastric acidity and GI motility
Atherosclerosis and decreased capillary blood flow
Thin, easily traumatized skin
Decreased activity secondary to motor and balance problems
Impaired host defense mechanisms
Inadequate nutrition and hydration
Lack of recent immunization against preventable diseases
Neuropsychologic diseases and mental deterioration
Chronic use of medications
Chronic diseases (diabetes, cardiac disease, renal disease, alcoholism)
Previous exposures to hazardous materials (asbestos, chemicals, dusts)
Hospitalization and residence in long-term care facilities
Invasive devices (urinary catheters, nasogastric tubes)

From Alder WH, Nagel JE. Clinical immunology and aging. In: Hazzard WR et al eds. *Principles of Geriatric Medicine and Gerontology* 3rd ed. McGraw Hill, New York, NY. 1994:70–76. Reproduced with permission of McGraw-Hill, Inc.

The chief presenting complaint with infection may be anorexia, excess fatigue, unexplained weight loss, new incontinence, falls or mental confusion.

Infections in the elderly population often present atypically. An acute decline in functional status should raise a suspicion of underlying infection. Such non-specific symptoms and signs as anorexia, excess fatigue, unexplained weight loss, new incontinence, falls, and mental confusion may be the primary clinical manifestations of infection in elderly persons. Whereas fever in children and younger adults often accompanies relatively benign illnesses, fever in elderly persons often indicates a serious infection and one that is more frequently bacterial than viral. However, infection without fever is also common in the elderly population. As many as 30% of elderly patients presenting with bacteremia, pneumonia, UTI, intraabdominal infection, or tuberculosis are not febrile.[1,6,7]

30% of elderly patients presenting with bacteremia, pneumonia, UTI, intraabdominal infection, or TB are afebrile.

The emergency physician must distinguish among different subgroups that exist within the growing elderly population to appreciate how variable susceptibility to infection can be (Table 14–2). Infections in the independent, community-dwelling individual differ from those in nursing home residents and those who have recently been hospitalized. For example, respiratory infections are most common among community-living elderly and include influenza, bronchitis, and pneumonia. Urinary tract infections follow next in frequency and then intraabdominal infections, including cholecystitis, diverticulitis, and appendicitis. In contrast, 70% to 80% of infections in nursing home residents can be accounted for by the acronym *pus*: *p*neumonia, *u*rinary tract infections, and *s*oft tissue infections. The nursing home resident is also more likely to contract tuberculosis, hepatitis, and infectious diarrhea.[1,2,5]

Making a decision as to whether to treat an elderly patient with infection as an outpatient or an inpatient often can be difficult. Many factors must be considered, including (1) the patient's clinical status, comorbid conditions, functional status, and social and economic support and (2) the confidence of the emergency physician in timely, ap-

Table 14–2 **Differential Diagnosis of Infection in Older Adults by Functional Status or Level of Care**

Functional Status or Level of Care	Types of Infection	
	Primary Considerations	Secondary Considerations
Independent, healthy individual living in community	Bacterial pneumonia and other respiratory tract infections UTI Intraabdominal infections (cholecystitis, diverticulitis, appendicitis)	Infective endocarditis Tuberculosis Septic arthritis Meningitis
Hospital patient	UTI Pneumonia Surgical wound infections	Septic thrombophlebitis Drug reactions* Pulmonary emboli* Hepatitis
Nursing home resident	Pneumonia UTI Decubitus ulcer	Tuberculosis Drug reactions* Intraabdominal infection Gastroenteritis

*Noninfectious disorders simulating an infection or causing fever.
From Yoshikawa TT. Approach to the diagnosis and treatment of the infected older adult. In: Hazzard WR et al eds. *Principles of Geriatric Medicine and Gerontology* 3rd ed. McGraw Hill, New York, NY. 1994:1160. Reproduced with permission of McGraw-Hill, Inc.

propriate follow-up. If the patient was referred from a nursing home facility it is important to consider the level of care the facility is able to provide. It is often most prudent to err on the side of hospitalization. Hospitalization may result in more rapid recovery with less potential for complications and prolonged disability, which can translate ultimately into considerable savings.

AGING AND RESISTANCE TO INFECTION

Physiologic changes in the immune system were discussed in Chapter 2. To summarize, almost every aspect of immune function is affected by aging (Table 14–3). Mucocutaneous barriers to infection deteriorate. Mechanical defenses such as the cough reflex and swallowing may become less coordinated and predispose to aspiration and pneumonia. Urinary retention and incontinence are common and contribute to the increased occurrence of complicated UTIs. Specific immunity imparted by T- and B-cell activity and immunoglobulin production is diminished with aging, although non-specific immunity imparted by neutrophil, complement, and opsonization activity remains largely intact. However, decreased production of pyrogenic lymphokines by the monocyte/macrophage system attenuates the febrile response to infection. Declines in marrow volume and hematopoietic potential contribute to a diminished white blood cell (WBC) response to infection. Indeed, an abrupt decline in white cell count is a common response to sepsis in elderly patients.

Table 14–3   **Summary of Changes in Immune Function in Elderly Persons**

Decreased production of thymic hormones
Diminished in vitro responsiveness to interleukin II
Decreased cell proliferation in response to mitogenic stimulation
Decreased cell-mediated cytotoxicity
Enhanced cellular sensitivity to prostaglandin E_2
Increased synthesis of antiidiotype antibodies
Decreased levels of specific antibody response
Increased presence of autoimmune antibodies
Increased incidence of serum monoclonal immunoproteins
No change in natural killer cell function
Decreased representation of peripheral blood B lymphocytes in men
Diminished delayed hypersensitivity
No change in numbers of peripheral blood lymphocytes
Enhanced ability to synthesize IFN-gamma, interleukin VI, and TNF-alpha

From Alder WH, Nagel JE. Clinical immunology and aging. In: Hazzard WR et al eds. *Principles of Geriatric Medicine and Gerontology* 3rd ed. McGraw-Hill, New York, NY. 1994:70–71. Reproduced with permission of McGraw-Hill, Inc.

Nutrition plays an important role in maintaining immune competence throughout life, and protein malnutrition, common in the elderly population, contributes to lymphoid tissue involution and increased susceptibility to infection. Probably the most important generalization that can be made about the aging immune system is the concept of "too little, too late." By the time the senescent immune system has mobilized against an infection, the infection may be well established and overwhelmingly systemic.[4,5,8–11]

ANTIBIOTIC CHOICES

Antibiotic choices are discussed below in the treatment of specific infections. A few generalizations can be made regarding antibiotic use in the elderly. It is important to appreciate the differences in pathogens that cause infections in the elderly in contrast to children and younger adults. It is often more difficult to isolate a specific pathogen in the older patient for a variety of reasons, including poor sputum production, changes in normal bacterial flora, colonization with multiple potential pathogens, and generalized debility that may prevent the aggressive pursuit of culture specimens. The aging immune system is frequently slow to respond to infection, making established and systemic infection more common on first presentation. Therefore, the empiric application of antibiotics when infection is suspected is preferred to a more nihilistic approach of culture-and-wait. Empiric antibiotic therapy should at first be directed broadly until a specific pathogen is identified and, when possible, bactericidal drugs should be chosen over bacteriostatic. Care should be taken to consider the impact of diminished renal function or hepatic insufficiency on antibiotic dose and dosing interval. When possible, aminoglycoside antibiotics should be avoided because of the increased potential for nephrotoxicity and ototoxicity.

COMMON INFECTIONS

PNEUMONIA

Pneumonia remains the leading cause of death from infection in Americans older than 65 years. Atypical presentations are common, with approximately one third of patients presenting without altered sputum production or fever and one half presenting without cough. Acute functional decline or altered mental status accompanied by tachypnea is a common presentation. On physical examination signs of consolidation are frequently absent. Chest radiographs are occasionally non-diagnostic, particularly when acute illness is accompanied by dehydration.[12-16]

Community-acquired pneumonia is caused predominantly by *Streptococcus pneumoniae* (50%) followed by *Haemophilus influenzae* (15%) and gram-negative bacilli (15%). The remaining 20% are caused by *Staphylococcus aureus*, B. *catarrhalis*, *Legionella* species, chlamydia, mycoplasma, anaerobes, and influenza. Mortality in streptococcal pneumonia is as high as 15% to 20%, rising to 30% to 50% for those with bacteremia. In nursing home residents, gram-negative bacilli are more frequent (30%-45%) than *Streptococcus pneumoniae* (20%-30%), and anaerobes are more commonly isolated (30%-35%).

Gram-negative pneumonia is far more common in recently hospitalized persons or in residents of nursing homes and chronic care facilities than in community-dwelling persons. Risk factors for gram-negative pneumonia, presumably caused by microaspiration, include the presence of neuromuscular disease, depressed sensorium, and the use of nasograstric tubes. In these cases gram-negative colonization of the oropharynx and upper respiratory tract occurs. Predominant organisms include *Pseudomonas aeruginosa* and *Klebsiella pneumoniae*. Other less frequent pathogens include *Enterobacter, Proteus, Escherichia coli, Actinobacter,* and *Serratia marcescens.*

Anaerobic pulmonary infections accompany aspiration pneumonia and the secondary complications of empyema and lung abscess. Anaerobic infections commonly involve lower lung segments in the clinical setting of aspiration. These infections are more likely than aerobic infections to have an indolent course with symptoms evolving over weeks and months before becoming clinically apparent—the so-called walking pneumonias. The subacute presentation of empyema, lung abscess, or putrid-smelling sputum suggests anaerobic infection.

Staphylococcus aureus is present in 10% to 30% of nosocomial pneumonias, including both hospitalized and nursing home patients. *Staphylococcus aureus* is also common when bacterial infection complicates influenza. Most strains produce beta-lactamase and require the use of penicillinase-resistant synthetic penicillins or cephalosporins. However, methicillin-resistant *Staphylococcus aureus* is found in 30% to 40% of isolates from nosocomial infections and is becoming more common in community-acquired infections as well. Vancomycin should be considered when initial therapy appears ineffective and culture results are unavailable or pending.

Haemophilus influenzae follows *Streptococcus pneumoniae* as the bacterial pathogen most commonly isolated from elderly patients with com-

Atypical presentations of pneumonia are common with approximately 1/3 presenting without altered sputum production or fever, and 1/2 without cough.

Mortality in streptococcal pneumonia is as high as 15% to 20%, rising to 30% to 50% for those with bacteremia.

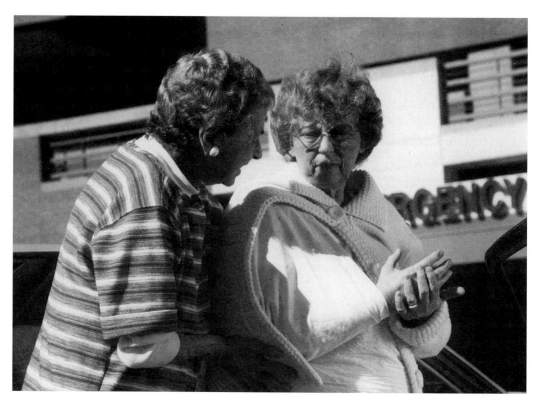

Pneumonia remains the leading cause of death from infection in Americans over the age of 65.

munity-acquired pneumonia. These organisms are also the most likely cause of exacerbations of bronchitis seen in patients with chronic lung disease. In the United States 25% to 30% of *Haemophilus influenzae* isolates are resistant to ampicillin, and more reliable therapy includes amoxicillin-clavulanate (Augmentin), a second- or third-generation oral cephalosporin or trimethoprim-sulfamethoxazole.

From its first description in the Philadelphia outbreak of 1976, Legionnaires' disease, caused by *Legionella pneumophila*, was recognized as having the greatest impact on elderly patients. Although uncommon, *Legionella* pneumonia carries a high mortality in the elderly population. *Legionella* species may account for 15% of community-acquired pneumonias requiring hospitalization and, in periods of epidemic, up to 40% of nosocomial infections. Outbreaks are more likely to occur in summer months when pneumonia in general is less common. *Legionella pneumophila* proliferates in standing water and is disseminated in aerosols produced by air-cooling equipment used most heavily in warm weather. Symptoms often include high fever and non-productive cough with a variable prodrome or accompanied by chills, malaise, myalgia, anorexia, and headache. In established infections the chest radiograph generally shows bilateral infiltrates and involves multiple lobes. The drug of choice remains intravenous erythromycin at a dose of 4 g/day. Rifampin is added when patients are severely ill.

Recent studies have implicated *Chlamydia pneumoniae* in 5% to 10% of atypical pneumonias occurring in elderly persons requiring hospitalization and in 5% to 10% of all nosocomial pneumonias. It is diffi-

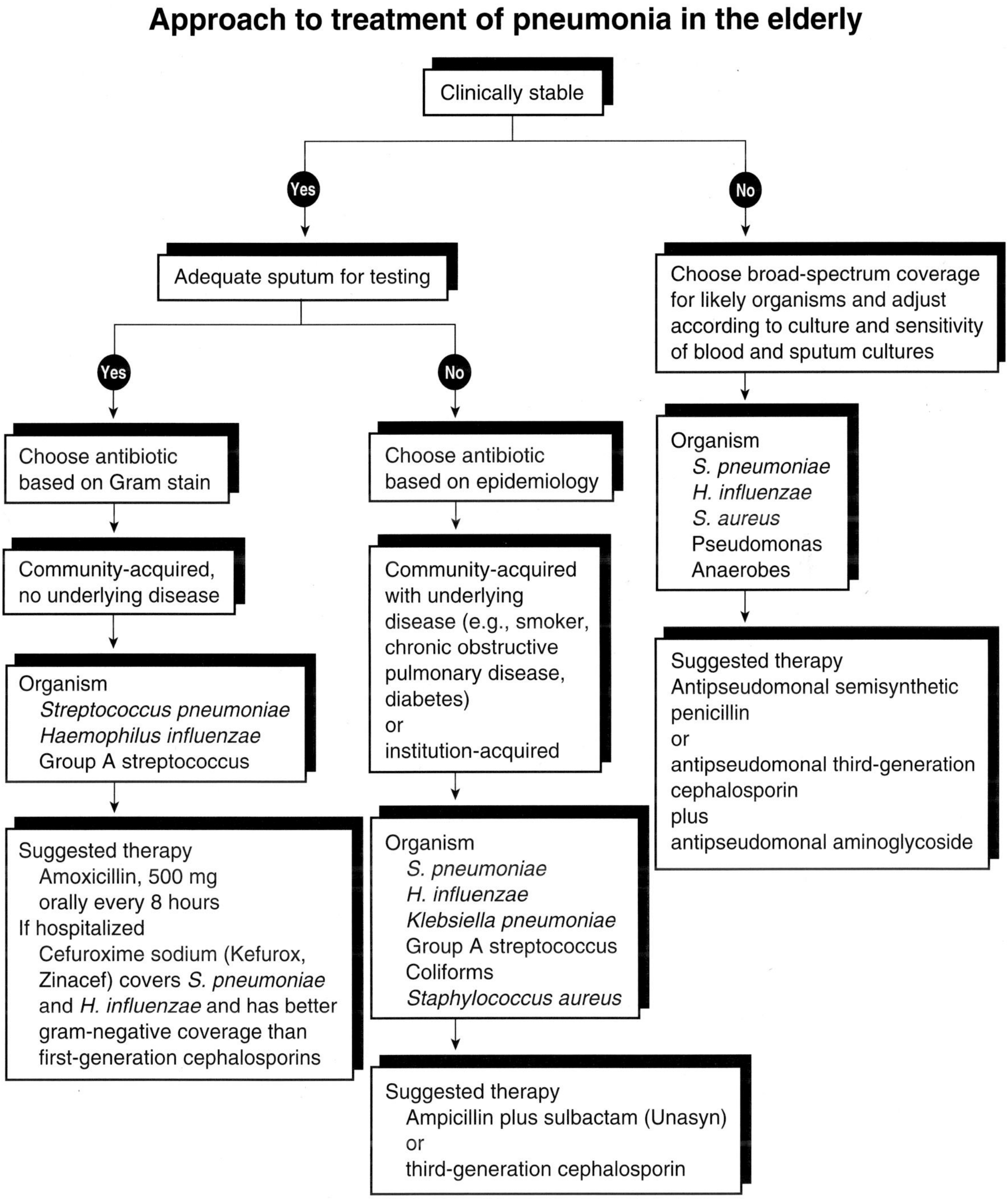

Approach to treatment of pneumonia in the elderly

Clinically stable

Yes →

No →

Adequate sputum for testing

Choose broad-spectrum coverage for likely organisms and adjust according to culture and sensitivity of blood and sputum cultures

Yes / **No**

Organism
 S. pneumoniae
 H. influenzae
 S. aureus
 Pseudomonas
 Anaerobes

Choose antibiotic based on Gram stain

Choose antibiotic based on epidemiology

Community-acquired, no underlying disease

Community-acquired with underlying disease (e.g., smoker, chronic obstructive pulmonary disease, diabetes)
or
institution-acquired

Suggested therapy
Antipseudomonal semisynthetic penicillin
or
antipseudomonal third-generation cephalosporin
plus
antipseudomonal aminoglycoside

Organism
 Streptococcus pneumoniae
 Haemophilus influenzae
 Group A streptococcus

Suggested therapy
 Amoxicillin, 500 mg
 orally every 8 hours
If hospitalized
 Cefuroxime sodium (Kefurox, Zinacef) covers *S. pneumoniae* and *H. influenzae* and has better gram-negative coverage than first-generation cephalosporins

Organism
 S. pneumoniae
 H. influenzae
 Klebsiella pneumoniae
 Group A streptococcus
 Coliforms
 Staphylococcus aureus

Suggested therapy
 Ampicillin plus sulbactam (Unasyn)
 or
 third-generation cephalosporin

FIGURE 14-1 From McClure CC. Common infections in the elderly. *Am Fam Physician.* 1992;45:2692.

cult to demonstrate this organism by conventional testing, which further supports the use of erythromycin or doxycycline to treat the atypical pneumonias of the elderly.

Important viral causes of respiratory tract infections in the elderly population include influenza, parainfluenza, and respiratory syncytial virus. Of these, influenza carries the highest overall morbidity and mortality. The major complications of influenza infection are influenza

Table 14–4 **Recommendations for Treatment of Specific Types of Pneumonia**

Organism	Agent*	Alternative (Comments)
Bacteria		
S. pneumoniae	Penicillin	Cephalosporins, erythromycin, clindamycin
S. aureus		
Methicillin-sensitive	Penicillinase-resistant penicillin*	Cephalosporins (1st or 2nd generation), clindamycin, vancomycin
Methicillin-resistant	Vancomycin	Sulfa-trimethoprim
Klebsiella†	Cephalosporin	Aminoglycoside, piperacillin, imipenem
Pseudomonas†	Aminoglycoside + antipseudomonad penicillin*	Aminoglycoside + imipenem, ceftazidime, cefoperazone, ciprofloxacin, or aztreonam
Gram-negative bacilli (other)†	Aminoglycoside, cephalosporin, ampicillin, or antipseudomonad penicillin	
H. influenzae†	Ampicillin (ampicillin-sensitive strains), cefuroxime, third-generation cephalosporins	Tetracycline, chloramphenicol, sulfa-trimethoprim
Anaerobes	Penicillin or clindamycin	Tetracycline, chloramphenicol, antipseudomonad penicillin, imipenem, metronidazole + penicillin, beta-lactam beta-lactamase inhibitor
Nocardia	Sulfonamides	Sulfa-trimethoprim, minocycline, doxycycline
Legionella	Erythromycin	Erythromycin + rifampin, sulfa-trimethoprim + rifampin
Mycoplasma	Erythromycin or tetracycline	
C. pneumoniae	Tetracycline	Erythromycin
Fungi		
Histoplasma, blastomycosis, coccidioidomycosis	Ketoconazole	Amphotericin B (histoplasmosis and coccidioidomycosis confined to lung are usually not treated)
Candida, Aspergillus	Amphotericin B ± 5-fluorocytosine	
Phycomycetes *(Mucar)*	Amphotericin B	
Viruses		
Herpes simplex	Acyclovir	
Varicella-zoster	Acyclovir	
Influenza A	Amantadine	

*Antipseudomonad penicillins: ticarcillin, piperacillin, and mezlocillin, usually considered equally effective; in vitro testing facilitates choice.
Penicillinase-resistant penicillins: nafcillin, oxacillin, and methicillin.
Cephalosporins: in vitro testing determines choice.
Aminoglycosides: in vitro testing facilitates choice among tobramycin, gentamicin, and amikacin.
†CNB: in vitro testing required.
From Bartlett JG. Pneumonia. In: Hazzard WR et al eds. *Principles of Geriatric Medicine and Gerontology* 3rd ed. McGraw-Hill, New York, NY. 1994:571. Reproduced with permission of McGraw-Hill, Inc.

pneumonia and secondary bacterial infections that accompany the paralysis of respiratory macrophage activity. The most common bacterial pathogens in this setting are *Streptococcus pneumoniae* and *Staphylococcus aureus.* Influenza vaccine is recommended annually for all elderly persons. Amantadine has proven efficacy in the treatment of influenza A if given within 48 hours of symptom onset. Amantadine can also be used as a preventive medication, although it carries a relatively high rate of central nervous system side effects, which limits its general application.

Management of pneumonia in the ED includes routine laboratory tests and radiographs as well as arterial blood gas determinations, blood cultures, and sputum Gram stain and culture (Figure 14–1). The decision to hospitalize the patient is made on the basis of overall clinical status and comorbid conditions, as well as an assessment of the patient's functional status, social support, and confidence in timely and adequate follow-up. A clinically stable and otherwise healthy patient with a community-acquired pneumonia and no signs of respiratory compromise may be treated as an outpatient.[17]

Choice of antibiotics depends on several factors (Table 14–4). Community-acquired pneumonia can be treated empirically with a second-generation cephalosporin (i.e., cefuroxime, cefoxitin) or trimethoprim-sulfamethoxazole (TMP/SMX). For seriously ill patients with community-acquired pneumonia a combination of erythromycin and cefuroxime (or cefamandole) or erythromycin and trimethoprim-sulfamethoxazole is a reasonable choice when no specific pathogen has been identified. For the nursing home resident or elderly patient with chronic disease (i.e., diabetes, chronic obstructive pulmonary disease, congestive heart failure, cerebrovascular accident or alcohol abuse) coverage should be broadened. In this population adequate coverage of gram-negative bacilli, anaerobes, and gram-positive cocci can be achieved with third-generation cephalosporins: ticarcillin-clavulanic acid (Timentin), ampicillin-sulbactam (Unasyn), or clindamycin and aztreonam (Azactam) in combination.[18] Aminoglycoside antibiotics should be avoided when possible because of the increased potential for nephrotoxicity and ototoxicity seen in the elderly population.

URINARY TRACT INFECTIONS

UTIs are the most common type of infection in the elderly and the most frequent source of bacteremia. Women experience UTIs more commonly than men; however, with aging the disparity between the sexes narrows somewhat. The elderly are at higher risk for UTI for a variety of reasons. Anatomic and functional abnormalities such as bladder prolapse with cystocele in women and prostatic hypertrophy in men can cause urinary obstruction and incomplete bladder emptying. Atrophic changes in the genital and urinary tract in women result in a decline in natural defenses to infection and promote colonization with pathogenic bacteria. In men prostatic enlargement and changes in prostatic fluid production and composition predispose to chronic prostatitis. The elderly are more likely to undergo instrumentation of the lower tract and have chronic indwelling urinary catheters. The incidence of urinary incontinence, neurogenic bladder, vesicoureteral reflux, and kidney stones increases with aging and predisposes to infectious complications.[19–24]

The microbiology of urinary pathogens further complicates infections in the elderly population. Chronic and recurrent infections are not uncommon. The presence of multiple organisms and antibiotic resistance

Distinguishing lower from upper UTI may be complicated by the absence of characteristic flank pain with pyelonephritis.

50% to 60% of uncomplicated UTIs in the elderly are caused by E. coli.

makes diagnosis and treatment further perplexing. *Escherichia coli* accounts for 50% to 60% of uncomplicated UTIs in the elderly population. However, infection with *Proteus, Klebsiella, Enterobacter,* and *Citrobacter* species, *Serratia marcescens,* and *Pseudomona aeruginosa* is not uncommon and should be considered when faced with recurrent infection. Indwelling urinary catheters predispose to colonization by multiple organisms and the development of multidrug resistance. Resistant group D streptococci may be especially problematic in this setting. The finding of asymptomatic bacteriuria is common in elderly persons. Most authorities recommend against treatment unless there has been recurrent symptomatic infection or chronic urinary obstruction as in prostatism.[24,25]

Diagnosis of UTI can be difficult in the elderly patient, especially when there is significant concurrent disability. Elderly persons are less likely to exhibit a febrile response to infection or demonstrate an elevated WBC count. Distinguishing lower from upper tract infection may be complicated by the absence of characteristic flank pain with pyelonephritis. In older men chronic prostatitis is more common than acute infection and may present with persistent low back pain and vague perineal discomfort in the absence of urinary urgency, urinary frequency, or prostate tenderness. A history of frequent or recurrent UTI is helpful, as is knowledge of recent instrumentation or the presence of kidney stones. A complete urinalysis should be performed with a specimen sent for culture and antibiotic sensitivity. Catheter-derived specimens will provide more reliable data. A urinalysis of specimens obtained before and after prostate massage may be helpful in making a diagnosis of chronic prostatitis. In the febrile elderly patient with suspected UTI a serious bacterial infection should be assumed and blood cultures obtained before starting parenteral antibiotics.[19]

Indwelling urinary catheters predispose to multiple organism colonization and multidrug resistance.

Choice of antibiotic therapy is ideally based on the results of urine culture. However, without culture results the following guidelines are reasonable for empiric therapy (Table 14–5). Simple lower tract infections (e.g., uncomplicated urethritis or cystitis) can be treated by a 7- to 10-day course of TMP-SMX, amoxicillin–clavulanic acid, or ce-

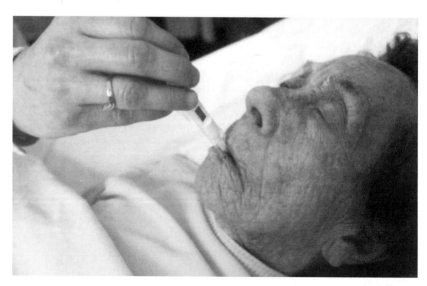

Elderly persons are less likely to exhibit a febrile response to infection or demonstrate an elevated WBC count.

Table 14–5 **Dosages of Selected Oral Antimicrobial Agents for Use in UTIs***

Antimicrobial Agent	Dosage and Dosing Interval
Amoxicillin-clavulanate	250–500 mg q8h
Amoxicillin	250–500 mg q8h
Cephalexin	250–500 mg q6h
Ciprofloxacin	250–500 mg q12h
Norfloxacin	400 mg q12h
Ofloxacin	200–300 mg q12h
Trimethoprim	100 mg q12h
Trimethoprim-sulfamethoxazole	160 mg/800 mg q12h

*Patients with normal renal and hepatic function. Dosage adjustment may be needed in elderly patients because of deterioration of renal function.
From Tunkle AR, Kay D. Urinary tract infections. In: Hazzard WR et al eds. *Principles of Geriatric Medicine and Gerontology* 3rd ed. McGraw-Hill, New York, NY. 1994:630. Reproduced with permission of McGraw-Hill, Inc.

fadroxil. Single-dose or short-course therapy is less likely to be effective in the elderly population and should be used only with close follow-up. When infection in an ambulatory patient is complicated by a history of frequent or recurrent UTI, recent instrumentation or hospitalization, or an indwelling urinary catheter, the fluoroquinolones (norfloxacin, ofloxacin, ciprofloxacin, and others) may be effective. Chronic prostatitis is difficult to cure and calls for prolonged treatment with either ciprofloxacin (500 mg twice daily) or norfloxacin (400 mg twice daily) for 4-6 weeks. Alternately, TMP-SMX (one double-strength dose twice daily) for 3 months has been demonstrated to be effective.[3,18]

Patients requiring hospitalization for serious infection should be treated with parenteral antibiotics that provide broad coverage of urinary pathogens (Table 14–6). A reasonable first choice is ampicillin or cefazolin plus aztreonam or an aminoglycoside. Alternate choices include a third-generation cephalosporin: ticarcillin-clavulanate, ampicillin-sulbactam, TMP-SMX, or imipenem-cilastatin.[18]

INTRA-ABDOMINAL INFECTIONS

Diagnosis of intraabdominal infection can be challenging in any age group. In the elderly, a high index of suspicion must be maintained, because classic presentations are uncommon. Abdominal pain may be vague and poorly localized. Fever and elevated WBC count are less likely to be present. Delayed diagnoses are common, and elderly patients often have complications of peritonitis, bowel perforation, gangrene, and evolving sepsis at first presentation. The elderly tolerate sepsis very poorly and suffer a high mortality. Early consultation with a surgeon is of primary importance.[1,2,8]

Cholecystitis is a common disease in the elderly population. At least 20% of the US population older than 60 years has gallstones. An elderly patient presenting with cholecystitis will often give the valuable history of similar, although less severe, attacks in the past. The elderly patient is more likely to present with ascending infection (cholangitis),

Delayed presentation is common with intra-abdominal infection, and the elderly often have complications of peritonitis, bowel perforation, gangrene, and evolving sepsis at first presentation.

Table 14–6   **Dosages of Selected Intravenous Antimicrobial Agents
for Use in Hospitalized Patients with Upper Urinary
Tract Infections***

Antimicrobial Agent	Dosage and Dosing Interval
Ampicillin	1–2 g q4h
Ampicillin-sulbactam	1.5–3 g q6h
Aztreonam	1–2 g q8h
Cefotaxime	1–2 g q6h
Ceftizoxime	1–2 g q8h
Ceftriaxone	1–2 g q24h
Ciprofloxacin	200–400 mg q12h
Gentamicin[†]	1–1.7 mg/kg q8h
Mezlocillin	3 g q4h
Piperacillin	3 g q4h
Trimethoprim-sulfamethoxazole	4–5 mg/kg q12h[‡]
Vancomycin[†]	1 g q12h

*Patients with normal renal and hepatic function. Dosage adjustment may be needed in
elderly patients because of deterioration of renal function.
[†]Need to monitor serum peak and trough concentration.
[‡]Dosage based on trimethoprim component.
From Tunkle AR, Kay D. Urinary tract infections. In: Hazzard WR et al eds. *Principles of
Geriatric Medicine and Gerontology* 3rd ed. McGraw Hill, New York, NY. 1994:630.
Reproduced with permission of McGraw-Hill, Inc.

perforation, gangrene and abscess, and a paucity of classic signs. Acal-
culous or ischemic cholecystitis may accompany major illness in elderly
patients, such as myocardial infarction, congestive heart failure, sepsis,
and dehydration. Pain and tenderness generally localize to the right
upper quadrant, and frequently deep inspiration is arrested while palpating below the right costal margin (Murphy's sign). Diagnosis may
be aided by emergent ultrasound and occasionally radionuclide scan.

Management requires surgical consultation, appropriate fluid resuscitation, nasogastric intubation for intractable vomiting, and parenteral antibiotics. Antibiotics chosen must achieve adequate billiary
penetration and broadly cover Enterobacteriaceae, enterococci, and
Bacteroides and *Clostridium* species. First-choice therapy could be mezlocillin in combination with metronidazole, or ticarcillin-clavulanate,
ampicillin-sulbactam, or imipenem-cilastatin alone. Alternate therapy
includes cefoxitin plus an aminoglycoside or aztreonam, or a third-generation cephalosporin combined with either metronidazole or clindamycin.[18]

Diverticulitis is a complication experienced by 10% to 20% of patients with the common condition of diverticulosis. Symptoms range
from minimal abdominal discomfort to frank peritonitis. There is
often a history of similar, although less severe, episodes in the past.
Pain and tenderness commonly localize to the left lower quadrant, and
a palpable mass may be appreciated. Occasionally brisk rectal bleeding
may complicate the presentation. A differential diagnosis should include bowel ischemia, appendicitis, UTI, pelvic disease, colon cancer,
inflammatory bowel disease, and fecal impaction. The diagnostic study
of choice is an intravenous contrast-enhanced abdominal computed to-

mography (CT) scan. Even a limited barium enema study should be avoided because of the real potential for bowel perforation.

Surgical consultation should be sought early and parenteral antibiotics begun (see preceding discussion of cholecystitis). As a rule, the elderly individual with suspected diverticulitis should be admitted to the hospital for parenteral antibiotics, hydration, and bowel rest. There is a subset of otherwise healthy and robust individuals with an uncomplicated presentation, minimal symptoms, and the clinical diagnosis of diverticulitis who may be considered for management as outpatients. Such a decision should be made in concert with a surgical consultant. A reasonable outpatient antibiotic regimen would be TMP-SMX or ciprofloxacin in combination with metronidazole. Outpatients must have ready access to close follow-up. Discharge instructions should describe a clear liquid diet and the exhortation to return to the ED immediately for worsening symptoms.[8,18]

Approximately five percent of all cases of *appendicitis* occur in individuals older than 60 years; however, these patients suffer the majority of related fatalities. Again, delayed diagnosis secondary to the frequency of atypical presentation and lack of classic signs results in a higher rate of gangrene and perforation found at surgery. Early surgical consultation, fluid resuscitation in anticipation of shock, and appropriate antibiotics are key elements to survival.[8,18]

> *Age-related changes in heart valves and a higher incidence of prosthetic valves are major predisposing factors for bacterial endocarditis.*

BACTERIAL ENDOCARDITIS

Fifty percent of all new cases of bacterial endocarditis occur in individuals older than 60 years. Age-related changes in heart valves, atherosclerosis, and a higher incidence of prosthetic valves are major predisposing factors. The elderly are more likely to undergo instrumentation that can cause transient bacteremia and the potential for inflammation at affected heart valve sites. The older patient has a lower rate of infection by *Streptococcus viridans* and a higher rate of infection by group D streptococci (i.e., enterococcus and *Streptococcus bovis*). *Staphylococcus aureus* accounts for 20% to 40% of endocarditis in the elderly population and is often fulminant at presentation.

In subacute infections symptoms may be minimal and fever is often absent. Successful diagnoses are made by maintaining a high index of suspicion.[1,26]

MENINGITIS

As with young children, the diagnosis of meningitis can be elusive in the elderly secondary to the paucity of classic signs. Headache, photophobia, and neck stiffness may not be prominent. Some degree of cognitive impairment is a relative constant, and seizures are not uncommon. As with all serious infections in the elderly, a fever or elevated WBC count cannot be relied on. Meningitis in the elderly population is more frequently bacterial in origin than viral. *Streptococcus pneumoniae* and *Neisseria meningitidis* are found most frequently, but *Haemophilus influenzae,* *Listeria monocytogenes,* and the Enterobacteriaceae must also be considered in elderly patients. Therapy should include high-dose penicillin G or ampicillin in combination with ceftriaxone or cefotaxime. An alternative for penicillin-allergic persons is aztreonam plus TMP-SMX.[16,18]

> *Meningitis is often difficult to diagnose in the elderly, as classic signs such as headache, neck stiffness, and photophobia may not be obvious.*

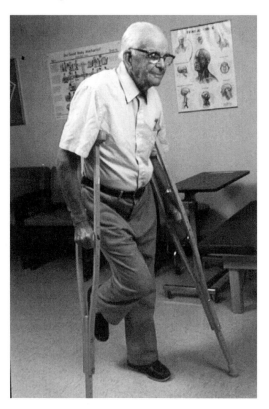

Prosthetic joints are more common in elderly persons, and infection may have a benign presentation.

35% to 50% of all nongonococcal bacterial joint infections occur in individuals 60 years and older.

CUTANEOUS INFECTIONS

Immobility, degenerative changes in the skin, and loss of cutaneous fat pads predispose the elderly to cutaneous infection. Diabetes, peripheral vascular disease, and chronic lower extremity edema are additional important factors.

Decubitus ulcers are present in 35% of nursing home patients in the US and are often overlooked as important sources of infection and bacteremia. Principal isolates include groups A, C, and D *streptococcus* species, anaerobes, and gram-negative bacilli. Initial management includes debridement and wound cultures. Appropriate x-ray studies should be obtained to rule out osteomyelitis when ulcers overlie bony prominences.

After debridement, uncomplicated ulcers can be treated locally with topical silver sulfadiazine. When systemic illness or surrounding cellulitis is present, hospitalization and parenteral antibiotics are indicated. Cefoxitin plus an aminoglycoside or aztreonam, or ticarcillin-clavulanate, ampicillin-sulbactam, or imipenem-cilastatin are reasonable antibiotic choices. Alternate therapy could include ciprofloxacin plus clindamycin, or a combination of ampicillin, aminoglycoside, and clindamycin.[18,27,28]

Erysipelas is an infection of the superficial layers of the skin that occurs primarily in children and elderly persons. It is caused by group A streptococci and very occasionally *Staphylococcus aureus*. The face is the primary site of involvement, and the condition is characterized by a bright red, warm, tender, raised, indurated eruption with sharply defined borders. Localized lymphadenopathy is common, and vesicles or bullae may form as well. Fever and systemic illness are common; however, bacteremia is not. Hospitalization is usually indicated for older patients, and parenteral penicillin or nafcillin is the antibiotic of choice.[18]

Cellulitis is an infection involving deeper layers of the skin and commonly affects the elderly as a complication of chronic venous stasis and edema in the lower extremities. Because of the depth of infection and potential for bacteremia, hospitalization for parenteral therapy is often indicated. *Staphylococcus* and group A *Streptococcus* are the predominant infecting organisms, and a synthetic penicillin active against *Staphylococcus aureus* is appropriate coverage. However, when cellulitis complicates a chronic ulcer, especially in diabetic patients, coverage should be broadened to include anaerobes and enteric gram-negative bacilli (see recommendation for treatment of complicated decubitus ulcer above).[18,27,28]

JOINT INFECTIONS

Septic arthritis is not common in elderly persons; however, 35% to 50% of all nongonococcal bacterial joint infections occur in individuals 60 years and older. Prosthetic joints are more prevalent in elderly persons, and infection may have a benign presentation. Natural joint infections are more common in elderly persons with preexisting joint disease, including osteoarthritis, rheumatoid arthritis, gout, and pseudogout. The older patient is less likely to have fever or systemic illness and often presents simply with pain and loss of movement at the affected joint. The hips and knees are most often affected. There is usually increased warmth, tenderness, an effusion on palpation, and decreased range of motion. An attempt should be made to aspirate joint fluid for cell count, culture, and Gram stain. Infected fluid will typically have WBC counts in excess of 50,000 cu/mm, with neutrophils predominating. Crystal analysis may be helpful in distinguishing gout or pseudogout from infection. However, antibiotics and hospitalization are indicated until infection can be ruled out. *Staphylococcus aureus* is the most common pathogen, and streptococci and gram-negative bacilli are not infrequent isolates. Ticarcillin-clavulanate or ampicillin-sulbactam is a reasonable antibiotic choice. Vancomycin in combination with an aminoglycoside or aztreonam is alternative therapy with penicillin allergy or when resistant *Staphylococcus aureus* is suspected (i.e., postoperative infection).[8,29–31]

BACTEREMIA AND SEPSIS

Bacteremia and sepsis can accompany and complicate any of the previously discussed infections in the elderly. In general hospital experience, 40% to 60% of blood cultures positive for bacteria occur in patients aged 60 years and older. In a study of nursing home patients with bacteremia, gram-positive cocci were isolated in 24% with an accompanying mortality of 50%. Gram-negative bacilli were isolated in 67% with a mortality of 25%. Primary sources of infection were urinary tract (56%), skin (14%), and respiratory tract (10%).[1,6,20]

40% to 60% of blood cultures positive for bacteria occur in patients 60 years and older.

TUBERCULOSIS

Tuberculosis is on the rise in the United States and is often equated with the evolving acquired immunodeficiency syndrome (AIDS) epidemic. However, 28% of newly diagnosed cases of tuberculosis are found in persons aged 65 years and older. Eighty-five to ninety percent of these cases are found in the general community. The majority of cases may involve reactivation of latent disease, which is a reflection of the impaired immune surveillance that accompanies aging. Tuberculosis in the elderly may be as vague as a general failure to thrive or may be discovered at the end of a workup of fever of unknown origin. Further complicating diagnosis is the frequency of cutaneous anergy in elderly persons, making a negative tuberculin skin test of limited value. Serologic tests for active mycobacterial disease are under development and may be available in the near future.[32,33]

28% of newly diagnosed cases of TB are found in patients 65 years and older.

VACCINATIONS

A complete evaluation of the elderly patient in the ED includes a vaccination history. All persons aged 65 years and older, nursing home patients, and patients with chronic medical conditions should receive

All persons 65 years and above should receive a yearly influenza vaccine between October and December.

yearly influenza vaccine administered between the months of October and December. Pneumococcal vaccine is also recommended for elderly persons and has been shown to prevent serious pneumococcal infection in 45% to 60% of this population. The pneumococcal vaccine is typically administered once. Repeat vaccination is recommended at 6-year intervals after splenectomy and in patients taking immunosuppressive drugs or with renal failure and nephrosis. Although rare in the United States, the majority of tetanus cases involve elderly persons and are frequently spontaneous occurrences unrelated to apparent trauma. Elderly patients are less likely to have had primary tetanus immunization or regular boosters.[2,34–36]

SUMMARY POINTS

- The presentation of acute infection in an otherwise healthy elderly individual may not differ appreciably from that of a younger adult. In such cases diagnosis and treatment of the infection should be straightforward with the proviso that elderly patients are often host to a different spectrum of pathogens and their immune systems may not mobilize as quickly or effectively as their younger counterparts.
- Elderly persons with significant concomitant illness are at special risk of infection. Their diagnoses are frequently delayed by atypical presentations and the absence of cardinal signs and symptoms of infection. Because of delays in diagnosis, compromised immunity, and a general decline in organ reserve capacity, these persons are prone to much higher morbidity and mortality from infection.
- It is important for emergency physicians to appreciate the features that distinguish infectious disease pathophysiology, microbiology, and pharmacology in the elderly population.
- It is equally important that the possibility of occult infection be considered when evaluating any elderly patient presenting with an acute functional decline.

CHAPTER AUTHOR

Rawden Evans, PhD, MD

REFERENCES

1. Jacobs LG. Geriatric emergency care: infectious disease emergencies in the geriatric population. *Geriatr Med.* 1993;9:559–575.
2. McClure C. Common infections in the elderly. *Am Fam Phys.* 1992;45:2691–2698.
3. Norman DC, Santiago DT. Infections in elderly persons: an altered clinical presentation. *Clin Geriatr Med.* 1992;8:713–719.
4. Phair JP, Hsu CS, Hsu YL. Ageing and infection. *Ciba Found Symp.* 1988;134:143–154.
5. Plewa MC. Altered host response and special infections in the elderly. *Emerg Med Clin North Am.* 1990;8:193–206.
6. Gleckman RA, Hilbert D. Afebrile bacteremia: a phenomenon in geriatric patients. *JAMA.* 1982;248:1478.
7. Keating HJ III, Klimek JJ, Levine DS, et al. Effect of aging on the clinical significance of fever in ambulatory adult patients. *J Am Geriatr Soc.*

1984;32:282.

8. Ben-Tehuda A, Weksler ME. Host resistance and the immune system. *Clin Geriatr Med.* 1992;8:701–711.

9. Chandra RK. Nutritional regulation of immunity and risk of infection in old age. *Immunology.* 1989;67:141–147.

10. Haddy RI. Aging, infections and the immune system. *J Fam Pract.* 1988;27:409–413.

11. Terpenning MS, Bradley SF. Why aging leads to increased susceptibility to infection. *Geriatrics.* 1991;46:77–80.

12. Esposito AL. Community acquired bacteremic pneumococcal pneumonia: effect of age on outcome. *Arch Intern Med.* 1984;144:945.

13. Marrie TJ, Durant H, Yates L. Community-acquired pneumonia requiring hospitalization: 5 year prospective study. *Rev Infect Dis.* 1989;11: 586–599.

14. McFadden JP, Price R, Eastwood HD, et al. Raised respiratory rate in elderly patients: a valuable physical sign. *Br Med J.* 1982;284:626.

15. Niederman MS, Fein AM. Pneumonia in the elderly. *Clin Geriatr Med.* 1986;2:241.

16. Sims RV. Bacterial pneumonia in the elderly. *Emerg Med Clin North Am.* 1990;8:207.

17. Gleckman RA, Bergman MM. Bacterial pneumonia: specific diagnosis and treatment of the elderly. *Geriatrics.* 1987;42:29.

18. Sanford JP. *Guide to antimicrobial therapy 1992.* Dallas, TX: Antimicrobial Therapy, Inc., 1992.

19. Gleckman RA. Urinary tract infection. *Clin Geriatr Med.* 1992;8:793–803.

20. Jerkeman M, Braconier JH. Bacteremic and non-bacteremic febrile urinary tract infection: a review of 168 hospital-treated patients. *Infection.* 1992;20:143–145.

21. Measley RE Jr, Levinson ME. Host defense mechanisms in the pathogenesis of urinary tract infection. *Med Clin North Am.* 1991;75:275–286.

22. Morgan MG, Brumfitt W, Hamilton-Miller JM. Treatment of urinary tract infection in the elderly. *Infection.* 1990;18:326–331.

23. Mulholland SG. Urinary tract infection. *Clin Geriatr Med.* 1990;6:43–53.

24. Nicolle LE. Urinary tract infection in the elderly: how to treat and when. *Infection.* 1992;4:261–265.

25. Abrutyn E, Boscia JA, Kaye D. The treatment of asymptomatic bacteriuria in the elderly. *J Am Geriatr Soc.* 1988;36:473–475.

26. Cantrell M, Toshikawa TT. Aging and infective endocarditis. *J Am Geriatr Soc.* 1983;31:216.

27. Kertesz D, Chow AW. Infected pressure and diabetic ulcers. *Clin Geriatr Med.* 1992;8:835–852.

28. Lipsky BA, Pecoraro RE, Larson SA. Outpatient management of uncomplicated lower extremity infections in diabetic patients. *Arch Intern Med.* 1990;150:790–797.

29. Bradley SF. Methicillin-resistant Staphylococcus aureus infection. *Clin Geriatr Med.* 1992;8:853–868.

30. Cooper C, Cawley MID. Bacterial arthritis in the elderly. *Gerontology.* 1986;32:222–227.

31. Klein RS. Joint infection, with consideration of underlying disease and sources of bacteremia in hematogenous infection. *Clin Geriatr Med.* 1988;4:375–394.

32. Dutt AK, Stead WW. Tuberculosis. *Clin Geriatr Med.* 1992;8:761–775.

33. Umeki S. Comparison of younger and elderly patients with pulmonary tuberculosis. *Respiration.* 1989;55:75–83.

34. Gareau AB, Eby RJ, McLellan BA, et al. Tetanus immunization status and immunologic response to a booster in an ED geriatric population. *Ann Intern Med.* 1990;19:1377.

35. Noah ND. Vaccination against pneumococcal infection. *Br Med J.* 1988;297:1351–1352.
36. Siddins M, Downie J, Wise K, O'Riley M. Prophylaxis against postsplenectomy pneumococcal infection. *Aust N Z Surg.* 1990;60:183–187.

SELECTED READINGS

Balsano N, Cayton CG. Surgical emergencies of the abdomen. *Emerg Med Clin North Am.* 1990;8:399–410.

Sloan RW. Principles of drug therapy in geriatric patients. *Am Fam Phys.* 1992;45:2709–2718.

Wispelwey B, Tunkel AR, Scheld WM. Bacterial meningitis in adults. *Infect Dis Clin North Am.* 1990;4:645.

Woodson CE, Sachs GA. Prevention, diagnosis, and management of infection in the nursing home. *Clin Geriatr Med.* 1988;4:507–525.

15 Cerebrovascular Accident

LEARNING OBJECTIVES

1. Explain the clinical significance of a transient ischemic attack in the elderly patient.
2. Explain the rationale for avoiding attempts to lower blood pressure in the initial stabilization phase of ED management.
3. Identify clinical features that aid in differentiating an ischemic stroke from a hemorrhagic stroke.

Cerebrovascular accident (CVA), or stroke, is the third leading cause of death among adults[1] and results in a significant amount of disability. A 33% decline in the incidence of stroke between 1975 and 1986 is attributed to improved identification and treatment of risk factors. However, despite this remarkable progress, the American Heart Association estimated in 1986 that approximately 500,000 strokes still occur annually, with a resulting 150,000 fatalities. Among survivors, sufficient disability results to account for more than 2 million individuals requiring long-term care.[1]

Until recently, the primary focus of treatment for stroke was rehabilitation; however, modalities for intervention during the acute phase are being developed and studied in the hope of providing methods to preserve damaged neural tissue, prevent ischemic tissues from forming infarcts, and reestablish blood flow to ischemic areas. Timely and appropriate intervention by the emergency health care professional remains pivotal in helping to minimize the patient's neurologic injury and improve the eventual functional outcome.

TYPES OF STROKE

Stroke is a clinically defined syndrome of rapidly developing symptoms and signs of focal or global cerebral impairment (Table 15–1) lasting longer than, or leading to death within, 24 hours and having a presumed vascular pathogenesis.[1]

ISCHEMIC STROKE

Ischemic strokes are usually caused by occlusion of a cerebral artery by an embolus or thrombus. They account for roughly 85% of acute strokes[2] and may result from primary thrombosis in an artery or occur secondary to occlusion of the vessel by an embolus. Ischemic strokes may be atherothrombotic, lacunar, or cardioembolic, or they may result from less common causes, including migraine, hematologic abnormalities (thrombocytosis, polycythemia, sickle cell anemia, leukemias), and vascular abnormalities (dissecting aortic aneurysm, arteritis). Approximately 75% occur in the territory of the middle cerebral artery, 15% in the vertebrobasilar territory, and 10% in the border zones between the territories of two major arteries.[2]

Among the most common of the cerebrovascular lesions, a *lacunar infarct* is typically a small lesion, usually less than 5 mm in diameter, that occurs in the distribution of short penetrating arterioles in the basal ganglia, pons, cerebellum, anterior limb of the internal capsule and, less commonly, the deep cerebral white matter.

A lacunar infarct may be associated with poorly controlled hypertension or diabetes and has been found in conjunction with several clinical syndromes, including contralateral pure motor or pure sensory deficit, ipsilateral ataxia with crural paresis, and dysarthria with clumsiness of the hand. The neurologic deficit may progress over 24-36 hours before stabilizing.

Lacunar infarcts are sometimes visible on computed tomography (CT) scan as small, punched-out, hypodense areas, but in other patients no abnormality is seen. Conversely, patients with symptoms suggesting lacunar infarct are sometimes found on CT scan to have severe

Table 15–1 **Useful Clinical Signs of Stroke**

Perceptual impairments	place
Sensory inattention	Cognitive impairment
Clock-face drawing	Disorientation (time, place,
Visual inattention test	person)
Tactile agnosia	Memory loss
Visual field loss	Reading, writing, arithmetic ability
Motor impairment	impaired
Gait pattern	Speech impairment
Drift of outstretched arms	Nominal dysphasia
Poor sitting balance	Dysarthria
Flat nasolabial fold	Tongue apraxia
False teeth difficult to keep in	

From Ebrahim S. *In:* Evans JG, Williams TF, Eds. *Oxford textbook of geriatric medicine.* Oxford: by permission of Oxford University Press; 1992:314.

hemisphere infarction. The prognosis for lacunar infarction is usually good, with partial or complete resolution occurring over the 4-6 weeks following the acute episode.

HEMORRHAGIC STROKE

Hemorrhagic strokes account for approximately 15% of strokes[2] and are the result either of primary intracerebral hemorrhage or hemorrhage secondary to aneurysmal rupture. The majority are intracerebral, although approximately one third are subarachnoid. Hemorrhagic transformation of an ischemic stroke occurs in up to 20% of patients, more commonly with an embolic stroke than with other types of ischemic stroke.

Intracerebral hemorrhage is frequently a complication of hypertension, although an increasing number of cases in the elderly are recognized as secondary to amyloid angiopathy.[2] Other causes include bleeding in association with berry aneurysms, mycotic aneurysms, arteriovenous malformation, arteritis, and neoplasms (particularly glioblastoma multiforme and melanoma). The frequency of deep ganglionic intracerebral hemorrhage is falling, and this has been attributed to improved control of hypertension in the community.

More superficial lobar hematomas, particularly in elderly demented patients, may be secondary to amyloid angiopathy.[2]

Hemorrhagic infarct is hemorrhage into an area of ischemic infarct, usually caused by reperfusion of damaged tissue. Anticoagulation and thrombolytic therapies often play a role.

TRANSIENT ISCHEMIC ATTACKS

Transient ischemic attack (TIA) is a transient episode of focal neurologic deficit of acute onset. It usually lasts a few minutes, although it can persist for up to 24 hours. TIAs represent a heterogeneous group of phenomena that have been attributed to embolus, thrombus, intracranial small vessel disease, and disturbance in blood viscosity. TIAs generally tend to be embolic (30%), most

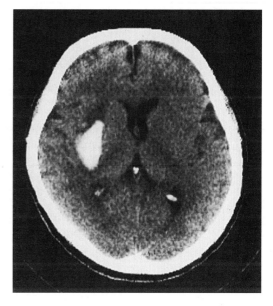

CT scan demonstrating right cerebral hemorrhage due to hypertension

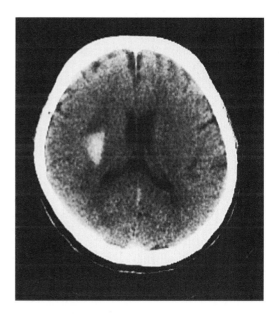

CT scan demonstrating right cerebral hemorrhage with edema

commonly from ulcerated plaques in the internal carotid arteries. The heart is the second most common site of origin, and the embolus may result from atrial fibrillation, myocardial infarction (MI) or fibrocalcific valves. The next most common cause of TIAs is atherothrombosis within large- and medium-sized arteries.

TIAs are usually mild, generally without such findings as total hemiplegia, global aphasia, or forced eye deviation. Symptoms such as light-headedness, isolated vertigo, syncope, or confusion are not focal symptoms and therefore do not, in the absence of definitive findings, constitute sufficient evidence for a diagnosis of TIA.

TIA often serves as a warning sign of stroke and may precede stroke in up to 20% of patients. However, only 33-40%[1] of patients with TIAs progress to stroke, and it is important to note that TIAs also may herald an impending MI or sudden death. Twenty-five percent of patients with TIAs actually have evidence from neuroimaging of cerebral infarction.[3]

REVERSIBLE OR RESOLVING ISCHEMIC NEUROLOGIC DEFICIT

The term reversible or resolving ischemic neurologic deficit (RIND) has been applied to syndromes similar to TIAs, although they may last 24-96 hours. RIND may leave a minor neurologic deficit or resolve completely (usually within 3 weeks). Only an estimated 9% of TIAs and RINDs are actually witnessed by physicians. In many cases, CT scan or magnetic resonance imaging (MRI) scan subsequent to resolution of symptoms has revealed an infarct. This has led to the designation of a third category, *cerebral infarct with transient symptoms (CITS)*.[4]

CRESCENDO TRANSIENT ISCHEMIC ATTACK

A crescendo TIA is a recurrent cerebral hemisphere or monocular TIA lasting several minutes to a few hours and increasing in frequency to several attacks per day.[4]

Studies of the natural history of TIAs have revealed a 4-10 times greater incidence of stroke in patients suffering TIAs than in the general population.[4] The incidence of stroke among patients who have experienced a TIA is 5%–6% per year, with the highest risk being in the first month after the initial TIA.[4]

TIAs precede stroke in up to 20% of patients; however, only 1/3 of patients with TIAs go on to stroke. TIAs also may herald an impending myocardial infarction or sudden death.

COMPLETED STROKE

Completed stroke is a stable and permanent neurologic deficit, usually consisting of weakness or paralysis. It may be sudden in onset or evolve to completion. It usually is lateralized; it results in permanent loss of neurologic function and is caused by a cerebrovascular ischemic or hemorrhagic event.

STROKE IN EVOLUTION

Stroke in evolution is the sudden onset of a neurologic deficit with progression over hours to days. It implies a dynamic process of neuronal ischemia and infarction resulting from the initial insult or its complications. Progressive stroke, or stroke in evolution, accounts for 15%–40% of all thromboembolic stroke syndromes.[4] Its diagnosis is suggested by a progressive or stuttering course over several hours, which is thought to be secondary to an enlarging intraarterial thrombus that can cause further obstruction or propagate to occlude collateral channels.

RISK FACTORS

Risk factors can be divided into treatable and nontreatable causes. Treatable causes include TIAs, hypertension, cigarette smoking, diabetes mellitus, hyperlipidemia, obesity, heart disease, and oral contraceptive use. Non-treatable causes include genetic predisposition and rising age, with the incidence of stroke more than doubling in each successive decade after 55 years of age.[1] Men suffer a 30% higher incidence of stroke than women.[1]

Hypertension is the primary risk factor for stroke of all types; however, any individual with evidence of impaired cardiac function is considered at significant risk for stroke even if blood pressure is normal. Such impairments may include coronary artery disease, congestive heart failure, atrial fibrillation, or cardiac enlargement.

PRE-HOSPITAL CONSIDERATIONS

Most patients brought to the ED by emergency transport personnel have completed strokes, and important assessments and interventions can be implemented during transport. The history is directed primarily toward obtaining the following information: nature of symptoms, time of onset and duration; risk factor profile; and medication history, including any known allergies. Physical assessments during transport should include airway status and adequacy of ventilation; vital signs and general appearance; level of consciousness, as measured by the Glasgow Coma Scale (GCS); pupil size, equality, and reaction to light; and any abnormal responses to stimuli such as paralysis, weakness, or posturing.

Concurrent with the assessment, certain interventions can be applied generally or in accordance with local protocol. Priorities include supplemental oxygen by nasal cannula or mask (4-6 L/min as tolerated); intravenous (IV) access; cardiac monitoring (up to 30% of patients with a new neurologic insult will have an abnormal cardiac rhythm); and dysrhythmia management by protocol or physician order.

INITIAL EMERGENCY DEPARTMENT ASSESSMENT AND STABILIZATION

The clinical significance of acute cerebral ischemia extends beyond the initial insult to include the pathophysiologic sequelae of reduced blood flow and supply of nutrients. Although precise mechanisms are not completely understood, the biochemical changes that result from energy deprivation consist of tissue acidosis, neurotransmitter dysfunction, abnormalities of cal-

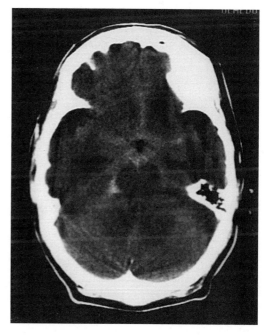

CT scan demonstrating subarachnoid bleed

cium transport, free radical production, cerebral edema, and microcirculatory obstruction.[3] The extent of damage and the potential for preservation of threatened neuronal tissue vary according to the depth and duration of the ischemic insult, the effectiveness of collateral circulation, and the secondary effects of metabolic derangements and cerebral edema.[3] Because of the complexity of this "ischemic cascade"[3] it is unlikely that any one modality will emerge for definitive acute management, and current priorities are to maintain oxygen and glucose supply[5] while conducting a thorough assessment and diagnostic evaluation.

Goals of the ED history and physical examination are as follows:

1. To differentiate a cerebrovascular occlusion from other causes of stroke
2. To establish the initial extent of the neurologic deficit
3. To anticipate and identify complications

The initial examination is repeated serially to detect any changing neurologic signs and symptoms.

On presentation to the ED any patient in whom acute cerebrovascular disease is suspected is brought immediately to a monitored bed in the ED, and the patient's current status is quickly reassessed. Parameters include the ABCs (airway, breathing, and circulation), level of consciousness, color and general appearance, patency of the airway and adequacy of ventilation, blood pressure, and adequacy of peripheral perfusion (Figure 15–1).

Key information to obtain about the patient's symptoms includes the following:

1. Exact onset, duration, and progression of symptoms
2. Nature of symptoms, for example, what the patient cannot do now that he or she could do before
3. Associated symptoms
4. History of similar symptoms and functional baseline

Every effort is made to determine the patient's activity at the onset of symptoms, the pattern of progression (e.g., maximum deficit immediately after onset, progressive course, or "stuttering" course), and symptoms accompanying the event (e.g., headache, loss of consciousness, palpitations, vomiting).

Essential data are confirmed with information from the paramedics or family members, and the patient is undressed, allowing full exposure for ongoing assessments. Cardiac monitoring and supplemental oxygen are continued, and the patency of the IV line is confirmed.

Attend to the ABCs and monitor oxygen with pulse oximetry if possible. A finger-stick glucose should be obtained promptly. Hypoglycemia may be treated (one ampule of D50 or 25-50 ml of 50% glucose by IV push); hyperglycemia may worsen the stroke patient's condition by producing lactic acidosis. If the patient does not already have an IV line, gain IV access. If the patient is malnourished or an alcoholic, administer thiamine (50-100 mg by IV line) before IV glucose. Naloxone (0.4-2.0 mg by IV push) can be given to patients with depressed consciousness who are suspected of narcotic overdose.

Emergency Department Management of CVA

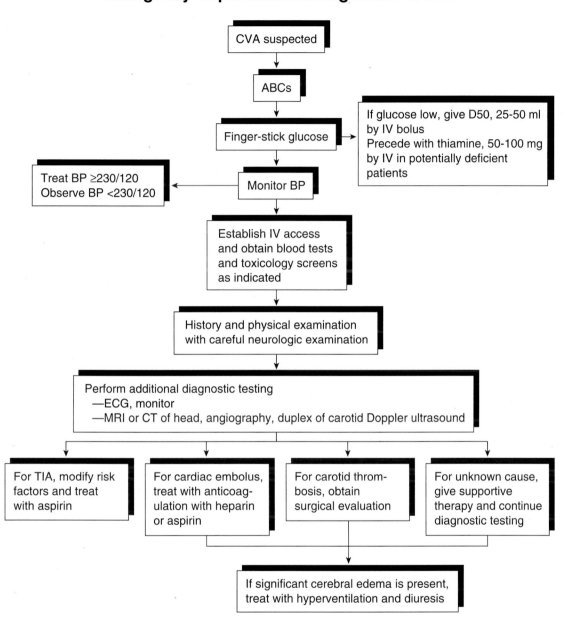

FIGURE 15–1

Evidence of cardiac or atherosclerotic vascular disease is investigated, and the presence of increased intracranial pressure or impending herniation syndrome is determined. Neurologic and functional baselines are established for future comparisons, and potential complications, including the following, are anticipated:

1. *Airway compromise.* If the stroke victim is having respiratory difficulties or cannot protect the airway, nasotracheal or endotracheal in-

tubation should be accomplished. Also, if respiratory rate suddenly slows, the potential for impending herniation must be considered.

2. *Dysrhythmias* can be a cause of stroke and should be treated if related to symptoms.

3. *Hypertension* is often seen in patients presenting with acute cerebrovascular disease. In acute situations, hypertension may be physiologic, allowing adequate cerebral perfusion during periods of increased intracranial pressure. Acutely lowering the blood pressure could result in failure of perfusion of a stenotic or thrombosed cerebral vessel and extension of the primary ischemic zone or creation of new ischemic territories. Therefore blood pressure should be lowered only to relieve excess burden caused by cardiac ischemia and insufficiency or by aortic dissection and acute renal insufficiency. Severe hypertension (systolic above 180-230 mm Hg or diastolic above 130-140 mm Hg), or hypertensive encephalopathy is treated with agents that relax smooth muscle in peripheral arterioles and reduce peripheral vascular resistance, such as nitroprusside. The diastolic pressure is gradually reduced to approximately 110 mm Hg while the patient is closely monitored. Do not aim for a diastolic pressure lower than 100 mm Hg, because this may result in overshoot and hypotension, again, posing a risk to collateral circulation and the potential for extension of the ischemic zone.

4. *Cerebral edema or herniation syndrome.* Acute herniation is uncommon in the early hours of a CVA, because it results from the cumulative mass effect of the initial insult and brain edema. The goal of management is to reduce intracranial pressure, and interventions include intubation and hyperventilation, elevation of the head of the bed, fluid restriction, and use of osmotic diuretics, such as mannitol or glycerol.

DIFFERENTIAL DIAGNOSIS

STROKE OR NON-CEREBROVASCULAR EVENT

1. *Subdural and epidural hematoma.* Both forms may manifest with lateralizing signs. Subdural hematoma is more likely than epidural hematoma to be confused with stroke.

2. *Postictal state with Todd's paralysis.* This condition is preceded by a history or physical findings consistent with seizure; it usually lasts 2-3 hours and has a rapidly improving neurologic pattern.

3. *Occult neoplasm.* Rarely, the onset is acute if a hemorrhage occurs within the tumor. More often there is an insidious onset associated with systemic symptoms, such as anorexia and weight loss.

4. *Drug toxicity.* Although lateralizing deficits are rare, stroke can be caused by abuse of narcotics or sedative/hypnotics. This diagnosis is usually supported by a characteristic toxidrome. It can also be a complication of drug abuse, because IV drug use increases the potential for brain abscess, septic emboli, and thrombotic stroke.

5. *Metabolic encephalopathy.* Stroke syndromes rarely occur in patients with hypoxia, hypoglycemia, or nonketotic hyperosmolar coma. Data gathering usually gives clues to these systemic diseases.

6. *Central nervous system (CNS) infections.* Meningitis, encephalitis, and brain abscess rarely present as a stroke. Other signs of infection, such as fever, elevated white blood cell (WBC) count, immunosuppression, meningismus, headache, or a prodromal history, may be present.
7. *TIA.* TIAs have their own differential signs, including focal seizures, migraine aura, syncope, and dysrhythmias.

INFARCT OR HEMORRHAGE

If the patient's presentation and current status are consistent with stroke, the differentiation of infarction from hemorrhagic stroke is essential for immediate management. Table 15–2 outlines the differential diagnosis based on characteristics of onset and clinical presentation.

However, it is important to note that a *clinical* differentiation of hemorrhage and infarction is not easily made, especially in the early acute phase. Table 15–3 lists possible errors in the diagnosis of stroke. Signs usually thought to be more common in cerebral hemorrhage are initial loss of consciousness, headache, vomiting, neck stiffness, and blood-stained cerebrospinal fluid (CSF). Signs of meningeal irritation only occur if blood leaks into the subarachnoid space, so small hemorrhages may be clinically indistinguishable from thromboses.[1] The site of the lesion generally determines the nature of signs and symptoms. Although hemisphere lesions are most common, and clinicians are familiar with speech and perceptual impairments that may occur in conjunction with hemiplegia, many patients with hemisphere damage also

Table 15–3 **Causes of Error in Diagnosis of Stroke**

False-negative diagnoses	False-positive diagnoses
Non-specific presentations	Mass lesions
Immobility	Primary tumors
Falls	Metastases
Incontinence of urine	Subdural hematoma
Social breakdown	Abscess
Impaired consciousness	Infection
Confusional states	Subacute bacterial endocarditis
Fractures	Meningitis
Neck of femur	Neurosyphilis
Humerus	Metabolic disturbances
After general anesthetic	Hypoglycemia
Previous stroke	Hyperosmolar states
Acute intoxication	Hyponatremia/hypernatremia
Alcohol	Previous stroke
Neuroleptics	Grand mal seizure
	Intercurrent illness
	Acute hypotension
	Cranial arteritis
	Severe anemia

From Ebrahim S. Diagnosis. *In:* Evans JG, Williams TF, Eds. *Oxford textbook of geriatric medicine.* Oxford: by permission of Oxford University Press; 1992:314.

Table 15-2 Stroke Symptoms—Differential Diagnosis*

	Presentation	Associated Symptoms	Risk Factors	Physical Examination	Useful Tests	Additional Aspects
TIA	Sudden onset of symptoms (vision or speech change, focal weakness) Short duration—minutes to hours (maximum 24 hr)	Numbness/sensory loss Vertigo (basilar TIA) Speech change (dysarthria, aphasia) Gait change—ataxia Vision change (diplopia, field cut, monocular or bilateral vision loss)	Age Male sex Smoking ASCVD Hyperlipidemia Heart disease Hypercoagulable states	Usually normal unless attack still in progress Funduscopic changes Cardiac examination (murmur) Carotid bruits	Good HX/PE Non-invasive carotid evaluation Carotid arteriogram	20-60% of TIA patients have a stroke within 2–5 yr
Stroke in evolution (progressive stroke)	Sudden onset of symptoms Duration > 24 hr Progressive neurologic signs and symptoms	Same as above Nausea and vomiting on occasion	Same as above	Hypertension/bradycardia typical Possible dysrhythmia Neurologic examination findings referable to involved area Funduscopic, carotid, and cardiac changes as above	Baseline laboratory studies CT scan of head Cerebral angiography	Seen in approximately 15–25% of stroke patients
Completed stroke	Sudden onset of symptoms Duration—permanent No progression or regression of symptoms	Same as above	Same as above	Same as above	Same as above	If thrombotic, may commonly develop during sleep with symptoms perceived on awakening in the morning resulting from low flow through stenotic area

Embolic	Sudden onset of symptoms Duration > 24 hr	Same as above	Same, especially heart disease, e.g., atrial fibrillation and cardiac mural thrombus	Same—emphasis on cardiac examination	Same as above	May occur at any time; often follows exertion Often responsible for hemorrhagic infarction; friable clot dissolves with perfusion through ischemic vessels May be acutely associated with seizures in up to 20% of patients
Subarachnoid hemorrhage	Sudden onset of symptoms Severe headache, syncope, and nuchal pain Focal neurologic signs, including cranial nerves	Nausea and vomiting Obtundation, sometimes comatose	None (aneurysms are congenital)	Hypertension/bradycardia Nuchal tenderness and rigidity to movement Fundi-subhyaloid hemorrhage or papilledema Dilated pupil if posterior communicating artery aneurysm Neurologic examination non-focal	Same as above Lumbar puncture considered if CT scan negative and if diagnosis still suspected	One third from anterior communicating artery aneurysms One fourth from middle carotid artery aneurysms One fifth from posterior communicating artery aneurysms
Intracerebral hemorrhage	Sudden onset of symptoms (dense hemiplegia, hemianesthesia, field cut, obtundation) Duration > 24 hr, usually permanent	Usually comatose Rapid progression to loss of consciousness Reticular activating system impairment	Hypertension (brain stem and basal ganglia) Anticoagulant therapy (frontal, parietal, temporal, and occipital lobes)	Usually comatose Cranial nerve findings, e.g., cranial nerve III palsy Hemiparesis/hemisensory loss, pinpoint pupils (pontine or cerebellar) Posturing Ataxia, vertigo, vomiting (cerebellar) Upgoing Babinski's sign	Same as above except lumbar puncture not done	Occurs in approximately 10–20% of stroke patients

*ASCVD, Atherosclerotic cerebrovascular disease; HX/PE, history and physical examination.

From Binder LS. Stroke. In: Hamilton G. Sanders AB, Strange GR, Trott AT eds. Emergency Medicine: An Approach to Clinical Problem Solving 1st ed. W.B. Saunders Co. Philadelphia, PA. 1991:884–885

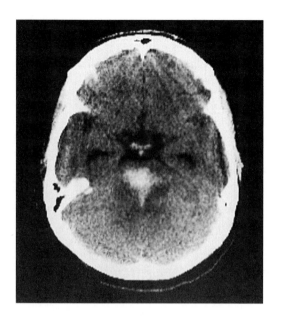

CT scan demonstrating pontine hemorrhage

may have impairment of lower cranial nerve functions, in particular swallowing.[1]

Generally speaking, the major criteria in making a diagnosis of embolic stroke are that the patient has a potential cardioembolic source and demonstrates a non-lacunar stroke syndrome (i.e., a cortical finding) and that the patient has no evidence of primary cerebrovascular disease.[4] Previous studies have tended to show that early coagulation reduces the chance of reembolus to about one third of the natural rate.[4] However, early hemorrhagic transformation of an infarct and long-term complications of anticoagulation continue to remain significant concerns. Once a decision in favor of anticoagulation has been made, the goal should be to achieve a partial thromboplastin time (PTT) of 1.5 times the control value.[4]

The emergency physician considers which manner of progression and overall pattern best fit the individual's clinical picture. The following questions can assist in this process:

1. Are the neurologic examination results normal or abnormal at this time? If the examination results have returned to normal, the diagnosis is most consistent with a TIA.
2. Is the clinical course progressive, constant, or fluctuating?
3. Are there potential sources of cerebral emboli? Most of these sources are cardiac in nature, and the patient should be evaluated for mural thrombus, atrial fibrillation, or valvular heart disease.
4. Most important, the possibility of intracranial hemorrhage must be considered. Factors supporting this diagnosis are a history of hypertension, anticoagulation therapy, or headache and findings of altered mental status, nuchal rigidity, or subhyaloid hemorrhage.

CAUSE AND SITE OF INSULT

Findings from the physical examination may help in localizing the site of the insult and in determining the underlying cause. The syndromes most commonly seen in the ED are listed below:

1. *Internal carotid syndrome.* This is a combination of hemiparesis, hemisensory deficit, aphasia, and hemianopsia.
2. *Middle cerebral artery syndrome.* Contralateral hemiparesis or hemiplegia, contralateral impairment of sensation, dysarthria, and expressive or receptive aphasia comprise this syndrome. The face and arm are more commonly affected than the leg.
3. *Anterior cerebral artery syndrome.* Contralateral lower extremity paresis or paralysis, contralateral lower extremity sensory defect, urinary incontinence, and abnormalities in behavior are the main features of this syndrome.

4. *Vertebrobasilar syndrome.* This is a combination of hemiparesis or quadriparesis, dysarthria, dysphagia, impaired sensation, vertigo, nausea, vomiting, nystagmus, diplopia, and internuclear ophthalmoplegia.
5. *Lateral medullary (Wallenberg's) syndrome.* Wallenberg's syndrome comprises vertigo, nausea, vomiting, nystagmus, dysphagia, ataxia, ipsilateral Horner's syndrome, and impaired sensation to the face ipsilaterally and contralaterally in the body.
6. *Lacunar infarct syndrome.* Patients are usually hypertensive and manifest isolated neurologic deficits. Lesions in the internal capsule produce pure motor hemiparesis; thalamic lesions cause contralateral sensory loss; and pontine infarcts produce ataxic hemiparesis.

DIAGNOSTIC TESTS

To reduce diagnostic error, more investigations are often needed for older patients than for younger patients, in part because of the more non-specific presentation of disease and because histories are often incomplete at the time of the acute event.

An electrocardiogram (ECG) is obtained immediately to assess the patient for an acute MI. Laboratory tests are generally ordered during the initial assessment. These include complete blood count (CBC), prothrombin time (PT), partial thromboplastin time (PTT), INR, and platelets to assess clotting function. Electrolytes, glucose, and a renal battery are often useful. Arterial blood gases may be helpful if there is suspicion of hypoxia or systemic acidosis.

Imaging studies should be considered to rule out lesions that may mimic stroke. A head CT scan is useful for ruling out hemorrhage; however, a normal CT scan of the head does not rule out an infarct. This is especially evident if the infarct is small, if it is located in the brain stem, or if the scan is obtained within 24 hours of a stroke. An MRI scan of the head is more sensitive than a CT scan for detection of most strokes (e.g., acute strokes, lacunar strokes, or strokes located in the brain stem), but the technology is not immediately available in most EDs at all times.

A normal CT scan of the head does not rule out an infarct, especially if the infarct is small, if it is located in the brainstem, or if the scan is obtained within 24 hours of a stroke.

ED MANAGEMENT

Management of the patient with stroke consists of appropriate supportive care. Airway control is always the first priority, together with maintenance of ventilation. Adequate cardiac output is essential, because there is loss of autoregulation of cerebral blood flow in ischemia areas, and hypotension and low cardiac output states can result in extension of the ischemic zone. As stated earlier in this chapter, elevated blood pressure should be treated only if an intracerebral hemorrhage is documented or if the pressure is extremely high.

The guidelines listed below provide an overview of current acute management strategies.

1. *Transient ischemic attack.* No acute intervention is needed. Acute anticoagulation therapy with either heparin or sodium warfarin is controversial and generally is not recommended by most authori-

Do not aim for a diastolic pressure lower than 100 mmHg because this may actually result in overshoot and hypotension affecting the collateral circulation.

ties. Both medications have unfavorable risk-benefit ratios. A regimen of daily aspirin is often started.

Assessment of the patient's carotid arteries may be important, although only 20%-30% of patients with TIAs will have significant disease. Carotid Doppler ultrasound can be ordered, followed by consult with a neurologist, neurosurgeon or primary care physician to determine further treatment. Current indications for carotid endarterectomy are symptomatic internal carotid artery stenosis involving 70%-99% of the arterial diameter.[3,5]

2. *Stroke in evolution.* Intravenous anticoagulant therapy is instituted following CT scanning if there is no evidence of bleeding.

3. *Completed thrombotic stroke.* Blood pressure is monitored, and the patient is observed for signs of developing cerebral edema. Because the deficit is complete, there is no need for anticoagulation.

4. *Embolic stroke.* Anticoagulation is indicated to promote mural thrombus resolution, prevent recurrences, and inhibit propagation of cerebral thromboemboli. A CT scan is performed to rule out hemorrhagic infarct before anticoagulation therapy is given. This therapy may be deferred if the stroke is massive.

5. *Subarachnoid hemorrhage.* Priorities include placing the patient in a dark, quiet room to reduce CNS stimulation and the potential for vasospasm, maintaining adequate arterial blood pressure, and treating cerebral edema appropriately. Early neurosurgical consultation is important. Intracranial pressure monitoring may be indicated.

6. *Intracerebral hemorrhage.* The mass effect caused by the intracerebral hematoma and associated cerebral edema is treated with selected use of hyperventilation, diuretics, and positional maneuvers. Acute neurosurgical intervention for evacuation of the hematoma is controversial.

DISPOSITION PLAN

Because of the risk of significant complications, including pulmonary embolus, aspiration pneumonia, myocardial infarction, recurrent stroke, and sudden death, patients diagnosed with acute stroke should be admitted for diagnostic evaluation, continued observation and early treatment. Patients should be monitored with serial neurologic examinations to detect further neurologic deterioration or improvement, and early institution of in-hospital rehabilitation should be implemented.

Disposition of the patient with a TIA is more controversial. Benefit may be gained by hospital admission to identify the source of an ischemic episode, but admitting every patient with a TIA would be not only costly and but also is not always conclusive. Patients who are sent home should be monitored closely by family members and the primary care physician for recurrence or further deterioration.

SUMMARY POINTS

- Cerebrovascular accident is an inclusive term representing several disorders. It is important to recognize the different presentations and etiologies of stroke to implement rapid evaluation and appropriate interventions.

- Do not lower blood pressure rapidly. An infarct may be extended, or the patient may suffer cardiovascular compromise.
- Do not administer intravenous glucose before thiamine in a potentially thiamine-deficient patient.
- Anticoagulation and thrombolytic therapy may cause hemorrhage and extend infarct size.
- A negative CT scan does not rule out stroke within the first 24 hours.
- Always check the glucose after assessing the ABCs.
- Cerebral edema peaks 2-3 days after a stroke and may cause hemorrhage or extension of the infarction.

CHAPTER AUTHORS

Lidia Pousada, MD, FACP
Darrin M. Fryer, MD

REFERENCES

1. Wolf PA, Cupples LA. Epidemiology of stroke. *In:* Evans JG, Williams TF, Eds. *Oxford textbook of geriatric medicine.* Oxford: Oxford University Press; 1992:304–313.
2. Hyman NM. Pathology of stroke. *In:* Evans JG, Williams TF, Eds. *Oxford textbook of geriatric medicine.* Oxford: Oxford University Press; 1992:297–303.
3. Sila CA. Prophylaxis and treatment of stroke: the state of the art in 1993. *Drugs.* 1993;45(3):329–337.
4. Barnaby W. Stroke intervention. *Emerg Med Clin North Am.* 1990;8(2):267–280.
5. Rose FC. Care of the acute stroke patient. *In:* Evans JG, Williams TF, Eds. *Oxford textbook of geriatric medicine.* Oxford: Oxford University Press; 1992:318–321.

SELECTED READINGS

Alberts MJ. Diagnosis of acute stroke: how to relate presentation to vascular anatomy. *Postgrad Med.* 1989;86(8):95–102.
Biller J, Love BB. Controversies in the management of cerebrovascular disease in older patients. *Geriatrics.* 1992;47(12):47–51.
Brass LM, Fayad PB, Levine SR. Transient ischemic attacks in the elderly: diagnosis and treatment. *Geriatrics.* 1993;47(5):36–50.
Bruno A. Ischemia stroke, part 1: early accurate diagnosis. *Geriatrics.* 1993;48(3):26–54.
Dyken ML. Controversies in stroke: past and present. The Willis Lecture. *Stroke.* 1993;24(8):1251–1258.
Ebrahim S. Diagnosis. *In:* Evans JG, Williams TF, Eds. *Oxford textbook of geriatric medicine.* Oxford: Oxford University Press; 1992:313–318.
Flegel KM, Hutchinson TA, Groome PA, Tousignant P. Factors relevant to preventing embolic stroke in patients with non-rheumatic atrial fibrillation. *J Clin Epidemiol.* 1991;44(6):551–560.
Koller RI. Prevention of recurrent ischemic stroke. *Postgrad Med.* 1991;90(8):81–84, 89–91, 96.
Young G. Cerebrovascular disease. *In:* Bosker G, Schwartz GR, Jones JS, et al, Eds. *Geriatric emergency medicine.* St. Louis: Mosby–Year Book; 1991:127–144.

16 *Dizziness*

LEARNING OBJECTIVES

1. Identify and define five types of dizziness.
2. Identify key characteristics of dizziness to be determined from the patient's description of symptoms.
3. Demonstrate key elements of the neurologic examination, and explain their role in the evaluation of dizziness.
4. Apply knowledge of characteristic presentations to establish an appropriate differential diagnosis in the ED setting.

The vague complaint of dizziness is a frequently encountered and often challenging ED presentation. Sorting through a wide-ranging differential diagnosis requires well-honed clinical skills. A correct diagnosis will result from a careful history, a directed physical examination, and a clear understanding of the subtleties of this perplexing complaint with particular attention to those conditions seen most commonly in elderly persons.

Dizziness is a particularly common complaint in the elderly. One study revealed 47% of men and 61% of women older than age 70 experience dizziness.[1] It is the most common presenting complaint in patients over age 75.[2] Dizziness predisposes the elderly to falls and fractures, and 20% of all elderly people living at home fall each year. Falls contribute to two thirds of all accidental deaths in the elderly population, and only one half of elderly fall victims who are hospitalized are still alive one year later[1] (see Chapter 10.).

The thorough evaluation of dizziness in the elderly patient is often rewarding, because the older patient is more likely than a younger in-

One study revealed that 47% of men and 61% of women over age 70 experience dizziness.

dividual to be manifesting an early symptom of a potentially treatable or preventable disorder. Some patients will need emergent management; others require referral to appropriate primary care providers; and yet others need only gentle reassurance that their condition is benign and self-limited.

DEFINITIONS

Numerous authors over the past 30 years have attempted to devise a logical framework from which to examine the complaint of dizziness. The landmark article by Drachman and Hart in 1972 identified four basic types of dizziness[3]:

1. *Vertigo*: an illusion of motion or rotation of the environment or of the body
2. *Pre-syncope*: a sensation of impending faint or loss of consciousness
3. *Disequilibrium*: an unsteadiness, an imbalance of gait, the feeling of an imminent fall
4. *Light-headedness*: a non-specific complaint, occasionally described as internal spinning or whirling within the head or a floating, swaying, giddy feeling

An additional category has relevance to the ED:

5. *Post-traumatic (acute or remote) dizziness*

Keeping these five categories in mind will facilitate the examiner's review of the differential diagnosis. The distinctions between these groupings, however, are not absolute, and often a particular lesion will fit into more than one category.

INITIAL EMERGENCY DEPARTMENT ASSESSMENT

Dizziness is a general colloquial term an ill patient may use to describe a variety of sensations. Initial ED assessment focuses on ruling out the most serious and potentially life-threatening causes. These include cardiac pathologic conditions, acute blood loss, and central neurologic lesions. If the patient sustained trauma, it must be clarified whether the dizziness was the cause or the result of trauma. A focused history and physical examination, orthostatic vital signs, hematocrit, electrocardiogram (ECG), and altered mental status reversal (from naloxone, [Narcan], thiamine, dextrose) may be critical. The majority of cases of dizziness, however, are not acutely life threatening, and a more structured review may be subsequently initiated.

HISTORY

The examiner initiates the interview with the intent of better understanding the patient's concept of dizziness. One should first ask the patient to describe his or her complaint without using the term *dizziness*. Key historical questions include the following:

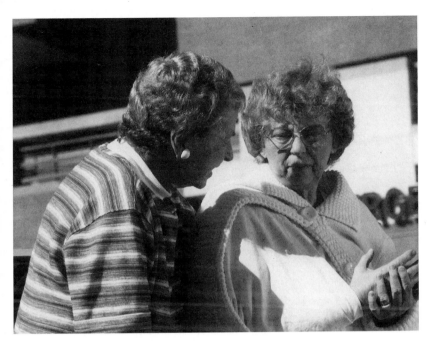

If the patient sustained trauma, it must be clarified whether the dizziness was the cause or the result of trauma.

- Has there been a history of trauma?
- Is there a rotational component (i.e., sense that the environment is spinning or the patient is spinning within the environment)?
- Is the dizziness affected by head or body position or change of position?
- Is the dizziness continuous or episodic?
- Was the onset of dizziness abrupt or gradual?
- Have any other neurologic changes been noticed, such as headaches, hearing loss, tinnitus, slurred speech, visual disturbances, ataxia, motor weakness, sensory loss, or peripheral paresthesias?
- Does the patient usually rely on a cane, a hearing aid, or glasses?
- What medications is the patient currently using (including alcohol)?
- Does the patient have cardiovascular risk factors?
- Is there a history of chest discomfort, palpitations, worsening dyspnea on exertion, peptic ulcer disease, melena, or diabetes mellitus?
- Has the patient noted increased psychologic stressors, anxiety, or depression?

PHYSICAL EXAMINATION

In addition to the routine assessment of the elderly patient, including mental status examination (see Chapters 7 and 8) and functional assessment (see Chapter 9), the physical examination will focus on specific causes of dizziness.

General

Estimate general severity of symptoms, and review vital signs. Is the patient hyperventilating? Is there an orthostatic change in blood pressure

The older patient is more likely than younger individuals to be manifesting an early symptom of a potentially treatable or preventable disorder.

and pulse? Is there a blood pressure difference between arms (suggests aortic dissection or subclavian steal syndrome)?

Head

Inspect and palpate for signs of trauma. Mild, often forgotten head injuries may cause a subdural hematoma in elderly persons.

Eyes

An exacting eye examination is vital in the dizzy elderly patient. Visual acuity should be checked. Are cataracts present? Visual deficits are often correctable and may contribute to multisensory deficit syndrome.

A careful extraocular motor examination is important, because abnormalities may be quite subtle and when present can often give clues to the cause of dizziness. Close examination of the eyes, aided by keeping the patient's lids open during down gaze, may demonstrate a variety of nystagmoid movements. Although horizontal nystagmus on lateral gaze is usually benign, asymmetric findings on vertical gaze nystagmus are never normal and suggest brain stem disease. After the full range of eye movements has been examined, saccadic movements should be tested. The patient performs horizontal, back-and-forth saccades while the examiner looks at the bridge of the nose (permitting the study of conjugate eye movements). If either eye is slow in adduction, the patient has an internuclear ophthalmoplegia (INO). An INO is significant because it indicates a midline pontine lesion. An INO is suggestive of vascular infarction in the elderly patient and of multiple sclerosis in the younger patient. Other important eye findings include visual field testing and ophthalmoscopic examination looking for absent venous pulsations or papilledema, both signs of increased intracranial pressure.

Ears

Check hearing. If the patient is able to hear a faint whisper with the opposite ear covered or masked, hearing is probably normal. If hearing is abnormal, Weber and Rinne testing may help distinguish sensorineural from conductive deficits. Look for middle ear pathologic findings, cerumen impaction, or infection.

Throat

Check palatal movement, gag reflex, and clarity of speech, any of which may be abnormal with lower brain stem lesions.

Neck

Check for the presence of bruits or thyroid enlargement. Also keep in mind that patients with

A blood pressure difference between arms may suggest aortic dissection or subclavian steal syndrome.

cervical spondylosis may develop spinal compression leading to gait instability and dizziness.

Cardiac and pulmonary systems

Arrhythmias and pump failure may lead to pre-syncopal symptoms.

Rectal examination

A rectal examination and a stool Hemoccult test are done.

Neurologic Examination

The elderly patient with dizziness deserves a thorough neurologic examination with special attention to the cranial nerves, cerebellum, and gait. A detailed cranial nerve examination may reveal subtle signs of stroke (facial palsy, palatal weakness) or evidence of increasing intracranial pressure (pupillary dilation or lateral abducens palsy) or of an acoustic neuroma expanding in the cerebellopontine angle (loss of corneal reflex).

The cerebellar examination is a key part of the neurologic exam. Cerebellar lesions produce lack of coordination, hypotonia, and ocular motor abnormalities. Incoordination may be manifested by abnormal finger-to-nose examination. The patient repetitively reaches out to touch the examiner's finger and then returns to the nose. The patient may overshoot the target (hypermetria). The patient may also develop a tremor in the horizontal plane that increases in amplitude as the finger approaches the target (intention tremor). The patient may have a resting tremor of the head (titubation) or have difficulty with rapidly alternating movements (dysdiadochokinesis). With the patient sitting, have the arm gently but rapidly come down from midchest level to strike the distal thigh. The patient should alternate dorsum of hand with palm each time. One author recommends the patient tap out a tune with the fingers. Arrythmokinesis (i.e., alterations in rhythmic timing and clumsiness) may be evident.[4]

Hypotonia may be apparent with acute cerebellar lesions. Passively flex and extend the patient's wrist and elbows to assess tone. Have the patient's forearms rest on a table with hands hanging over the edge. Hypotonia will result in the ipsilateral hand sagging lower than its normal counterpart. A dramatic, albeit potentially dangerous, test for hypotonia involves asking the patient to pull the fist toward the face with the examiner resisting this movement. If the examiner releases the patient's fist, the hypotonic triceps muscle may not be able to react quickly and the face may be struck. Naturally, the examiner should take precautions to block this potentially damaging lack of a check reflex. Less dramatically, have the patient stretch out the arms with eyes closed. The examiner taps on the wrists. The hypotonic arm will swing through a wider than normal arc.

Eye movements may also be impaired in cerebellar disease. Analogous to limb movement abnormalities, extraocular motor activity is also incoordinated and tremulous. Have the patient saccade back and forth between two visual points. This voluntary gaze is accomplished with jerky movements that may overshoot the intended visual target (saccadic dysmetria). The ill patient also may be unable to maintain a steady point of lateral gaze and thus make continuous small adjusting saccades to maintain visual contact (gaze-paretic nystagmus).

Finally, the patient's gait may be analyzed by having the patient walk across the room. Cerebellar ataxia may be striking. The patient demonstrates a wide-based stance, taking small, irregular steps and lurching unsteadily toward the affected hemisphere. Limbs and trunk lack coordination as described earlier. Elderly patients with presbyastasis (multisensory deficit dizziness syndrome) may be unsure and hesitant in gait. These patients improve markedly with the addition of a cane or the minimal reassurance of an ambulation assistant.

Patients with severe peripheral neuropathy have difficulty walking, since the walking surface cannot be fully sensed. These patients often lean forward, watching and directing their feet in motion.

Patients with vertigo of peripheral origin may have extreme difficulty walking. They may become nauseated and vomit and resist attempts to walk. They may veer sharply to one side but, as opposed to cerebellar ataxia, do not demonstrate ataxia or clumsiness within individual limb or trunk movements.

SPECIAL PHYSICAL EXAMINATION TESTS

The *Barany maneuver* (Figure 16–1) is a test for positional vertigo and nystagmus. If nystagmus is induced it should be observed closely. Key characteristics to record include the following:

- Direction (named by fast component)
- Lag time (latency) before onset
- Duration: greater or less than 1 minute
- Fatigability on repeated testing

The Barany maneuver should be avoided in cases of suspected vertebrobasilar insufficiency, since an atheromatous plaque may be dislodged.

For the *hyperventilation challenge* the patient is asked to hyperventilate for 3 minutes. Are symptoms reproducible?

Carotid sinus stimulation (10 seconds) may be used in patients without bruits and without signs of new central nervous system (CNS) lesions. This vagal maneuver, which may cause a profound depression of pulse rate, will direct the examiner to a possible cardiac source of dizziness if symptoms are reproduced.

The *fistula test* is used to evaluate post-traumatic dizziness. Air is introduced into the ear canal with the otoscope insufflator. A positive test resulting in nystagmus and vertigo indicates the presence of a perilymphatic fistula.

DIFFERENTIAL DIAGNOSIS

The complaint of dizziness comprises a vast array of diagnostic possibilities (Table 16-1). The following discussion elaborates on the elements of an algorithmic approach outlined in Figure 16–2 and defined earlier.

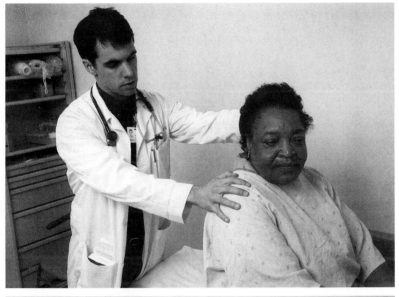

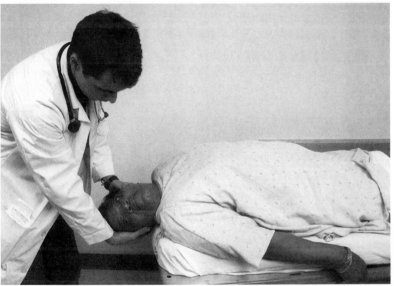

FIGURE 16–1 Barany Maneuver. **A.** The patient is seated on the examination table with head turned 45 degrees to one side. **B.** The patient is then assisted to quickly assume (less than 2 seconds) the supine position with head hanging 30 degrees below the plane of the table.

VERTIGO

Initial evaluation is directed at differentiating peripheral (within temporal bone) lesions from CNS lesions.

Peripheral causes of vertigo (85% of cases) are more likely than central lesions to have the following characteristics:

1. Onset of symptoms is acute.
2. Symptoms, especially nausea and vomiting, are severe.
3. A positional component causes the patient to be fearful that particular head or eye movements will worsen symptoms.

Table 16–1   **Diagnostic Pearls**

- It may be difficult to differentiate a small cerebellar stroke from a peripheral vestibular lesion. A thorough understanding of the cerebellar examination may uncover subtle findings useful in making this distinction.
- A younger patient complaining of new-onset vertigo who appears very sick, perhaps lying in bed, nauseated, vomiting, and afraid to move, is likely to have a peripheral cause of vertigo.
- In elderly patients, sudden inability to stand and walk suggests an acute cerebellar lesion.[10]
- Truncal ataxia is a distinguishing feature of dizziness caused by a cerebellar cerebrovascular accident.
- Vertical nystagmus is always abnormal and strongly suggests a central lesion.
- Induced hyperventilation may result in non-specific dizziness.
- Absence of latency during Barany testing should alert the examiner to a potential central neurologic lesion.
- "Top shelf vertigo" (episodic vertigo when reaching up) suggests vertebrobasilar insufficiency or benign positional vertigo.
- Dizziness associated with rolling over in bed strongly suggests benign positional vertigo.

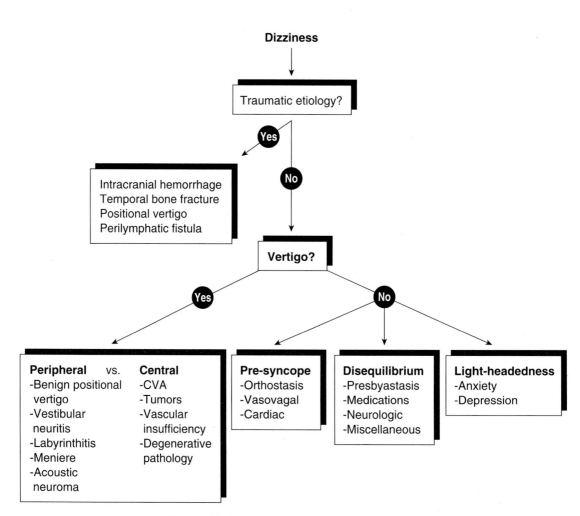

FIGURE 16–2   Differential diagnosis of dizziness.

4. Hearing loss with cochlear (hearing) and vestibular (balance) symptoms occurring together suggest a peripheral lesion affecting both parts of the eighth cranial nerve.
5. Nystagmus induced by the Barany maneuver will have a significant lag of onset (3-30 seconds), short overall duration (less than 1 minute), and fatigue on repetition. The nystagmus may be horizontal or rotatory, never vertical or disconjugate.
6. Nystagmus is enhanced by eliminating visual fixation.

Peripheral lesions include benign positional vertigo, vestibular neuritis, labyrinthitis, Meniere's syndrome, and acoustic neuroma.

Benign positional vertigo is the most common cause of vertigo. Generally, episodic, short-lived (less than 1 minute) bouts of severe symptoms are associated with position changes but without hearing loss. Benign positional vertigo may follow head trauma. It usually resolves in 6-12 months but may recur.

Vestibular neuritis is the sudden unilateral loss of vestibular function. It is generally not associated with a positional component or with hearing loss. Recently 18 patients ages 52-74 with a clinical diagnosis of vestibular neuritis were subjected to intensive cerebral imaging. Four of eighteen (22%) demonstrated infarction of the cerebellum.[5] The subtle distinctions between these two clinical entities will be discussed later.

Labyrinthitis (otitis interna) usually has an associated hearing loss and may follow an upper respiratory tract infection, otitis externa, or otitis media or result from drug toxicity (most commonly aminoglycosides). Symptoms persist for days and may occur as outbreaks within a community. It is most common in the middle-aged population. Rarely, labyrinthitis may be associated with secondary syphilis.

Meniere's syndrome is the idiopathic overaccumulation of endolymphatic fluid resulting in a feeling of ear fullness and characterized by a classic triad of episodic vertigo, fluctuating low-frequency hearing loss, and tinnitus. These symptoms may occur together or separately and generally persist for hours. The syndrome may have periods of remission for years.

Acoustic neuroma is progressive unilateral hearing loss with nonepisodic tinnitus and vertigo. Unilateral tinnitus is generally the earliest symptom and may precede other findings by months or years. Check for neighboring symptoms caused by compression of local structures by the enlarging tumor, particularly decreased corneal reflex and facial palsy. High clinical suspicion may lead to early diagnosis and surgical removal before irreversible damage occurs.

Older patients are much more likely than younger patients to have a central neurologic lesion.

Central causes of vertigo (15% of cases) are more likely than peripheral causes to have the following characteristics:

1. Associated neurologic deficits
2. Lesser severity of symptoms
3. Nystagmus with no lag, long duration (greater then 1 minute), and no fatigability on Barany maneuver (Nystagmus, if present, may be disconjugate and of any direction, including vertical.)
4. Nystagmus enhanced by visual fixation

Central lesions include tumors, vascular insufficiency, strokes, vertebrobasilar migraine, and degenerative and demyelinating pathologic

Primary cardiac disease may present as central vascular insufficiency in the elderly.

conditions (see discussion under "Disequilibrium"). Older patients are much more likely than younger patients to have a central neurologic lesion. Patients with a history of prior stroke or cardiac risk factors are particularly at risk. Primary cardiac disease may present as central vascular insufficiency in the elderly. One study of nearly 600 elderly patients with acute myocardial infarction (MI) revealed 5% presented with vertigo.[6]

One of the great challenges of the emergency physician is to search diligently for evidence that may point to a central lesion. A subtle unilateral cerebellar deficit may, for example, be the only indication of stroke.

The blood supply to the cerebellum, labyrinth, eighth cranial nerve, and vestibular nuclei originates from the vertebrobasilar circulation. Vertigo caused by transient ischemia, infarction, or hemorrhage in this territory is likely to be accompanied by focal neurologic findings. Four specific vascular syndromes that may cause vertigo are cerebellar infarction, lateral medullary infarction, labyrinthine infarction, and subclavian steal syndrome.

Cerebellar infarction may be difficult to differentiate from acute vestibular neuritis or labyrinthitis and thus is often misdiagosed. It may be associated with vomiting, truncal and gait ataxia, incoordination, dysmetria, hypotonia, and dysarthria. The patient may appear relatively comfortable lying in bed but be unable to stand and walk. The physical findings may be overt or extremely subtle. The nuances of the cerebellar examination must be familiar to the emergency physician.

Small, unrecognized cerebellar infarctions may, over 24–72 hours, result in edematous swelling and death.

It is vital to consider and rule out this diagnosis, since small unrecognized cerebellar infarctions may, over 24-72 hours, result in edematous swelling and death. Early recognition and intensive management may decrease mortality. The overall most common cause of stroke in the elderly is atherosclerotic vascular disease. It is interesting to note, however, that a recent study of patients with isolated cerebellar infarction without concomitant brain stem or occipital infarct revealed associated cardioembolism in 67% of cases.[7] Although the number of patients in this review was small, the surprising results are important to bear in mind.

Lateral medullary infarction (Wallenberg's syndrome) involves a posterior inferior cerebellar artery (PICA) lesion. It is characterized by nausea, vomiting, hiccups, prominent vertigo, and ipsilateral Horner's syndrome. The patient also loses pinprick and temperature sensation of ipsilateral face and contralateral body.

Labyrinthine infarction involves an anterior inferior cerebellar artery (AICA) lesion. It is characterized by sudden unilateral deafness and vertigo.

Subclavian steal syndrome is a relatively unusual cause of vertebrobasilar insufficiency, but it is readily treated when correctly diagnosed. The patient has an obstruction (usually atherosclerotic in the elderly population) of the proximal subclavian artery. When the arm is exercised, demand for oxygen increases. Since flow is limited by subclavian obstruction, blood is "stolen" from the ipsilateral vertebral artery. These patients often have differing blood pressure in their arms. A bruit may occasionally be noted over the area of blockage.

PRE-SYNCOPE

With pre-syncope the patient may sense visual blurring with decreased light perception and a fading level of consciousness. The three basic antecedents of pre-syncope are orthostasis, a vasovagal cause, or a cardiovascular cause.

Orthostasis, a postural syndrome, is a very common cause of dizziness and falls in elderly persons and may be suggested by a careful history. These patients may have a systolic blood pressure drop of 20 mm Hg or pulse increase of 20/min or more with postural change. Orthostatic dizziness may result from hemorrhage (consider gastrointestinal blood loss, abdominal aortic aneurysmal leak), dehydration (vomiting, diarrhea), early sepsis, medications, or prolonged bed rest. Up to 10% of elderly hospitalized patients have postural hypotension caused by deficient baroreceptor reflexes.

Vasovagal pre-syncope usually results from fear, anxiety, or visceral irritation (pain, micturition, cough, or defecation).

Cardiovascular pre-syncope involves arrhythmias, congestive heart failure, ischemia, valvular disease, carotid sinus hypersensitivity, or pulmonary embolism.

DISEQUILIBRIUM

The causes of disequilibrium resulting in dizziness can be categorized into four groups: (1) multisensory deficit dizziness syndrome, (2) neurologic syndromes, (3) medications, and (4) miscellaneous causes.

Multisensory deficit dizziness syndrome is also known as presbyastasis. Dizziness results from deficiencies within several sensory modalities. This condition is most commonly seen in the elderly. In one study of 740 patients over 65 years of age referred to an otolaryngologist, only 21% were found to have a specific cause of dizziness. The remaining 79% were diagnosed with presbyastasis.[8] This study focused on a subspecialty practice. Presbyastasis will be diagnosed much less frequently in an ED. It is vital, however, to recognize in the elderly that deficits, including poor visual acuity, proprioceptive loss, and mild vestibular dysfunction, may combine to create a sense of disequilibrium and dizziness.

The following specific *neurologic syndromes* also need to be considered with disequilibrium.

Peripheral neuropathy may contribute to presbyastasis. It can result from alcoholism, diabetes mellitus, or vitamin B_{12} deficiency (patient complains of "walking on cotton wool").

Parkinson's disease is characterized by cogwheel rigidity, bradykinesia, "pill-rolling" tremor, and shuffling gait. It is seen in approximately one percent of the population over 55 years of age. These patients may develop an intrinsic postural instability and orthostatic blood pressure changes.

Although it is unusual for multiple sclerosis (MS) to occur for the first time after the sixth decade, 10% of cases in elderly patients may present with disequilibrium or vertigo. Internuclear ophthalmoplegia is highly suggestive of MS. Intention tremor, optic neuritis, memory loss, cranial nerve signs, and bladder dysfunction are other common findings.

Poor visual acuity proprioceptive loss, and mild vestibular dysfunction may combine to create a sense of disequilibrium and dizziness in the elderly.

Normal pressure hydrocephalus generally develops subacutely over weeks to months and is characterized classically by the triad of gait imbalance, incontinence, and dementia.

A brain tumor, especially acoustic neuroma (discussed under "Vertigo") and posterior fossa mass lesions, can affect equilibrium.

Subdural hematoma may be a result of remote, unrecognized, or forgotten trauma and be associated with fluctuating levels of consciousness.

Seizure disorder may result in disequilibrium. Look for other clues of this episodic disease, such as incontinence, post-ictal confusion, or paralysis.

Medications can cause disequilibrium in the elderly, because they are particularly susceptible to pharmaceutical side effects. Many medications have been reported to cause dizziness. Common offenders include the following:

1. Psychotropics
2. Sedatives
3. Aminoglycoside antibiotics
4. Salicylates
5. Quinine
6. Diuretics
7. Anticonvulsants
8. Antihypertensives
9. Vasodilators
10. Tricyclic antidepressants
11. Antiparkinsonism medications

Miscellaneous causes of disequilibrium are hypothyroidism, heavy metal poisoning, metabolic derangements, and alcoholism.

LIGHT-HEADEDNESS

Light-headedness, a non-specific complaint, may have a psychiatric basis. The examiner probes for indications of external stress, anxiety, and depression. The history may also reveal an exaggerated fear of passing out or dying. Hyperventilation testing may reproduce these symptoms along with possible headache, chest pain, shortness of breath, palpitations, and paresthesias of hands, mouth, and legs. Caution, however, must be advised in diagnosing this condition. Provocative hyperventilation may also reproduce dizziness from other unrelated causes.

POST-TRAUMATIC DIZZINESS

Mild blunt head trauma without skull fracture can produce dizziness and vertigo.

Dizziness may result from major or seemingly minor trauma. Significant head trauma may result in intracranial hemorrhage and cervical spine injuries. Sudden deceleration injuries as seen in motor vehicle accidents or falls may fracture the temporal bones. This condition is clinically diagnosable when blood is seen at the tympanic membrane or in the external canal following head trauma at a site distant from the affected ear. A cerebrospinal fluid (CSF) leak may not be readily discernible, but direct communication with the subarachnoid space probably exists and appropriate precautions should be taken. Use sterile otoscopic equipment if available. The temporal bone fracture may damage the vestibular portion of the inner ear, eighth cranial nerve, brain stem, or cerebellum. Nystagmus and vertigo may result.

Mild blunt head trauma without skull fracture may also produce dizziness and vertigo. This "labyrinthine concussion" may be associated with permanent neurologic hearing loss. The resulting positional vertigo may be intense but generally resolves spontaneously within 6 weeks.

Head trauma may also rupture the oval window of the inner ear. The perilymphatic fistula created may cause a Meniere's type of syndrome with episodic vertigo and hearing impairment. This condition may be surgically correctable. The fistula test is useful in diagnosing this condition.

EMERGENCY DEPARTMENT MANAGEMENT AND DISPOSITION

Initial ED evaluation is geared to distinguish emergent, life-threatening causes of dizziness from the more common, relatively benign forms. Patients with acute bleeding, cardiac pathologic conditions, and potentially unstable central neurologic lesions are stabilized in the ED and admitted. An elderly patient with suspected new-onset vertebrobasilar insufficiency is admitted to observe for progression of symptoms and for possible anticoagulation. A patient with a new cerebellar stroke may rapidly develop edema leading to herniation of the cerebellar tonsils or fourth ventricle compression and hydrocephalus. This patient may become increasingly somnolent in the ED and require intubation, hyperventilation, diuresis, and immediate neurosurgical evaluation for possible decompression or shunt placement.

Suspected new-onset vertebrobasilar insufficiency warrants admission for monitoring and possible anticoagulation therapy.

If a cardiac arrhythmia is suspected, 24-48 hours of continuous cardiac monitoring may establish the cause of symptoms. Patients with evidence of head trauma should undergo emergent CT scanning. Patients with temporal bone skull fractures should not be treated prophylactically with antibiotics but are usually admitted for observation. Patients are advised not to blow their nose, since there is a potential communication between the subarachnoid space and the nasopharynx.

Presbyastasis may be managed by initiating a multidisciplinary review. Visual and auditory testing may reveal remediable lesions. A cane may lessen the effects of proprioceptive loss. A home visit by a health care professional to assess environmental hazards and the need for assistive devices may be useful if coordinated through the primary care physician (See Chapter 10, Table 10–4).

Some patients with peripheral vestibular dizziness may benefit from antihistaminic medications such as meclizine or diphenhydramine (Benadryl®). Benign positional vertigo in the older population, however, is episodic, and thus continuous use of suppressive medication may be inappropriate and sedating side effects may be harmful. Several authors recommend the use of postural desensitization therapy.[9] These maneuvers place the patient repetitively in positions that stimulate symptoms. In time this technique may result in diminished intensity or, less commonly, resolution of symptoms. Meniere's disease may respond to the use of a diuretic or dietary salt restriction. Treatment of other causes of dizziness depends on the individual cause.

The emergency physician may give definitive treatment for dizziness if a particular offending agent such as a medication is identified. More commonly, however, dizziness may be difficult to treat. All patients will need a primary care provider (general medicine, neurology, cardiology, or psychiatry) for continued long-term management.

An elderly person with new dizziness is usually worried. ED evaluation may lead to a better understanding of this disturbing symptom. If potentially life-threatening causes are ruled out, reassurance that a condition is benign, self-limited, or treatable, or that natural compensatory mechanisms will eventually diminish the symptom is a vital part of management.

SUMMARY POINTS

- Dizziness is a common and often vaguely described complaint. A directed history and physical examination keeping the specific categories of dizziness in mind will lead to a diagnosis in up to 75% of cases.
- Dizziness is a particularly common complaint in the elderly population.
- The older patient is more likely than a younger individual to be manifesting an early symptom of a potentially treatable or preventable disorder.
- A careful extraocular motor examination is important, because abnormalities may be quite subtle and, when present, can often give clues as to the cause of dizziness.
- Special physical examination tests, including the Barany maneuver, hyperventilation challenge, carotid sinus stimulation, and fistula test, may be helpful depending on the patient's presenting symptoms.
- Elderly patients are much more likely than younger patients to have a central neurologic lesion.
- The three basic antecedents of pre-syncope are orthostasis, a vasovagal cause, or a cardiovascular cause.
- Medications can cause disequilibrium in the elderly, because they are particularly susceptible to pharmaceutical side effects.

CHAPTER AUTHOR

Richard S. Hartoch, MD

ACKNOWLEDGMENT

The author would like to thank Daniel H. Bobker, MD, for comments on the manuscript.

REFERENCES

1. Luxon L. Disturbances of balance in the elderly. *Br J Hosp Med.* 1991;45:22.
2. Baloh RW. Dizziness in older people. *J Am Geriatr Soc.* 1992;40:713.
3. Drachman DA, Hart CW. An approach to the dizzy patient. *Neurology.* 1972;22:323.
4. Walker H. *Clinical methods.* 3rd ed. Butterworths; 1990.

5. Magnusson M, Norrving B. Cerebellar infarctions as the cause of "vestibular neuritis." *Acta Otolaryngol Suppl (Stockh)*. 1991;481:258–259.
6. Rossman I. *Clinical geriatrics*. 3rd ed. 1986
7. Bogousslavsky J et al. The etiology of posterior circulation infarcts. *Neurology*. 1993;43:1528.
8. Belal A, Glorig A. Disequilibrium of aging (presbyastasis). *J Laryngol Otol*. 1986;100:1037.
9. Paparella M et al. Otolaryngology. 3rd ed. Philadelphia, PA: WB Saunders Co; 1991.
10. Venna N. Dizziness, falling and fainting: differential diagnosis in the aged: parts I and II. *Geriatrics*. 1986;41(6,7).

SELECTED READINGS

Adams RD, Victor M. *Principles of neurology*. 5th ed. 1992.
Alberti PW, Ruber RJ. *Otologic medicine and surgery*. 2nd ed. 1988.
Brandt T. *Vertigo: its multisensory syndromes*. Springer-Verlag; 1991.
Droller H, Pemberton J. Vertigo in a random sample of elderly people living in their homes. *J Laryngol Otol*. 1953;22:689.
Edmeads J. Understanding dizziness. *Postgrad Med*. 1990;88:255.
Herr RD et al. A directed approach to the dizzy patient. *Ann Emerg Med*. 1989;18:664.
Jenkins HA et al. Disequilibrium of aging. *Otolaryngol Head Neck Surg*.
Jonsson P, Lipsitz L. Dizziness and syncope. *Principles of geriatric medicine and gerontology*. 2nd ed. 1990.
Madlon-Kay D. Evaluation and outcome of the dizzy patient. *J Fam Pract*. 1985;21:109.
Magerian G. Hyperventilation syndromes: infrequently recognized common expressions of anxiety and stress. *Medicine*. 1982;61:219.
Olsky M, Murray J. Dizziness and fainting in the elderly. *Emerg Med Clin North Am*. 1990;8:295.
Pearson BW, Barber HO. Head injury: some otoneurologic sequelae. *Arch Otolaryngol*. 1973;97:81–84.
Rosen P, Barkin R. *Emergency medicine concepts and clinical practice*. 2nd ed. 1992.
Warner E et al. Dizziness in primary care patients. *J Gen Intern Med*. 1992;7:454.

Index